AF530554

From Western Medicine to Global Medicine

New Perspectives in South Asian History 27

The **New Perspectives in South Asian History** series publishes monographs and other writings on early modern, modern and contemporary history. The volumes in the series cover new ground across a broad spectrum of subjects such as cultural, environmental, medical, military and political history, and the histories of 'marginalised' groups. It includes fresh perspectives on more familiar fields as well as interdisciplinary and original work from all parts of South Asia. It welcomes historical contributions from sociology, anthropology and cultural studies.

Series Editors

SANJOY BHATTACHARYA *Reader in History, The Wellcome Trust Centre for the History of Medicine at University College London*

PETER CAIN *Professor of History, School of Cultural Studies, Sheffield Hallam University*

MARK HARRISON *Professor, History of Medicine, and Director, Wellcome Unit for the History of Medicine, University of Oxford*

MICHAEL WORBOYS *Director, Centre for the History of Science, Technology and Medicine, and Wellcome Unit for the History of Medicine, University of Manchester*

Editorial Advisory Committee

Clive Dewey *Formerly Reader, Department of Economic and Social History, University of Leicester*

Paul Greenough *Professor of History and of Community and Behavioral Health, Director, South Asian Tsunami Research Program, University of Iowa*

Biswamoy Pati *Reader, Department of History, Sri Venkateswara College, University of Delhi*

Douglas M. Peers *Professor of History, and Dean of Graduate Studies, York University*

Peter Robb *Pro-Director and Professor of the History of India, School of Oriental and African Studies, University of London*

Tan Tai Yong *Associate Professor of History, National University of Singapore*

From Western Medicine to Global Medicine
The Hospital Beyond the West

Edited by

MARK HARRISON
MARGARET JONES
HELEN SWEET
University of Oxford

Orient BlackSwan

ORIENT BLACKSWAN PRIVATE LIMITED

Registered Office
3-6-752 Himayatnagar, Hyderabad 500 029 (A.P.), India
E-mail: centraloffice@orientblackswan.com

Other Offices
Bangalore, Bhopal, Bhubaneshwar, Chennai,
Ernakulam, Guwahati, Hyderabad, Jaipur, Kolkata,
Lucknow, Mumbai, New Delhi, Patna

© Orient Blackswan Private Limited 2009

First Published 2009

Series cover and book design
© Orient Blackswan Private Limited 2009

ISBN 978 81 250 3702 6

Typeset by
OSDATA, Hyderabad 500 029
in Bembo (Aldine) 10.5/12.5

Printed at
De Unique
New Delhi

Published by
Orient Blackswan Private Limited
1/24 Asaf Ali Road, New Delhi 110 002
E-mail: delhi@orientblackswan.com

The publishers gratefully acknowledge the financial support received for this volume from the Wellcome Trust

Contents

Acknowledgements

This volume has been compiled from a selection of papers given at the conference "From Western Medicine to Global Medicine: The Hospital Beyond the West", 18–19 March 2004, organised by the Wellcome Unit for the History of Medicine, University of Oxford. The Editors wish to express their gratitude to the Wellcome Trust for their generous support in funding this project. We would also like to thank Carol Brady and Belinda Michaelides for their invaluable administrative support.

Abbreviations

AGA	Assistant Government Agent
ANY	Archives Nationales du Cameroun, Yaoundé
Bara PR	Baragwanath Public Relations Department Archive
BL	British Library
CMC	China Medical Commission
CMS	Church Missionary Society
CMU	China Medical University
CO	Colonial Office
CPC	Centre Pasteur du Cameroun
CPC	Correspondance Politique et Consulaire
CSO	Colonial Secretary's Office
DMF	Department of Medicine Files
ELCSA-SER	Evangelical Lutheran Church in Southern Africa South East Region
FCS	Free Church of Scotland
FIDES	Fond d'Investissement pour le Développement Economique et Social
GA	Government Agent
GES	Afrikaans Gesondheid
GFSG	Government of Fort St George (Madras)
GH	Government House
GOI	Government of India
HSF	Hôpital de la Sainte Famille
HEIC	Honourable East India Company
IMPM	Institut de Recherche Médicale et des Plantes Médicinales
IPC	Institut Pasteur du Cameroun
IRMCAM	Institut de Recherches Médicales du Cameroun
J. J. Hospital	Jamsetjee Jejeebhoy Hospital
KCM	Killie Campbell Museum

KZN	KwaZulu Natal
LMF	Lutheran Medical Foundation
LMS	London Missionary Society
MB	Bachelor of Medicine
MMC	Moukden Medical College
MO	Medical Officer
MSA	Maharashtra State Archives
NAR	National Archives Repository
NBB	Natal Blue Book
NGA	Natal Government Asylum
NLCA	Norwegian Lutheran Church in America
NLS	National Library of Scotland
NS	Nouvelle Série
OIOC	Oriental and India Office Collections
ORSTOM	Office de la Recherche Scientifique et Technique Outre Mer
PAR	Pietermaritzburg Archives Repository
PC	Pietermaritzburg Corporation
PCMO	Principal Civil Medical Officer
PMO	Prime Minister's Office
PRO	Public Record Office
PUMC	Peking Union Medical College
RCN	Royal College of Nursing
RG	Record Group
RHO	Rhodes House Oxford
RN	Registered Nurse
RSC	Registrar Supreme Court
RU	Rhodes University
RVE	Ruznâmeh-ye Vaqâye'-e Ettefâqiyyeh
SAMDC	South African Medical and Dental Council
SAMJ	*South African Medical Journal*
SANA	South African National Archives
SHMP	Service d'Hygiène Mobile et de Prophylaxie
SLNA	Sri Lanka National Archives
SMR	South Manchuria Railway
Sr	Sister
TNA	The National Archives

TPA	Transvaal Provisional Administration
UMCA	Universities' Mission to Central Africa
UMN	United Mission to Nepal
USOP	United States Operating Mission
vdH	van den Heever
WHO	World Health Organization
WHSL	Wits Health Science Library

Introduction

Mark Harrison

For many non-Western countries—especially the former European colonies—there is an extensive literature on the history of disease and public health,[1] but we know relatively little about how Western medicine came to be the dominant form of medicine around the world.[2] To understand this process we must examine far more closely the institution which has, more than any other, come to symbolise Western medicine—the modern hospital. In most countries, the hospital has become the main focus for the dissemination of Western medicine and plays a major—albeit contested—role in health care systems; not only on account of their curative functions, but also as centres of teaching and research. Just as in the West, the hospital has become a familiar institution and often serves as a focal point for local culture and as a symbol of community pride. But the history of hospitals beyond the West cannot be easily subsumed within a narrative generated from within the West and which pertains mainly to Europe and North America. While sharing many similar features, the development of hospital medicine in non-

[1] For example, David Arnold, *Colonizing the Body: State Medicine and Epidemic Disease in Nineteenth-Century India* (Berkeley: University of California Press, 1993); John Farley, *Bilharzia: A History of Imperial Tropical Medicine* (Cambridge: Cambridge University Press, 1991); Maryinez Lyons, *A Social History of Sleeping Sickness in Northern Zaire, 1900–1940* (Cambridge: Cambridge University Press, 1992); Lenore Manderson, *Sickness and the State: Health and Illness in Colonial Malaya, 1870–1940* (Cambridge: Cambridge University Press, 1996).

[2] See Michael Worboys, "The Spread of Western Medicine", in *Western Medicine: An Illustrated History,* ed. Irvine Loudon (Oxford: Oxford University Press, 1997), 249–63.

Western countries differs in several important respects. In many of the countries considered in this volume, hospitals were established and began to develop within a colonial framework, which in some cases provided very different structures of funding and administration, as well as a more complex professional hierarchy affected by notions of race. Suspicion of colonial motives may also have served to heighten fears about institutional care,[3] while in independent or nominally independent countries the rise of the hospital was generally part of a self-conscious effort to emulate the West, though not necessarily to the exclusion of indigenous medical traditions.

Modernisation, then, was by no means synonymous with Westernisation. Some countries, such as Japan, progressed along recognisably Western lines, while others, including many Islamic countries, continued or increased support for non-Western medical traditions at the same time as establishing Western-style hospitals. But there were notable differences within the Islamic world, too: between the increasingly Western orientation of Turkey, for example, and the bifurcated approach to modernisation evident in Iran or some of the Indian princely states. In other parts of the world, the position of hospitals within health care systems has also varied according to policies. Most obviously, perhaps, from the 1950s to the 1980s China consciously downgraded large-scale institutions in favour of primary health care; a tension that remains at the heart of medical care provision in many poorer countries.[4]

In writing the history of hospitals outside the developed world, we are not therefore writing a history of "the West and the rest" (and we should bear in mind that the Western experience is far from monolithic) but a history of societies and institutions that often differed as much from each other as from those of Europe and North America. And, while it is still possible to conceive of the dissemination of Western medicine through the institution of the hospital, this process did not represent a uniform trend towards medical

[3] Arnold, *Colonizing the Body*, 213–14.

[4] Gill Walt, "Health Care in the Developing World, 1960–2001", in *Caring for Health: History and Diversity*, ed. Charles Webster (Milton Keynes: Open University Press, 2001), 253–94; K. Newell, *Health by the People* (Geneva: WHO, 1975).

modernity, but sometimes a process of accommodation with local, non-Western modernities and traditions. But this is not to say that patterns cannot be discerned or that generalisations are impossible; our aim here is to identify commonalities and differences, which may pave the way for an understanding of the development of hospitals on a global basis.

Perhaps the most obvious starting point is to determine the importance of hospitals in health care systems in the non-Western world. Have they a central place in health care delivery as in Western countries, or has their role been subordinated for economic or cultural reasons? It is also, of course, necessary to examine the ways in which hospitals have developed in colonial (and, later, post-colonial) countries, and in countries such as Japan or Iran, which retained their independence from colonial rule. Comparisons between these different contexts may help us to gauge the impact of colonial rule on the development of health care. We also need to gain a clear impression of the main stimuli to hospital development and how far these differed from those in the West and in different non-Western countries. Did the professional aspirations of physicians, for example, play a lesser role and government a stronger role, than in most European countries or North America? Were the needs of political economy and social control more or less evident, or did they merely take different forms? Similarly, it may be useful to look at the ways in which hospitals have been organised into health-care systems. Do we find the regional hierarchies that exist in Britain and North America, for instance,[5] or more fragmented structures reflecting differences in funding, planning and so forth? More importantly, it is vital to establish the degree of success with which hospital-based health care systems have met the needs and expectations of peoples living in non-Western countries.

The form of the hospital is likely to be another fruitful area of enquiry. How far do hospitals—as physical entities—differ from those in the West? What do differences in architectural style and spatial organisation tell us about the influence of locality and culture on

[5] Daniel M. Fox, *Health Policies, Health Politics* (Princeton: Princeton University Press, 1986).

medical modernity? And last, but not least, we need to look at the hospital as a centre of research and teaching, at its role in the emergence of medical and nursing professions, and at relations between hospital medicine and non-Western medical traditions. Has hospital medicine displaced indigenous practices or have they adopted the institution as their own?

The Colonial Clinic

The list of questions is endless but it is as well to begin this volume by asking the most fundamental question of all: what do we mean by a hospital? The first hospitals established by Europeans outside Europe predated the emergence of modern infirmaries in the West by several centuries; likewise, many non-Western countries possessed at some point in their history institutions akin to medieval hospitals in Europe. Institutions of a charitable nature, offering refuge for the sick and the poor, were very much part of the Islamic, Jewish, Buddhist, Hindu and Jain traditions.[6] Are these in some sense precursors to modern hospitals, or are they fundamentally different types of institution? If we take the history of the hospital in the West as our guide, it is likely that there are threads of continuity with the "medieval" past, not least the continuing importance of the charitable imperative.[7] Yet many historians have insisted that hospitals were progressively "medicalized", their main function

[6] See Peregrine Horden, "The World of the Hospital: Comparisons and Continuities", in *The Impact of Hospitals, 300–2000*, ed. John Henderson, Peregrine Horden and Alessandro Pastore (Oxford: Peter Lang, 2007). Also see Peregrine Horden, "The Earliest Hospitals in Byzantium, Western Europe, and Islam", *Journal of Interdisciplinary History* 35, no. 3, 2005, 361–89.

[7] Sandra Cavallo, "Charity, Power, and Patronage in Eighteenth-Century Italian Hospitals: The Case of Turin", in *The Hospital in History*, ed. Lindsay Granshaw and Roy Porter (London: Routledge, 1989), 63–92; J. Barry and C. Jones, eds., *Medicine and Charity before the Welfare State* (London and New York: Routledge, 1991); Nobert Finzsch and Robert Jütte, eds., *Institutions of Confinement: Hospitals, Asylums, and Prisons in Western Europe and North America, 1500–1950* (Cambridge: Cambridge University Press, 1996).

shifting from charitable relief to the cure of the sick.[8] This distinction is problematic, partly because of the persistence of palliative or poor relief in some modern hospitals (hospices and fever hospitals, for example[9]) and partly because the point at which 'modern' institutions emerge depends largely on the eye of the beholder. Do we take as our starting point the new infirmaries of Enlightenment Europe and the advent of clinical teaching at the bedside,[10] or ought we to locate the origins of the modern hospital in the institutions of revolutionary Paris, and the emergence of clinico-anatomical medicine?[11]

[8] Prominent examples include: Henry Sigerist, "An Outline of the Development of the Hospital", *Bulletin of the History of Medicine* 4, 1936, 573–81; N. Jewson, "The Disappearance of the Sick Man from Medical Cosmology, 1770–1870", *Sociology* 10, 1976, 225–44.

[9] On fever hospitals and the poor, see John V. Pickstone, "Dearth, Dirt and Fever Epidemics: Rewriting the History of British 'Public Health', 1780–1850", in *Epidemics and Ideas: Essays on the Historical Perception of Pestilence,* ed. T. Ranger and P. Slack (Cambridge: Cambridge University Press, 1992), 125–48; John V. Pickstone, "Ferriar's Fever to Kay's Cholera: Disease and Social Structure in Cottonopolis", *History of Science* 22, 1984, 401–19; John V. Pickstone, *Medicine and Industrial Society: A History of Hospital Development in Manchester and Its Region, 1752–1946* (Manchester: Manchester University Press, 1985). On the hospice movement, see David Clark, ed., *Cicely Saunders: Founder of the Hospice Movement; Selected Letters, 1959–1999* (Oxford: Oxford University Press, 2005).

[10] Günther B. Risse, *Hospital Life in Enlightenment Scotland: Care and Teaching at the Royal Infirmary of Edinburgh* (Cambridge: Cambridge University Press, 1986); Günther B. Risse, *Mending Bodies, Saving Souls: A History of Hospitals* (New York: Oxford University Press, 1999); Susan C. Lawrence, *Charitable Knowledge: Hospital Pupils and Practitioners in Eighteenth-Century London* (Cambridge: Cambridge University Press, 1996); Laurence Brockliss and Colin Jones, *The Medical World of Early Modern France* (Oxford: Clarendon Press, 1997).

[11] Erwin H. Ackerknecht, *Medicine at the Paris Hospital, 1794–1848* (Baltimore: Johns Hopkins University Press, 1967); Michel Foucault, *The Birth of the Clinic: An Archaeology of Medical Perception* (London: Routledge, 1997 [1963]); David Vess, *Medical Revolution in France, 1789–1796* (Gainesville: University Presses of Florida, 1975); Dora Weiner, *The Citizen-Patient in Revolutionary and Imperial Paris* (Baltimore: Johns Hopkins University Press, 1993); Jacalyn Duffin, *To See with a Better Eye: A Life of R. T. H. Laennec* (Princeton: Princeton University Press, 1998).

Some historians of eighteenth-century medicine have difficulties with the notion of a sharp discontinuity between the "old" clinics of Leiden, Vienna and Edinburgh, and the "new" ones of revolutionary Paris.[12] These earlier hospitals were, perhaps, breaking away from established bodies of knowledge and practice well before the 1790s. It is possible that the early history of hospitals beyond the West may shed some light on this and on the more general problem of what constitutes a modern hospital. If nothing else, it alerts us to the fact that modern hospital practices had multiple origins, some of which lay beyond Europe; indeed, some of the features of what Michel Foucault dubbed clinico-anatomical medicine were flourishing in the European colonies some years before they appeared in revolutionary Paris. However, the history of hospitals beyond the West over the last half millennium serves as an antidote to the incipient Whiggism of much hospital historiography.[13] The continuing vitality and importance of Christian mission hospitals in many African countries reminds us that medicalisation is not synonymous with modernity. We, too, see the persistence or, more often, the revival of hospitals within other religious traditions. And even if we do choose to view the history of hospitals in terms of medicalisation, integrating this within a more general history of Western 'expansion' is far from easy, not least because the first hospitals established by Europeans in their colonies preceded the infirmaries of Revolutionary Paris by nearly three centuries.

The history of European hospitals beyond the West begins in 1501, with the foundation of a hospital on the Spanish Caribbean island of Santo Domingo. Soon after the conquest of the Aztecs, another such institution opened in 1524, in what was to become

[12] For example, Brockliss and Jones, *Medical World of Early Modern France*, 689–700; Othmar Keel, "The Politics of Health and the Institutionalisation of Clinical Practices in Europe in the Second Half of the Eighteenth Century", in *William Hunter and the Eighteenth-Century Medical World,* ed. W. F. Bynum and Roy Porter (Cambridge: Cambridge University Press, 1985), 207–58; Othmar Keel, *L' Avènement de la Medicine Clinique Moderne en Europe, 1750–1815: Politiques, Institutions et Savoirs* (Montreal: Les Presses de l'Université de Montreal, 2001).

[13] See Horden, "The World of the Hospital".

Mexico City and, in the Portuguese colony of Goa, a hospital was founded soon after the creation of the colony in 1510. These institutions were intended primarily for the use of Europeans, who were mostly soldiers and sailors.[14] However, the evangelical dimension of Iberian colonialism soon became manifest with the opening of hospitals for indigenous peoples, with the hope that the exercise of Christian charity would win conversions. To this end, another hospital was opened in Mexico City in the early 1530s—the Hospital Real de San José de los Naturales—especially for the treatment of "poor Indians"; several provincial institutions followed from the 1540s.[15] Like the hospital in Goa, these hospitals also trained indigenous peoples in Western medicine, with the hope of weaning them away from medical practices that were considered barbaric and idolatrous. In some cases, such as Portuguese Goa, there were even ill-fated attempts to curb traditional medical practice.

During the 1600s other European countries began to establish hospitals overseas. In the early seventeenth century, the Dutch East India Company built hospitals in some of its main trading centres, as did the English and French East India companies from the 1660s. By the early 1700s, as imperial rivalry between the British and French intensified, these hospitals were enlarged and supplemented by separate institutions run by the armed forces.[16] The creation of hospitals overseas was seen as essential to the morale of men working and fighting far from their home, as had been recognised for some time in Europe itself—the Spanish Army in Flanders having established a hospital at Mechelen in 1585 to placate its

[14] F. da Silva Gracias, *Health and Hygiene in Colonial Goa, 1510–1961* (New Delhi: Concept Publishing, 1994).

[15] Gordon Schendel, *Medicine in Mexico: From Aztec Herbs to Betatrons* (Austin and London: University of Texas Press, 1968), 89–95; Hernando Ruiz de Alarcón, introduction to *Treatise on the Heathen Superstitions that Today Live among the Indians Native to this New Spain,* trans. and ed. J. R. Andrews and R. Hassig (Norman: University of Oklahoma Press, 1984 [1629]), 32.

[16] The first hospitals established by the English East India Company in India opened in Madras in 1664, Bombay in 1676, and Calcutta in 1707. See D. G. Crawford, *A History of the Indian Medical Service* (London: Thacker and Co., 1913), 1: 392, 400, 418.

disaffected soldiers.[17] However, there were other reasons to create hospitals in the colonies, the most important of which was to stem the loss of manpower from disease. By the eighteenth century, as the commitment of European forces became more extensive, there was mounting unease about the economic costs of colonial warfare, both in terms of the loss of well trained men and the constant drain of manpower from agriculture and manufacturing. The British military surgeon Donald Monro, for example, declared, "In a commercial Country like our own, where Numbers of Hands are constantly wanted for the carrying on [of] our Manufactories, we have a strong political Argument to add to that drawn from the Dictates of Humanity, why the Life of every individual should be most carefully attended to."[18]

Whether hospitals did much to stem such losses is doubtful, but at the time it was widely believed that they could, if properly constructed and managed. Writing of his experiences in the Caribbean, the physician Benjamin Moseley insisted: "As the restoring [of] soldiers speedily to health is of the first consequence, in climates where a short illness renders them useless, where their place cannot be supplied, and where diseases are inevitable, convenient and proper hospitals are of the utmost importance. The cost of a good hospital is nothing in the scale of expense. . . . A bad hospital may deprive the state in a few months, of as many men, whose value would amount, in political calculation, to a sum sufficient to build a good one".[19] Even when practitioners felt themselves powerless to stop the ravages of tropical diseases, they could at least begin to understand them, with the hope of finding more effective remedies

[17] Geoffrey Parker, *The Army of Flanders and the Spanish Road, 1567–1659* (Cambridge: Cambridge University Press, 2004 [1972]), 141–44. Also see Eric Gruber von Arni, *Hospital Care and the British Standing Army, 1660–1714* (Aldershot: Ashgate, 2006).

[18] Donald Monro, *An Account of the Diseases Which Were Most Frequent in the British Military Hospitals in Germany, from January 1761 to the Return of the Troops to England in March 1763* (London: A. Miller, D. Wilson and T. Durham, 1764), ix.

[19] Benjamin Moseley, *A Treatise on Tropical Diseases; on Military Operations; and on the Climate of the West Indies* (London: T. Cadell, 1789), 155–56.

in future. From the early seventeenth century, European practitioners such as Jacobus Bontius, working at the Dutch East India Company's hospital in Batavia, began the systematic investigation of the diseases of that region, viewing them in relation to their environment, and seeking to understand their pathology by conducting post-mortem dissections.[20]

By the mid-eighteenth century some of the hospitals established by the armed forces of the European powers in Asia and the Americas were in the vanguard of medical innovation and practically all the main features of clinical medicine as defined by Foucault were present. In the hospitals of the English East India Company post-mortem dissections were being carried out regularly by the 1750s and, within two decades, medical texts show that morbid anatomy was becoming the principal basis of medical knowledge and practice in the region's military and naval hospitals. High death rates in the colonies meant that there was a plentiful supply of cadavers, and there were no restrictions preventing dissection of the dead, or at least of lower ranking soldiers and sailors. For this reason, colonial practitioners were able to make important contributions to the pathology of diseases such as fevers and hepatitis, their work informing the publications of even the most eminent physicians back at home.[21]

Colonial hospitals were also centres of therapeutic innovation, subjecting to systematic trial a range of botanical and chemical remedies either pioneered in the colonies, or adopted from indigenous traditions. These included some exotic preparations like the controversial bezoar stone and other remedies for snake-bite as well as many local febrifuges. Indeed, it is notable that colonial hospitals were normally situated close to markets or bazaars, from which

[20] Harold J. Cook, "Global Economies and Local Knowledge in the East Indies: Jacobus Bontius Learns the Facts of Nature", in *Colonial Botany: Science, Commerce, and Politics in the Early Modern World,* ed. Londa Schiebinger and Claudia Swan (Philadelphia: University of Philadelphia Press, 2005), 100–18; J. Bontius, *Medicina Indorum* (Batavia: Franciscum Hackium, 1642), section 4.

[21] See Mark Harrison, *A Great Independence of Mind: British Medicine in an Age of Commerce and Empire, c.1660–1830* (in preparation).

surgeons could easily obtain local remedies or ingredients to supplement their meagre supplies from abroad.[22] Apart from the use of various local remedies, surgeons working in colonial military and naval hospitals also experimented freely with novel therapies including the use of chemicals. One good example is the use of mercury to treat hepatic disorders and bilious fevers: a practice begun in India in the 1750s and which subsequently became widespread throughout the East Indies and the Caribbean. Another is the use of nitrous acid as a cure for venereal and some other complaints. This practice was first developed at the East India Company's military hospital in Bombay by Dr Helenus Scott and was later propounded by Dr Thomas Beddoes and others in Britain.[23]

However, it is important to bear in mind that early colonial hospitals tended to have an ephemeral existence. Many were flimsy structures and liable to collapse during heavy rains or high winds, and they frequently shifted from site to site. Moreover, for every colonial hospital that was well run, there were many more that were poorly disciplined, filthy and dilapidated. Benjamin Moseley, for example, was appalled by the numbers of men who perished in British military hospitals in Jamaica,[24] while Robert Jackson, writing of his experiences as a surgeon in North America and the Caribbean during the American War of Independence, complained that most general hospitals overseas suffered from lax discipline and poor hygiene on account of the inferior quality of their commanding officers, who were combatant officers rather than medical men.[25] Ramshackle hospitals were to be found in the French colonies, too. On

[22] Pratik Chakrabarti, "'Neither meete nor drinke but what the Doctor Alloweth': The Hospital Amidst War and Commerce in Eighteenth-Century Madras", *Bulletin of the History of Medicine* 80, no. 1, Spring 2006, 1–38; Londa Schiebinger, *Plants and Empire: Colonial Bioprospecting in the Atlantic World* (Cambridge, MA: Harvard University Press, 2004).

[23] Mark Harrison, "Science and Medicine in Early Colonial India, *c.*1750–1820", in *The Oxford Companion to the History of the British Empire: India,* ed. Nandini Gooptu and Douglas M. Peers (Oxford: Oxford University Press, forthcoming).

[24] Moseley, *Treatise on Tropical Diseases*, 156.

[25] Robert Jackson, *A Treatise on the Fevers of Jamaica, with Some Observations on the Intermitting Fever of America, and an Appendix, Containing Some Hints on the*

arriving on the island of Martinique, *en route* to China, the French traveller P. Savary found the hospital and its patients in a truly appalling condition.[26]

Colonial Hospitals and Colonial Subjects

Apart from religious institutions in Latin America, and the small hospitals established for slaves in American plantations and in Asian colonies like the Dutch East Indies,[27] early colonial hospitals were primarily for the use of Europeans. Even where growing numbers of indigenous peoples found employment with Europeans—as in the massive armies of the English East India Company—medical care was normally provided outside of hospitals and by indigenous practitioners. An exception to this appears to be a separate hospital established for the use of sepoys in Ghireti near Calcutta in about 1742, although very little is known about it.[28] Hospital treatment for the sick and wounded of so-called native forces in most European colonies was sporadic until the twentieth century,[29] but in the course of the nineteenth century there were numerous attempts to provide modern hospital care for civilians. From the 1790s some European philanthropists established charitable infirmaries similar to those found in many Western countries.[30] However, they differed from their European counterparts in that private donations

---

Means of Preserving the Health of Soldiers in Hot Climates (London: J. Murray, 1791), 419–20.

[26] P. Savary, "Journal au Voyage de France au Chine", 38–39, MS 6065, Wellcome Library for the History and Understanding of Medicine, London.

[27] G. T. Haneveld, "From Slave Hospital to Reliable Health Care: Medical Work on the Plantations of Sumatra's East Coast", in *Dutch Medicine in the Malay Archipeligo, 1816–1942,* ed. G. M. van Heteren et al. (Amsterdam & Atlanta: Rodopi, 1989), 73.

[28] Crawford, *Indian Medical Service*, 422.

[29] Mark Harrison, "Disease, Discipline and Dissent: The Indian Army in France and England, 1914–1915", in *Medicine and Modern Warfare,* ed. Roger Cooter, Mark Harrison and Steve Sturdy (Amsterdam and Atlanta: Rodopi, 1999), 185–204.

[30] See, for example, Ann Borsay, *Medicine and Charity in Georgian Bath: A Social History of the General Infirmary, c.1739–1830* (Aldershot: Ashgate, 1999).

tended to be reinforced with assistance from government. The Native Hospital built in the Indian holy city of Benares, for example, was funded by a combination of private funding (Rs 50,000 in private subscriptions) and a recurring monthly grant of Rs 600 from the Government of Bengal. This institution appears to have flourished and the old building was replaced by a new hospital and dispensary after 1811.[31]

Several other hospitals were established at around the same time in the larger towns of British India,[32] but there were no similar provisions in the Dutch East Indies, for example. When it came to hospital provision, British India bore more similarity to French Algeria, where medical care of indigenous peoples was offered soon after the colonial occupation. By the 1840s there was a formal health service, including hospitals and dispensaries for the use of the local population, in addition to separate civilian and military hospitals for Europeans. As in India, one of the main objectives behind these moves was to present colonial rule as beneficent so that the population would be "controlled not only by military force" but "tied to the benefits of civilization", as one French doctor put it.[33]

In many instances, however, the foundation of hospitals was linked overtly to the requirements of European colonisers. In the course of the nineteenth century and into the twentieth, hospitals and dispensaries were established by plantation owners, and by mining and railway companies, to meet the health needs of their workforce. In many colonies the stimulus to the provision of hospitals was the end of formal slavery and the labour shortage it engendered. Free medical treatment, along with housing and food,

[31] Extract of public letter from Bengal, 28 July 1811, enclosing letters of 12 August 1793, 14 February 1807 and 5 April 1811, Oriental and India Office Collections (henceforth OIOC), Bengal Public (Home) Proceedings F/4/364, British Library (henceforth BL).

[32] For example, the Native Hospital in Calcutta, which admitted 3,681 outpatients in 1802–1803. See Crawford, *Indian Medical Service*, 424–31.

[33] Quoted in Anne Marcovich, "French Colonial Medicine and Colonial Rule: Algeria and Indochina", in *Disease, Medicine, and Empire: Perspectives on Western Medicine and the Experience of European Expansion,* ed. Roy MacLeod and Milton Lewis (London: Routledge, 1988), 105.

provided additional incentives to labourers, which in many cases had to be brought from overseas; such measures also aimed to increase labour productivity. In the Dutch East Indies, where there had been few medical facilities until the abolition of slavery in 1860, hospitals were established on many plantations, such as those in Sumatra, which depended almost entirely on labour imported from China and Malaya. Planters agreed collectively to provide medical care in order to stem losses from disease and to give an incentive to labourers. Medical care thus became part of the indenture agreement, whereby labourers were bound to work the duration of their contract, in return for a fixed wage and certain welfare provisions, including the small hospitals that were found on most plantations. These institutions were normally run on a day-to-day basis by Malays or Chinese, with the Company doctor visiting every week or so. The drawbacks of this system soon became obvious and, by the end of the century, these small estate hospitals were replaced or supplemented by larger and more permanent institutions, which became increasingly important in staving off criticism of high death rates in plantations.[34]

A similar pattern occurred in other colonies. Plantation hospitals were established in the tea gardens of Assam in British India, for example, and in Ceylon, as Margaret Jones shows in her chapter. There, plantation hospitals were established in response to criticism of the wretched state of the indentured labourers brought from southern India but these institutions were themselves found to be highly deficient, prompting growing government involvement.[35] The catalyst for change, here and in other British colonies, was a survey of hospitals across the British Empire in the 1860s; itself a response to the exposure of the shocking condition of medical institutions in Jamaica. Hospitals were also established for similar reasons by the owners of large industrial enterprises, such as the jute

[34] Haneveld, "From Slave Hospital to Reliable Health Care".

[35] C. G. Uragoda, "The British Period", in *A History of Medicine in Sri Lanka: From the Earliest Times to 1948* (Colombo: Sri Lanka Medical Association, 1987), chap. 6.

mills of Bengal and the cotton mills of Western India,[36] as well as by railway enterprises like the Manchurian Railway Company, described in Robert Perrins's chapter. The latter, however, was more an agency of the Japanese state than a traditional private concern.

Until the twentieth century, most hospitals for indigenous peoples in the colonies were essentially hospitals for the poor. As in most Western countries, prosperous patients continued to seek treatment from private practitioners in their homes, even if they solicited the attentions of a practitioner of Western medicine. Hospitals were generally institutions of last resort and care within the family seemed preferable to submission to unfamiliar and possibly demeaning regulations. To this may be added the perceived dangers of the hospital as a source of infection and disease. Such considerations deterred many people from entering hospitals in the West until the twentieth century, when their reputation began gradually to improve.[37] In colonial contexts additional factors served to limit their popularity: early colonial hospitals made few concessions to the requirements of caste and religion, for example, and in India most of those who attended appear to have been low caste or untouchables, some of whom had converted to Christianity. Even so, hospitals like those established for the poor in Calcutta and Benares were attracting several thousand in-patients each year by the early 1800s. One striking feature of admissions to these hospitals in their early years is that there were around three times as many in-patients as out-patients, which suggests that the hospitals were seen more as shelters for the indigent than as curative institutions, whatever the intentions of their founders and physicians.[38] By mid-century, however, it seems that hospital usage approximated more closely to Western institutions, with increasing demand for out-patient treatment. Thus the number of out-patients attending the Jamsetjee Jejeebhoy Hospital (J. J. Hospital) in Bombay rose from roughly equal

[36] Subho Basu, "Emergence of the Mill Towns in Bengal, 1880–1920: Migration Pattern and Survival Strategies of Industrial Workers", *The Calcutta Historical Journal* 18, no. 1, 1996, 97–133.

[37] Charles Rosenberg, *The Care of Strangers: The Rise of America's Hospital Sytem* (Baltimore: Johns Hopkins University Press, 1993 edn.).

[38] Extract of public letter from Bengal, 28 July 1811, BL.

with in-patients in the mid-1840s to become three times greater than in-patients by the 1850s.[39] The rising demand for out-patient care was also reflected in the growth of dispensaries in India, which were established by a variety of state (municipal and provincial) and private initiatives.[40]

This set the pattern for the development of medical institutions throughout the British Empire, which continued to evolve, as in Britain, through a mixture of private and public institutions. In the newer African colonies, however, the state never played so great a part in health care as it did in India or Ceylon, with missionaries having a much larger role in the running of hospitals. Other colonial powers, such as Germany and France, also permitted the establishment of mission hospitals alongside those of the state; on balance, however, it seems that government played a more important role in health care provision in German and French colonies than in British possessions. In the German Pacific colonies, for example, the state provided the first and only hospitals on the islands. Yet, it is important not to overstate the importance of such establishments: there was a huge difference between the comparatively well-resourced German African colonies and the often meagre facilities to be found in the Pacific.[41]

In some older colonies, where European notions of science and progress had begun to make in-roads into local culture, indigenous philanthropy was also beginning to play a part in the foundation of hospitals and dispensaries. From the middle of the nineteenth century, Indian magnates such as the Parsi businessman Jamsetjee Jejeebhoy and the Kutchi merchant Goculdas Tejpal endowed large

[39] Statement showing the annual admissions into the Jamsetjee Jeejeebhoy Hospital and the charges incurred for medicine, provisions, etc., from 1845 to 1855, Government of Bombay 43, 1855, General Department, Proceeding 911, Maharashtra State Archives (henceforth MSA).

[40] Mark Harrison, *Public Health in British India: Anglo-Indian Preventive Medicine, 1859–1914* (Cambridge: Cambridge University Press, 1994), 88–90.

[41] Wolfgang U. Eckart, *Medizin und Kolonialimperialismus: Deutschland, 1884–1945* (Paderborn: F. Schöningh, 1997); Wolfgang U. Eckart, "Medicine and German Colonial Expansion in the Pacific: The Caroline, Mariana, and Marshall Islands", in MacLeod and Lewis, *Disease, Medicine, and Empire*, 80–102.

institutions in Bombay.[42] Writing of English voluntary hospitals, Roy Porter once argued that such institutions put an idealised gloss on the relations between rich donors and the poor, and threw a "cloak of charity" over naked repression.[43] Allowing for the peculiarities of the English case, it is likely that the very visible form of philanthropy exercised in endowing or subscribing to a hospital performed similar functions in India and other countries undergoing industrialisation, with philanthropists aiming to create a sense of social solidarity in situations where bonds of customary obligation were becoming strained. Giving money to hospitals served to demonstrate the donors' benevolence and their credentials as community leaders. The decision by some Indian donors to associate themselves with Western medicine also indicates a growing commitment towards the West as the source of modernity and community renewal, although it rarely implied a wholesale rejection of traditional values.

Like some of their European counterparts, the Indian philanthropists mentioned above sought a guarantee from government about ongoing financial support before making a donation—an arrangement that was conducive to financial stability. The hospitals catered for Indians of all religions, treating a roughly equal number of Hindus and Muslims, for example. The number of all ethnic groups other than Europeans grew steadily and by 1891, nearly fifty years after it was established, the J. J. Hospital was treating a total of nearly fifty-four thousand patients per year. However, the J. J. Hospital, like some others, contained special wards for the use of the donor's community, signalling that hospitals could become important sources of community pride and identity. One striking feature of hospital admissions in the J. J. Hospital, as in other hospitals throughout India, was that the proportion of women to men patients changed little over this period, despite an overall increase

[42] Mridula Ramanna, *Western Medicine and Public Health in Colonial Bombay, 1845–1895* (London: Sangam Books, 2002), 48–82.

[43] Roy Porter, "The Gift Relation: Philanthropy and Provincial Hospitals in Eighteenth-Century England", in *The Hospital in History*, ed. Lindsay Granshaw and Roy Porter (London: Routledge, 1989), 149–78.

in numbers. In 1877, 23.8 per cent of J. J. Hospital's patients were women, and in 1891 the percentage was 21.4.[44]

This gendered difference in access to medical care was explained by the reluctance of women to submit to the attentions of a male doctor, for there were few hospitals in India or any other colony catering specially for women or staffed by women doctors. But this is not to say that women's health had been ignored altogether. From the 1840s a number of maternity hospitals were established in some of the larger Indian towns, some of which, like the Lying-in Hospital founded in Madras, were at least the equal of their counterparts in Europe. As Sean Lang suggests, the importance attached to these institutions—which were aimed at a population that had no direct bearing on colonial rule—may be explained by their symbolic function. As beacons of humanity and enlightenment, it was hoped that they would contrast sharply with the 'darkness' of Indian society and its treatment of women. The establishment of Lying-in Hospitals followed controversial moves to improve the lot of Indian women such as the attempt in 1829 to abolish *sati*, the immolation of Hindu widows.

Although their symbolic importance was considerable, hospitals for Indian women were few in number, and, by the 1880s, it was widely acknowledged that the Indian government had failed to live up to its presumed responsibilities. From the 1880s, the Lying-in Hospitals and missionary institutions catering for women were supplemented by hospitals staffed by female doctors from the semi-official Dufferin Fund (or the National Association for Supplying Female Medical Aid to the Women of India, to give it its proper name). The impetus behind the scheme was not simply the humanitarian desire to extend medical relief to Indian women (primarily of the higher castes), but to inculcate Western values, especially principles of hygiene. It was thought that women held the key to improving domestic sanitation and hygienic education of the population in general. But while these endeavours received official support, this seldom translated into hard cash. Medical care for Indian women was also offered on very traditional lines, which reinforced

[44] Arnold, *Colonizing the Body*, 271–73.

patriarchal structures of authority in Indian society.[45] From the early twentieth century, however, the medical care of women and children began to receive more attention in the colonies, in line with developments in the West.[46] Throughout the British colonies, for example, there was a concerted attempt to improve the welfare of women and children through a variety of measures ranging from the regulation of midwifery, through to the provision of specialist health units and hospitals. Behind these initiatives lay concerns over the effects of unfitness on imperial efficiency, but also the recognition that women had too often been neglected by colonial administrations.[47]

Another type of specialist hospital that is comparatively well served in accounts of medicine in the European colonies is the lunatic asylum. The historiography of Western asylums has made much of their function as institutions for the containment and reform of social deviance, and so one might expect them to be fertile ground for explorations of colonial power. Indeed, the colonial asylum seems promising as a case study of how the operation of power differed in colonial and non-colonial contexts. In her study of medicine in colonial East Africa, Megan Vaughan has claimed that

[45] Sarah Hodges, ed., *Reproductive Health in India: History, Politics and Controversies* (Hyderabad: Orient Longman, 2006); Ramanna, *Western Medicine and Public Health*, 194–202; Geraldine Forbes, "Medical Careers and Health Care for Indian Women: Patterns of Control", *Women's History Review* 3, no. 4, 1994, 515–30; Maneesha Lal, "The Politics of Gender and Medicine in Colonial India: The Countess of Dufferin's Fund, 1885–1888", *Bulletin of the History of Medicine* 68, Spring 1994, 29–66; Arnold, *Colonizing the Body*, 260–68.

[46] See, for example, Lara V. Marks, *Metropolitan Maternity: Maternal and Infant Welfare in Early Twentieth-Century London* (Amsterdam and Atlanta: Rodopi, 1991); Deborah Dwork, *War is Good for Babies and Other Young Children: A History of the Infant and Child Welfare Movement in England, 1898–1918* (London: Tavistock, 1987); Jane Lewis, *The Politics of Motherhood: Child and Maternal Welfare in England, 1900–1939* (London: Croom Helm, 1980).

[47] Margaret Jones, "Health Services for Women and Children: Imperialism or Welfare?" in *Health Policy in Britain's Model Colony: Ceylon,1900–1948* (Hyderabad: Orient Longman, 2004); Geraldine Forbes, "Managing Midwifery in India", in *Contesting Colonial Hegemony: State and Society in Africa and India,* ed. Dagmar Engels and Shula Marks (London: British Academic Press, 1994); Manderson, *Sickness and the State,* chap. 7.

colonial power operated in quite distinctive ways, observable in the treatment of the mentally ill and certain other categories of patient. The essential difference, according to Vaughan, was that colonial power worked solely through the process of objectification, operating at the level of groups rather than individuals, as Foucault maintained for Europe. In the colonial context distinctions between the mad and the sane, the normal and the pathological, were to some degree encapsulated within racial divisions, so that blackness itself became pathological. [48] There is some evidence to bear out this line of thought in colonial literature on madness in Africa, as the "primitive" state of African society was seen to be the root cause of mental and other diseases. Mental illness was often thought to result from an inability to adapt to modernity, while colonial insurgency was sometimes viewed as the expression of African mental pathology. As a result, some prominent rebel leaders were detained in psychiatric institutions. [49] Such perceptions undoubtedly reflected the prejudices and apprehensions of the colonisers rather than the reality of the situation, however. [50]

Yet in India, as James Mills reminds us, power operated in ways more reminiscent of Europe, with asylum superintendents using techniques such as 'moral management', just like their counterparts in Britain, with the aim of creating productive and self-disciplined individuals. [51] Furthermore, treatment regimes varied in accordance with perceived differences among patients, rather than crude generalisations about racial predispositions. Mills also takes issue with the view that asylums were merely places of detention, in which

[48] Megan Vaughan, *Curing Their Ills: Colonial Power and African Illness* (Cambridge: Polity, 1991).

[49] Sloan Mahone, "The Psychology of the Tropics: Conceptions of Tropical Danger and Lunacy in British East Africa" (DPhil diss., University of Oxford, 2004).

[50] Jonathan Sadowsky, *Imperial Bedlam: Institutions of Madness in Colonial Southwest Nigeria* (Berkeley: University of California Press, 1999).

[51] James H. Mills, *Madness, Cannabis and Colonialism: The 'Native-Only' Lunatic Asylums of British India, 1857–1900* (London: Macmillan, 2000).

socially disruptive elements were contained.[52] This does appear to have been the case with the first asylums established for Indians, like the Mangy asylum founded in 1795 for sepoys. As Seema Alavi has argued, this asylum was intended to contain disruptive soldiers and possibly those who had contracted venereal disease, to prevent them from spreading infection around the cantonment. Indeed, as Alavi points out, the foundation of this asylum coincided with the first 'lock hospitals' for the forcible treatment of venereal disease among prostitutes.[53] But while agreeing that the majority of those admitted to asylums were probably not mentally ill in the sense understood today, Mills argues that later asylums took their therapeutic role seriously. Recovery was said to have occurred when patients showed a capacity for self-regulation, but there was often a huge difference between intentions and results, with hospital discipline frequently undermined by Indian subordinate staff and patients.

Another issue that arises in relation to mental hospitals—as well as with infectious diseases and tuberculosis hospitals[54]—is the problematic relationship with the communities in which they were situated. The location of psychiatric institutions is always a controversial matter, but as Julie Parle shows, in colonial contexts, and still more in Apartheid South Africa, the location of such hospitals was rendered more sensitive by racial divisions. The number of people confined in lunatic asylums, however, was negligible, and proportionately much less than in most Western countries, which

[52] Waltraud Ernst, *Mad Tales from the Raj: The European Insane in British India, 1800–1858* (London: Routledge, 1991); Waltraud Ernst, "Idioms of Madness and Colonial Boundaries: The Case of the European and 'Native' Mentally Ill in Early Nineteenth-Century British India", *Comparative Study in Society and History* 39, no. 1, 1997; Shridhar Sharma, *Mental Hospitals in India* (New Delhi: Directorate General of Health Services, 1990).

[53] Seema Alavi, *The Sepoys and the Company: Tradition and Transition in Northern India, 1770–1830* (New Delhi: Oxford University Press, 1995), 146.

[54] Mark Harrison and Michael Worboys, "A Disease of Civilization: Tuberculosis in Britain, Africa and India, 1900–1939", in *Migrants, Minorities and Health: Historical and Contemporary Studies,* ed. Laura Marks and Michael Worboys (London: Routledge, 1997), 93–124; Randall Packard, *White Plague, Black Labour: Tuberculosis and the Political Economy of Health and Disease in South Africa* (Los Angeles: University of California Press, 1989), 93–124.

also speaks strongly of the limitations of these institutions as instruments of social control. Yet, like all hospitals, they provided rare and valuable opportunities for observing the subject population and were microcosms of each society, exhibiting its peculiar tensions and contradictions.

This was also true of institutions for the care of leprosy sufferers, which existed in most of the African and Asian colonies, and in large numbers in some independent nations such as Brazil and Japan.[55] Most colonial leprosaria began as private or missionary initiatives, some of which were later taken over by colonial governments. With its biblical overtones, the care of leprosy sufferers epitomised missionary endeavours, and also, by contrast, the callousness shown by some indigenous communities towards those afflicted with the disease. Although many indigenous societies in Africa and Asia were actually tolerant of those afflicted with leprosy, some were cast out from their homes and lived as vagrants dependent upon alms. The growing number of complaints about vagrant lepers in Indian towns may have been one of the main reasons why officials there began to take a more active interest in the subject. As Megan Vaughan points out, leprosaria also offered missionaries the possibility of engineering new communities, cut off from those features of traditional society that impeded the spread of Christianity.[56]

The emphasis on social engineering was evident in most missionary institutions, often generating tension between the mission hospitals and the societies in which they were located. In this volume, Walter Bruchhausen stresses the difficulty of separating medicine from religion in the missionary context: a mixture creating considerable confusion among both Africans and Europeans. However, missionary hospitals like the ones studied by Bruchhausen in Tanzania normally became assimilated into local society, becoming

[55] Sharma, *Mental Hospitals in India*; Susan L. Burns, "From 'Leper Villages' to Leprosaria: Public Health, Nationalism and the Culture of Exclusion in Japan", in *Isolation: Places and Practices of Exclusion,* ed. Carolyn Strange and Alison Bashford (London: Routledge, 2003), 104–18; Jane Buckingham, *Leprosy in Colonial South India: Medicine and Confinement* (London: Palgrave, 2002).

[56] Vaughan, *Curing Their Ills*, 79.

an integral part of local healing. Even the religious mission of these hospitals did not necessarily present an obstacle, with Muslim as well as Christian patients seeking admittance. Local healers have responded to such institutions not by setting themselves up in conflict with mission hospitals, but by carving out a distinct niche for themselves in natural and spiritual healing. Similar themes emerge in Anne Digby's chapter on Victoria Hospital, South Africa, which aimed to weaken the attachment of Africans to indigenous medicine and witchcraft, but which itself sent out ambiguous messages on account of the religious dimension of its work. Again, we see that mission medicine was more a supplement than an alternative to local healing practices, with patients usually not considering themselves cured until a local diviner had pronounced on the reason why the illness had struck and offered additional therapies. Indeed, as we see in Helen Sweet's chapter, it could take some time for mission hospitals to gain the trust and understanding of the local community.

In the case of Nepal, however, it was the very foreignness of mission hospitals that inspired confidence in them. Ian Harper draws an analogy between the almost magical power exerted by the "alienist" and the mission doctor, their esoteric knowledge and apparent command over nature inducing patients to surrender themselves for treatment. Patients viewed mission medicine as existing in a hierarchical relationship with local traditions, the foreign origins of both doctors and medicines giving them an authority that local traditions lacked.

Mission hospitals have continued to play an important part in health-care provision in a number of other countries, not least in many parts of Africa. In Kenya, for example, mission hospitals continue to provide the bulk of medical care available to the rural population. The large state hospitals are often inaccessible and the overall number of beds far fewer in proportion to the population than in Western countries. Also the hospital networks identified by Fox in Britain and America[57] are fully visible in Kenya only at a national rather than a regional level; regional hierarchies do exist—with referrals from small district to larger provincial hospitals—but the

[57] Fox, *Health Policies*.

more serious cases are usually referred to a single, central hospital in the capital, Nairobi. Thus, while there is some resemblance to the systems that have evolved in Britain and America, the regional system in Kenya has been modified on account of the scarcity of resources and the need to concentrate them.[58]

National and Professional Identity

At this point, it is instructive to draw some comparisons between the development of hospitals in the former European colonies and those non-Western countries that were not subjected to formal colonial rule. Some of these—like the Buddhist kingdoms of South East Asia and Islamic polities like the Ottoman Empire and Persia—had long traditions of hospital care, within institutions that resembled those of medieval Europe. In many cases these had fallen into disuse but their existence was often associated with a cultural golden age, and they lived on in folk memory and in the names of streets, for example. The introduction of the hospital—in the modern sense of the term—thus provides an important case study in tensions between modernity and tradition. In Qajar Iran, where no hospitals had survived from the medieval period, the first modern hospital was established during the nineteenth century. It was a military institution, created with the full support of physicians in the Islamic medical tradition, and modelled on institutions in the West, especially in terms of its sanitary design. Yet, as Hormoz Ebrahimnejad argues in his chapter, the Islamic hospital tradition was invoked to justify its construction. Traditional medicine also continued to be practised in the new hospitals, with doctors being trained in both Western and Islamic systems of medicine. In some other Islamic polities—like the semi-autonomous princely states of India—institutional medical care developed simultaneously for Western and indigenous medicine. In Hyderabad, as Guy Attewell has shown, its modernising ruler created hospitals for both unani-tibb and Western medicine, older Islamic institutions having decayed through neglect. He thereby attempted to resurrect the glories of

[58] George O. Ndege, *Health, State, and Society in Kenya* (Rochester, NY: University of Rochester Press, 2001), 135–37.

an early Indo-Islamic civilisation while attempting to modernise his domains.[59]

The Ottoman Empire's experience appears to have been different in several respects. Firstly, some old-style hospital institutions survived from medieval times and, second, the Empire consciously set aside traditional medicine—which lost state sponsorship—to endorse the Western model. As in the case of Iran, medical modernisation began with the army but by the 1870s, as Philippe Bourmaud shows in his chapter, Western hospitals had been founded in many parts of the Ottoman Empire, where they performed similar functions to hospitals in other colonial contexts. But there was one important difference: Western hospitals outside Turkey, in areas like Palestine, were run by French, German and other foreign organisations, such as Roman Catholic institutions. These organisations were given tremendous leeway by the Ottoman state, which very seldom intervened in the running of their hospitals. However, as Bourmoud shows, petitions sent to foreign consuls provide rare insights into local responses to the hospitals and their apparent deficiencies.

In other countries, such as Japan, hospitals evolved quite differently again. As is well known, modern Western medicine was introduced into Japan in the 1860s as part of the modernisation project that followed the Meiji Restoration of 1867.[60] From then, things progressed rapidly and, by 1913, Japan possessed 79 public general hospitals with 6,708 beds and 863 private general hospitals, with 28,395 beds, in addition to a number of specialist institutions. In order to meet the rapidly increasing demand for physicians, the Japanese government established Western medical education at the University of Tokyo and by 1884, at some thirty prefectural teaching hospitals. By 1938, there were over thirty thousand university graduates in medicine, together with almost as many graduates from

[59] Guy Attewell, "Authority, Knowledge and Practice in Unani Tibb in India, c.1890–1930" (PhD diss., University of London, 2004).

[60] A Portuguese hospital existed in Japan earlier, albeit briefly, during the period when it had been open to foreigners (1549–1639); see Jan van Alphen and Anthony Aris, eds., *Oriental Medicine: An Illustrated Guide to the Asian Arts of Healing* (Boston: Shambhala, 1995), 234.

medical colleges who possessed lower qualifications. By the eve of the Second World War, the numbers of those qualified in Western medicine dwarfed the rapidly dwindling number of traditional practitioners. Over time, these practitioners, though differently qualified, melded into one relatively homogenous medical profession, much as in America, although quite unlike Britain, where there was greater distinction between specialist doctors and general practitioners. Japan, however, was unique in that large numbers of medical graduates became physician-proprietors, owning as well as working in their own hospitals. As a result, the number of private hospitals expanded rapidly, reaching 2,955 providing 76,764 beds by 1940, some 92 per cent of all hospital beds in the country. [61]

Although the pattern of hospital development in Japan was distinctive, it was similar to many other non-Western countries in that the state was the driving force behind the establishment of teaching hospitals and medical education. Although the state was involved to some degree in professionalisation in many Western countries—more so in Germany, for example, than in Britain or America—the provision and content of medical education was far less dependent on government than in most non-Western countries. In Japan, which modelled itself closely on Germany, medical education remained substantially under state control until 1945. Following the German model, the Japanese government threw itself solidly behind Western medicine to the exclusion of other local medical traditions, in much the same way as the Ottoman Empire. In the colonies, indigenous medical professionals enjoyed what John Iliffe has described as an "ambivalent symbiosis" with the colonial administration. On the one had, the state provided them with training (through such institutions as Makerere Medical College and Mulago Hospital in Uganda); on the other, they saw themselves as locked in a struggle with government for professional recognition and equality with British doctors. [62]

[61] I am most grateful to Shuhei Ikai for allowing me to cite his unpublished paper, "Becoming Hospital Owners: The Evolution of Doctors Career Paths in Japan from the 1870s to the 1930s".

[62] John Iliffe, *East African Doctors: A History of the Modern Profession* (Cambridge: Cambridge University Press, 1998).

Hospitals such as Mulago ultimately grew into important teaching centres and, in the late-colonial era and after independence, began to produce more graduates who entered private practice. In other cases the teaching function of hospitals did not develop until after independence, and it was only on the eve of independence, in 1955, that Calabar hospital in south-eastern Nigeria appointed its first African doctor. However, in some British colonies education in Western medicine had been available for many years before independence. In India it began in the 1830s and clinical instruction was considered an important element from the very beginning. Although the majority of those who qualified in medicine initially entered government service—for instance, as military surgeons or municipal health officers—a growing number entered private practice and by the early twentieth century, Indian colleges were producing around four thousand new medical graduates each year, in addition to many who had dropped out of their studies but nevertheless described themselves as "doctors". This ultimately had an impact on the teaching of medicine in hospitals and on those who held senior posts. By the end of the First World War, private practitioners represented by organisations such as the Bombay Medical Union successfully negotiated rates of pay for government work and greater equality with British practitioners including access to consultancy posts in the major teaching hospitals.[63] Fighting shy of what would have been an extensive financial commitment, the government encouraged the development of an independent profession because it saw it as the only way of providing health care for all its subjects.[64]

63 Appointment of consulting staff for government hospitals in Bombay City for the year 1913 to 1914, Government of Bombay 81, 1913, General Department, Proceeding 604, MSA; Proposal to employ private medical practitioners in large hospitals in the mofussil, Government of Bombay 73, 1913, General Department, Proceeding 1/1324, MSA; Bombay Medical Union to Education and Health Secretariat, Government of Bombay, 21 November 1927, Government of Bombay, 1932, General Department, Proceeding 7090 (B), MSA.

64 A. Earle, Officiating Secretary to the Government of India, Home Department (Medical) to Secretary to the General Department, Government of

In some colonies, however, as well as in some independent countries, the origins of medical education lay not with government initiatives but with missionary organisations. In East Asia, one of the best known is the West China Union University, which evolved from a training programme established by missionaries from Canada. Now named the Sichaun Medical College, it became famous as the alma mater of Chiang Kai-shek.[65] The Mukden Missionary Hospital and Medical College in Manchuria was another fertile source of Western doctors. Founded in 1885 by the Scottish missionary Dugald Christie, the hospital and college grew to become one of the largest and most prestigious medical schools in the People's Republic of China. However, as Robert Perrins reminds us, the origins of the hospital and college are seldom acknowledged today for ideological reasons.

The development of nursing in non-Western countries has received very little attention by comparison with the medical profession. One thing that is clear is that the growth of hospitals outside of Europe and North America facilitated what has become known as a "nursing diaspora", with women from the USA, Great Britain, Holland, Germany, Scandanavia and North America working in a variety of missionary and state hospitals in the former colonies. As both Anne Digby and Helen Sweet show in their chapters, missionary nurses in South Africa tended to stay in their adopted communities, placing great emphasis on training local women, while those in the colonial services tended to remain overseas for just a few years, often leaving to get married.[66] In post-colonial South Africa, during the Apartheid period, the role played by nurses in their communities was far different, some becoming activists on behalf of their communities. In her chapter on Baragwanath Hospital in Soweto, Simonne Horwitz shows that nurses provided a bridge

Bombay, 22 February 1911, Government of Bombay 73, 1913, General Department, Proceeding 1/1324, MSA.

65 Karen Minden, *Bamboo Stone: The Evolution of a Chinese Medical Elite* (Toronto: University of Toronto Press, 1994).

66 See also Helen Sweet, "'Wanted: 16 Nurses of the Better Educated Type': Provision of Nurses to South Africa in the Late Nineteenth and early Twentieth Centuries", *Nursing Inquiry* 11, no. 3, 2004, 176–84.

between European doctors and local communities, and often acted as pressure groups for the betterment of conditions.

Elsewhere in the colonies nurses appear to have played an active part in education from the very beginning. In Ceylon, for example, some British nurses went out in the 1870s to initiate training programmes for local women, in what was referred to as "Scientific Nursing". Such moves appear to have furthered the spread of nursing in some colonial hospitals but the continued dominance of European women in nurse training served to inhibit local attempts to organise professionally. This situation contrasted markedly with the training of doctors in Ceylon, where the Ceylonese took a major role in medical education early on. The difference is exemplified by the fact that while doctors trained in Ceylon achieved registration by 1905 (before India) the nurses had to wait until 1949.[67] Thus, in Ceylon, nursing remained more subordinate than in Britain and the same appears to have been true of India. Doubts about the respectability of nursing as an occupation for women, coupled with often demeaning working conditions, meant that it was difficult to find sufficient nurses, particularly with adequate training, throughout the period of British rule. Nurses protested constantly about high-handed treatment by doctors and being forced to perform what they considered to be menial tasks.[68]

In independent states, the dynamics of professional development were of course very different. In Japan modern nursing developed as part of a general programme of medical Westernisation. Nursing was wholly alien to the Japanese, as patients were normally cared for at home. This meant that nursing was initially looked upon with some suspicion, as it entailed women (who made up the vast majority of the nursing profession) working away from the traditional domestic arena and having contact with male patients to whom they were not related. Doubts about respectability, together with the re-

[67] Margaret Jones, "Heroines of Lonely Outposts or Tools of Empire? British Nurses in Britain's Model Colony: Ceylon, 1878–1948", *Nursing Inquiry* 11, no. 3, 2004, 148–60.

[68] For example, Letter from twelve nurses to Lord Willingdon, 17 July 1913, Government of Bombay, 1913, General Department, Proceeding 2/271, MSA.

assertion of patriarchal values, meant that the development of nursing did not follow the same model as in the West, notwithstanding Japan's commitment to modernisation. The growth of the female nursing profession was, rather, circumscribed by having to conform to the traditional virtues normally associated with women, *viz.*, passivity and subordination. Japanese nurses lacked the autonomy of their counterparts in the West, although there were some opportunities to play a more prominent role. Nurses from the Japanese Red Cross participated in international forums, as well as in public health programmes under the auspices of the Rockefeller Foundation. In the sphere of nursing, Westernisation was therefore superficial: a case of "suffocated professionalism".[69]

One of the most important consequences of the growth of indigenous medical professions in non-Western countries was the effect it had upon the provision of hospitals and dispensaries. We see many examples of medical entrepreneurship driving the pace of specialisation, much as in Europe and North America.[70] Small and often specialised hospitals, like the hospital for eye and ear diseases established in Bombay by Dr J. A. Da Gama, with support from local philanthropists, became increasingly common from the turn of the twentieth century. This example is instructive because Da Gama appears to have solicited funds from the likes of J. N. Tata and other local magnates, rather than they seeking initially to endow a hospital.[71] In other words, this and other such initiatives were increasingly led by members of the medical profession; mirroring the shift that occurred in nineteenth-century Europe and America from paternalistic to professional control of hospitals.[72]

Another feature of these initiatives was that they were often intended to benefit particular communities. This was not the case in

69 Aya Takahashi, *The Development of the Japanese Nursing Profession: Adopting and Adapting Western Influences* (London: Routledge Curzon, 2004).

70 Lindsay Granshaw, "'Fame and Fortune by Means of Bricks and Mortar'? The Medical Profession and Specialist Hospitals in Britain, 1800–1948", in *The Hospital in History*, ed. Lindsay Granshaw and Roy Porter (London: Routledge, 1989), 199–220.

71 Ramanna, *Western Medicine and Public Health*, 77–8.

72 See Rosenberg, *The Care of Strangers*.

the hospital established by Da Gama but others were built in India for the use of particular castes and religions, and increasingly for high-caste Indians. This process began as a temporary provision during the plague crisis of the 1890s but became more common during the twentieth century as technological advances and better hygiene enhanced the reputation of hospital medicine. Some non-Western countries therefore followed the trend whereby prosperous and respectable sections of the population came to accept and even to demand hospital care. The hospital was becoming a potent symbol of modernity, readily embraced by those who considered themselves in the van of progress. However, there was normally some degree of accommodation with local culture, which was often demonstrated in the very architecture of hospitals, which retained elements of indigenous traditions while at the same time meeting the requirements of modern, hygienic buildings.

Many of the issues highlighted in histories of colonial hospitals, and those erected in independent countries, continue to be relevant today. Indeed, the question of whether earlier experiences and attitudes continue to shape health care in the non-Western world is taken up in many of the chapters in this book. Equally pertinent is the relationship of hospital medicine to other forms of health, particularly the question of whether high technology medicine has dominated medical provisions at the expense of primary health care? This matter has already generated extensive discussion,[73] but it is examined here by Reema Bhatia in relation to the contemporary Punjab. A host of other issues relating to contemporary health care may also profitably be examined from a historical perspective. For instance, to what extent have physicians, hospital managers and governments sought to alter the running of hospitals in the post-colonial era? Do hospitals serve the interest of affluent, globally-oriented professionals better than the people for whom they are intended? What is the

[73] For example, Imrana Qadeer, Kasturi Sen and K. R. Nayar, eds., *Public Health and the Poverty of Reforms: The South Asian Predicament* (New Delhi: Sage, 2001); Iliffe, *East African Doctors*; Manderson, *Sickness and the State*; Roger Jeffery, *The Politics of Health in India* (Berkeley: University of California Press, 1988); D. Morley, J. Rohde and G. Williams, *Practising Health for All* (Oxford: Oxford University Press, 1983).

relationship between global health strategies, such as those formulated by the World Health Organization (WHO), and the needs and realities of localities outside the West? What are the implications of the increasing role of NGOs in the provision of health care in some non-Western countries—particularly in Africa—not to mention an increasing reliance on missionaries, as states abdicate or are forced to abandon their commitments.

The chapters dealing with these issues explore a number of complementary avenues. Walter Bruchhausen, for example, considers the often strained relationship between hospital medicine and traditional healing, notwithstanding the World Health Organization's wish to integrate traditional practitioners into health care delivery. Indeed, it is possible that the WHO's strategy is designed largely to control traditional practitioners and to alter the way in which they operate. The continuing tension between different concepts of health and disease is also evident in James Mills's paper on the post-colonial asylum, a chapter which also explores the dilemmas of staff which inherited institutions and practices from a colonial regime. In some contexts, as Shahduz Zaman shows in his study of a hospital in Bangladesh, lines of authority between patients and practitioners are probably even starker today than they were in the colonial era. And last but not least, Guillaume Lachenal's paper on laboratory analysis in post-colonial Cameroon examines a dimension little studied in either the colonial or post-colonial eras: the hospital as a site of research. We know from other work, such as that of Iliffe on East Africa and Bell on the Sudan,[74] that hospitals became increasingly important as sites for research conducted by indigenous doctors trained in Western medicine. Lachenal examines the attempts by Cameroonian doctors and scientists to gain control of the Pasteur Centre of Cameroon, an institution founded during the colonial era and which continues to be associated with foreign influence and political privilege.

This book can claim only to represent a starting point for the analysis of the hospital 'beyond the West' but it is to be hoped that

[74] Heather Bell, *Frontiers of Medicine in the Anglo-Egyptian Sudan, 1899–1940* (Oxford: Clarendon Press, 1999); Iliffe, *East African Doctors*.

it will encourage others to look in greater detail at the history of these institutions. While it is possible to identify certain important themes—not least the peculiar cultural and economic factors affecting the growth of hospitals outside of Europe and North America—it is already clear that it is very difficult to generalise about the evolution of hospitals in those contexts. The development of hospitals was quite different in old colonies such as India than in the more recently established colonies of tropical Africa, for example. At the same time there were marked differences among independent countries, with Japanese medical modernisation taking a very different path from some Islamic countries, where vestiges of older medical systems were revived by the state. Whatever approaches scholars take to the study of these institutions in future, it is clear that the history of the hospital beyond the West offers great potential to illuminate the transformation of Western medicine into the global medical system that it has become.

1

The Indian Immigrant Worker and the Development of Hospital Provision in Nineteenth-Century Ceylon

Margaret Jones

Introduction

In 1890, Dr W. A. Kynsey, the Principal Civil Medical Officer (PCMO) of Ceylon reported that there were thirty-nine hospitals of various kinds operating in the island and a further nine either proposed or on the point of opening. These government funded hospitals along with the 126 outdoor dispensaries were intended to establish a "system of medical relief in those remote parts of the island where hitherto the people have had to depend on their own ignorant vederalas from the absence of European practice". This system would, Dr Kynsey confidently asserted, mean that there was "a Medical Officer and a dispensary within a reasonable distance" of all inhabitants of the colony.[1] Mere numbers admittedly give no indication of the therapeutic value of these hospitals but their number still represents a remarkable commitment by a colonial government to extend the perceived benefits of Western medicine to the indigenous population. Furthermore, hospital distribution in Sri Lanka today is very much shaped and formed by these early developments. The foundation of these hospitals is therefore an issue

I would like to thank the Wellcome Trust for funding the research for this paper and Rodney Lowe for comments on an earlier draft.

[1] Dr W. A. Kynsey to the Secretary of State, 24 May 1890, Public Record Office CO 54/587, The National Archives (henceforth PRO, TNA); *Annual Medical Report, 1890,* PRO CO 57/112, TNA. The population of Ceylon in 1890 was approximately 2.75 million.

of both historical and current importance. This chapter examines hospital foundation in relation to the needs of both the growing capitalist economy and an incipient indigenous medical profession.

There are three sections. The first outlines the political, economic and medical context. The second focuses on the major factor in the growth of a hospital system—the plantation economy and the health needs of the immigrant labour force. The third section links this with the developing medical profession within the colony and its desire to gain status and recognition. Charles Rosenberg, in his account of the rise of America's hospital system, has argued that one aspect of the hospital is that it "reproduces values and social relationships of the wider world".[2] This applies no less to the colonial society of Ceylon and its hospitals.

The Political, Economic and Medical Context

Ceylon became a unified crown colony of the British Empire in 1815. The Colebrook-Cameron reforms of 1833 imposed the superstructure of a *laissez-faire* state and set the pattern for crown colony governance within the empire. These reforms ushered in a period of rapid economic development on capitalist lines. From 1833 a policy of land sales and thus a land market, was introduced; this was greatly accelerated in 1840 by the Crown Land Encroachment Ordinance which laid down that all land not proved to have been granted previously was the property of the crown and could be sold.[3] Additionally, the abolition of the feudal system of compulsory labour—the *rajakariya*—in 1832 in the ancient Kandyan kingdom (incorporated into the colony in 1815) was intended to provide a free labour market. As K. M. de Silva has argued the thrust of this

[2] Charles E. Rosenberg, *The Care of Strangers: The Rise of America's Hospital System* (Baltimore: Johns Hopkins University Press, 1995), 4. Or to borrow John Pickstone's terminology, the 'political ecology' of Ceylon's hospitals, includes the political, economic and social structures not just of the colony but also of the British imperial system. John V. Pickstone, *Medicine and Industrial Society: A History of Hospital Development in Manchester and Its Region, 1752–1946* (Manchester: Manchester University Press, 1985), 2.

[3] Chandra Richard de Silva, *Sri Lanka: A History* (New Delhi: Vikas Publishing House, 1994), 161.

early legislation was to break down the "old conservative, aristocratic, status ridden and caste-oriented society" and replace it with "a new commercial and more egalitarian society".[4] These economic and constitutional changes had a direct impact, as will be seen, on the spread of hospital provision.

One of the accompaniments of imperial rule was the spread of Western medicine to the colonies. The hotly debated significance of this is outside the bounds of this chapter, although Ceylon provides an interesting case study of its complexity, to which it contributes.[5] The original medical imperatives as elsewhere in the empire were to protect the British administrators and the military. At the beginning of their rule the British established military hospitals in Colombo, Jaffna, Trincomalee and Galle, staffed by military doctors.[6] The control of epidemic disease and a certain humanitarian impulse also impelled the colonial government quickly to establish Leper and Lunatic Asylums, temporary isolation hospitals for smallpox and cholera victims and a general hospital at Colombo for the indigent sick.[7] The government also encouraged the foundation of Friend-in-Need Societies—charitable institutions, which set up hospitals for the general population in Kandy, Jaffna and Trincomalee.[8] However, the availability of Western medicine to the indigenous population was, up to the third quarter of the nineteenth century, severely limited.

Two pivotal events led to Western medical services becoming an integral part of the colonial state. The first was the creation of an independent civil medical department within the colonial administration in 1858. "Placing a civilian in charge of the principal hospitals", the Governor, H. G. Ward argued, "might facilitate the formation

4 Kingsley M. de Silva, *Social Policy and Missionary Organisations in Ceylon, 1840–1855* (London: Longmans, Green and Co. Ltd, 1965), 66.

5 See Margaret Jones, *Health Policy in Britain's Model Colony: Ceylon, 1900–1948* (New Delhi: Orient Longman, 2004).

6 C. G. Uragoda, *A History of Medicine in Sri Lanka: From the Earliest Times to 1948* (Colombo: Sri Lanka Medical Association, 1987), 82.

7 Uragoda, *History of Medicine in Sri Lanka,* 86–88.

8 Ibid., 90–92.

of medical classes and the extension of the simple branches of the healing art, to a much greater degree".[9]

The second crucial development was the foundation of a Medical School in Colombo in 1870. There had long been recognition of the need for non-military doctors in the colony. The government between 1839 and 1869 sent students to the Bengal Medical College (6 students left for Calcutta in the first year).[10] It also gave an annual grant to a medical school started by the American mission under Dr Samuel Green in Manipay in the north of the island.[11] Neither of these schemes met the deemed need for qualified indigenous practitioners in Western medicine. The Bengal scheme did not produce a sufficient flow of qualified men for the colony. Only those who failed to gain employment elsewhere, Dr W. P. Charsley (PCMO) complained in an 1866 letter to the Colonial Secretary, joined the government service.[12] In addition, by 1869 the "extended benefit" which had been "derived by the native population of the Northern Province" from Dr Green's school was about to end. The missionary's recent decision to confine the education at the school to the Tamil language would close the "source, from which a large class of useful Practitioners was derived".[13] At the same time there came a passionate plea for "the adoption of a plan of Medical education in the Island itself, for training an efficient class of medical Practitioners who will scatter themselves over the country, and displace the present class of ignorant quacks".[14]

[9] H. G. Ward to the Secretary of State, 27 August 1857, PRO CO 54/333, TNA.

[10] Uragoda, *History of Medicine in Sri Lanka* , 112.

[11] Ibid., 114–15.

[12] W. P. Charsley to the Colonial Secretary, W. C. Gibson, 13 February 1866, PRO CO 54/412, TNA.

[13] W. P. Charsley to the Colonial Secretary, 9 December 1869, PRO CO 54/448, TNA; W. P. Charsley to the Colonial Secretary, 9 September 1869, PRO CO 54/448, TNA. Dr Green's decision was made deliberately to preclude his graduates from joining the government service and thus deserting their villagers.

[14] Sessional Paper XIII, *Depopulation of the Vanni District,* Dr James Loos, Colonial Surgeon, Jaffna, 1868, 7, PRO CO 57/47, TNA.

These failures encouraged Dr Charsley to push again for a medical school first suggested to the Legislative Council by J. A. Stewart Mackenzie, the then Governor, in 1839.[15] With the exception of towns, Dr Charsley asserted, where there was already a hospital and thus a Medical Officer (MO) "I have no means whatever at my disposal for putting more efficient medical assistance within the reach of the people".[16] His initial limited aim was for an "Elementary School, capable of affording a sound and practical education of three years duration in the principles of Medicine and Surgery, and especially Midwifery, together with practical knowledge of Anatomy, Physiology, Materia Medica, Pharmaceutical Chemistry, and the Art of Dispensing". He had been convinced by the "number of respectable young men, chiefly of the Burgher Community, who voluntarily apply to be allowed to go round the Civil Hospitals of Colombo", that there was a "strong desire among the public" for such a school. The cost would be a modest £500 per annum.[17] The Medical School was opened in June 1870 with Dr James Loos as its first principal. The school was designated a College in 1880 and its course recognised in 1888 by the General Medical Council of Great Britain. In the first six years C. G. Uragoda noted 18 men in total had graduated from the school.[18]

[15] Uragoda, *History of Medicine,* 116.

[16] W. P. Charsley to the Colonial Secretary, 31 March 1869, PRO CO 54/448, TNA.

[17] W. P. Charsley to the Colonial Secretary, 9 September 1869, TNA. The Burghers were the Christian descendents of the Portuguese and Dutch colonists and were a highly Westernised group within the indigenous elites. See, for example, Kumari Jayawardena, *Nobodies to Somebodies: The Rise of the Colonial Bourgeoisie in Sri Lanka* (London and New York: Zed Books, 2002); and Kamalika Pieris, *The Medical Profession in Sri Lanka, 1843–1980* (Colombo:Visidunu Prakashakayo Ltd, 2001).

[18] Uragoda, *History of Medicine,* 117–18. Dr James Loos was himself a graduate of the Bengal Medical College and also of St. Andrews and Edinburgh. Clinical training at the School took place at the General Hospital, Colombo established in 1864 as a successor to the original civil hospital in Pettah, Colombo. C. G. Uragoda, "History of Teaching Hospitals in Sri Lanka: General Hospital Colombo (1)", *Ceylon Medical Journal* 36, no. 1, 1991, 27–32.

Thus the colony had started to produce a number of indigenous medical men who had a vested interest in expanding and extending the medical services of their country. The interests of this burgeoning indigenous professional class, in conjunction with their British colleagues, interacted with a pressing need for health care services created by the presence of an exploited labour force. The process by which these two factors coalesced with pressure from the imperial government to influence the spread of hospital provision is the focus of the next two sections.

Indian Immigrant Labour and the Plantation System

Capitalism came to Ceylon along with imperial rule. In the 1840s according to C. R. de Silva "the entire economy of the island was transformed by the rise of coffee plantations". This was due to the external factor of an increased demand for coffee in England and the internal factor of a colonial government which provided a favourable environment for producers. [19] As Asoka Bandarage has claimed the "colonial state was not a neutral observer of plantation development"; the "officials created the plantation economy". [20] Indeed until the civil service reforms of 1844–45 members of the administration and the British establishment were among the prime speculators. The Governor, the Colonial Secretary and lesser administrators, the military commander and members of the clergy all owned coffee estates. It was one way of supplementing their inadequate official salaries. [21] However, even after this direct involvement was prohibited in the mid-1840s, Bandarage has further argued that the "colonial state continued to serve the interests of the plantation economy by providing necessary legislation, infrastructure, tax

[19] De Silva, *Sri Lanka: A History*, 160–61. From the late 1870s the coffee industry came under threat from disease and by the 1890s it had been replaced by tea as the major export crop.

[20] Asoka Bandarage, *Colonialism in Sri Lanka: The Political Economy of the Kandyan Highlands, 1833–1886* (Berlin, New York and Amsterdam: Mouton Publishers, 1983), 274.

[21] H. A. J. Hulugalle, *British Governors of Ceylon* (Colombo: Arjuna Hulugalle Dictionaries, 2002), 68–69, 80.

policy and police protection".[22] The result of the economic concessions of the 1840s was a coffee boom.

The abolition of rajakariya had been intended to provide a free labour market but unfortunately the Kandyan peasant proved unwilling to work on the new plantations. However, as a pioneer coffee planter explained they had "their own paddy fields, their own cows, bullocks, their own fruit-gardens" which occupied all their attention and their "wants are easily supplied"; they therefore had no "inducement to work on the coffee plantations". In addition labouring for wages was in direct conflict with their culture.[23] The result, as summarised by the Colonial Secretary, Emerson Tennent in 1847 was that, despite having "an abundant population chiefly of that class that furnishes the supply of agricultural labour in every other country of the world", Ceylon presented the "anomaly of an actual dearth of labour". In order therefore to work their estates the coffee planters were forced to import their labour force from South India—the so-called "coolies".[24]

According to Hugh Tinker the word "coolie" may have originated in Ceylon; it was certainly given "wide currency by Portuguese captains and merchants", the first European colonisers of the island. By the nineteenth century it had come to be applied to those at the "lowest end of the industrial labour market"—the immigrant Indian labour force who could be found in many colonies of the British Empire.[25] The Indian immigrants to Ceylon came mainly from Madras, and initially their presence was seasonal. They were predominantly male workers who came for the picking season to earn money to take home at the end of the harvest. In general they were from the lowest echelons of Indian society and they came because of poverty and famine at home. Table 1.1 is a contemporary estimate of the extent and increasing levels of that immigration in the 1840s.

22 Bandarage, *Colonialism in Sri Lanka,* 274.

23 Quoted in De Silva, *Social Policy and Missionary Organisations*, 235–36.

24 Memorandum from Emerson Tennent to the Secretary of State, 21 April 1847, PRO CO 57/ 235, TNA.

25 Hugh Tinker, *A New System of Slavery: The Export of Indian Labour Overseas, 1830–1920* (London: Oxford University Press, 1974), 42–44.

TABLE 1.1 Number of Indian labourers arriving in northern parts of island, 1839–46

Year	Men	Women	Children
1839	1,971	182	90
1840	2,487	303	173
1841	3,461	362	162
1842	7,487	262	152
1843	3,149	81	119
1844	69,702	1,026	437
1845	66,557	642	79
1846	34,683	257	31
Total	189,497	3,115	1,243

Source: Tennent to the Secretary of State, 21 April 1847, TNA.

A graphic description of the difficulties of the journey undergone by these itinerant workers also survives. Only a few made the journey by sea to the ports of the western coast such as the capital Colombo. The majority in the 1840s crossed over by rice-boat from the southern tip of India to Talaimannar or Mannar. There were two routes from there. The one of lesser importance was from Mannar through what is now the Wilpattu National Park to Puttalam, Kurunegala and then the hill country. The main route was from Mannar to Mewdawachchiya and then south to Anuradhapura, Matale and then the hill country.[26] The Puttalam route took them about 70 miles over a "succession of low and barren sands . . . the passage at all times dreary and sometimes dangerous" through "one of the most desolate and inhospitable" parts of the island. From Puttalam there were two ways to reach Kandy and the plantations. The Puttalam to Kandy route, some 81 miles was "new and passable" and abounding in "water and forests which afford rest and shade". The other road via Anuradhapura crossed "a district once rife with population and still covered with the remains of tanks and

[26] I am grateful to Chris Uragoda for this information.

cultivation" and so was "not only unhealthy from malaria but desolate and solitary in the extreme".[27]

The sickness and death caused by the hardship of this journey, with workers often being left to die on the roadside, precipitated early medical intervention by the government. In 1841 W. Morris, the Assistant Government Agent (AGA) for Kurunegala, alerted the then Governor, Stewart Mackenzie, to the "wretched state of the coolies" and as a result rest houses were constructed along the Puttalam-Kandy road. Then in 1843 Morris's plea for a hospital at Kurunegala for those who became ill on the journey was put into effect.[28] Hospitals were eventually established at both ends of the line at government expense, in the coffee planting districts and on the route from Mannar to Puttalam and a subsidy was given to the Kandy Friend-in-Need Society Hospital. The cost to the government of these measures was estimated in late 1846 to be £3000 per annum.[29]

The sufferings of the immigrant labourer did not end once his/her destination was reached. Tinker has described the plantation as a "world apart . . . subject to the laws and whims of those in charge".[30] The colonial government was generally willing to allow the planters this level of autonomy but in this case it was hard for it to overlook the obvious suffering of sick labourers and the public health and order threat they presented. This disquiet between the professional and the entrepreneur, despite common economic interests, became increasingly apparent. Frederick Lewis (a coffee planter) noted later the "considerable gap between the sympathies of the planter . . . and

[27] Tennent to the Secretary of State, 21 April 1847, TNA. Also see Uragoda, *History of Medicine,* 97–98.

[28] Report of W. Morris, Police Superintendent, Colombo, 30 March 1847, PRO CO 57/235, TNA.

[29] Governor to the Secretary of State, 11 November 1846, PRO CO 54/227, TNA.

[30] Tinker, *A New System of Slavery*, 177. As Frederick Lewis, a planter and then member of the government Forestry Service put it, "[m]en regarded themselves as very supreme and any interference with their systems of control was naturally repugnant to them". Frederick Lewis, *Sixty-Four Years in Ceylon: Reminiscences of Life and Adventure* (New Delhi: Navrang, 1993), 6.

of the local administrators, whose ideas . . . were completely out of keeping with planting methods and ways."[31]

In the late 1840s open conflict between the government and the planting community erupted. The Planters' Memorial of 1846 was a call for greater government expenditure on medical care for the immigrant labourers but in describing so vividly the distress endured by their workers they scored something of an own goal.[32] Not only did the coolies die on the journey often on the roadside, the petitioners claimed, but those that survived arrived "so emaciated by disease" that they were unable to work and in many cases "absolutely die for want of shelter and food". Furthermore, the "humid-climate" contributed to much sickness and so, "utterly unable to earn their own subsistence", the unfortunate labourers became "the victims of beggary, disease and want". Returns from the Kandy Friend-in-Need Hospital were included in order to point out the high mortality rate of those admitted to the hospital, and illustrate the inadequacy of what was being done.

TABLE 1.2 Returns for the Kandy Friend-in-Need Hospital for June, July and August, 1846

	Admissions	Deaths	Remaining in Hospital
June	152	84	102
July	145	100	72
August	104	75	56

Source: Memorial of the Planters, 9 September 1846, PRO CO 54/227, TNA.

The purpose of the petition was to force the government to provide more medical care at its expense. The "distress', it argued, was of "such magnitude" that it was "quite beyond the control of the voluntary exertions of any class".[33]

31 Lewis, *Sixty-Four Years in Ceylon*, 6.

32 A Memorial was a petition to the Secretary of State through the Governor and was the accepted and common way in which the grievances and desires of colonial subjects, whether as individuals or groups, were brought to the notice of the Imperial Government.

33 Memorial of the Planters, 9 September 1846, PRO CO 54/227, TNA. This had 937 signatures including that of the Chairman, S. Butler.

However, the government had little problem in turning this argument on its head; the Planters' Memorial, it claimed, was evidence of their neglect of their own workforce. The response was a Governor's circular to magistrates in the planting districts requesting their observations. The magistrates' replies confirmed the Planters' testimony but laid the blame firmly, as might be expected, at their feet. For example, one police superintendent, J. S. Colepepper, had "no hesitation" in stating that "this class of population is in much worse condition in the Central Province than the Negro slave was described to be in the West Indies in former days". Few estates provided medical aid and sick 'coolies' were frequently driven from the estate "on a charge of idleness" to die by the roadside. When a coolie died on the estate he was buried with no inquiry or inquest.[34] A similar picture of total neglect emerged from the Matale magistrate E. J. Waring. "When they are sick their pay is stopped, there is no medical attendance, when they die they are buried by their friends" and sick workers "frequently wander away and are never heard of again".[35] The depositions which C. H. D. Sarum, the magistrate at Gampola took from six coolies recovering in the hospital there told the same tale. One described being "driven away from the estate like a dog". Sarum had no doubt where the responsibility lay: "I attribute the deaths on the bog road, bye paths and at the hospital as well as the great number of helpless beings seen daily lingering out a life of wretchedness and starvation to a want of the due care and attention on the part of the planter".[36]

Both planter and government thus accepted that the condition of the immigrant worker was appalling but each sought to blame the other. Both sides agreed that there was an urgent need for more medical services but who was to pay for the hospitals, the dispensaries and the medical care? The planters claimed that the economy of the whole island depended on the success of their industry. "It

[34] J. S. Colepepper, Police Superintendent, Central Province, 18 January 1847, PRO CO 57/235, TNA.

[35] E. J. Waring, Police Magistrate, Matale, 14 January 1847, PRO CO 57/235, TNA.

[36] C. H. D. Sarum, Police Magistrate, Gampola, 8 February 1847, PRO CO 57/235, TNA.

was self-evident", they argued, "that the prosperity of this colony depends upon its agricultural operations, and that the introduction of labour must contribute in every way to the public Revenue and benefit all classes, and not the Planters in particular".[37] Therefore medical care should be financed out of the general public revenue. Tennent on the other hand argued that "the whole body of the inhabitants of Ceylon are not dependent on the successful cultivation of one grand staple . . . on the contrary the vast mass of the population are supported by totally different pursuits". It would therefore "be a manifest injustice" for the "revenue raised by contributions from the entire community" to be used to support one sector alone.[38] Hence, in the late 1840s the government refused to increase its commitments beyond which was already in place.

Nevertheless, the problem was merely going to escalate and in the longer term could not be ignored. One of the first actions of Sir Christopher Elliot in 1858 on taking up his appointment as the first PCMO of the new civil medical department was to raise the issue once more with the government. The sufferings of the journey along the120 mile Northern Road from Mannar to Matale provoked his concern. Water was scarce in the dry season and the scanty population could not provide food and moreover it was "feared" that the coolies were often "robbed and otherwise ill-treated" on their way. According to Elliot they set off from home with a stock of cooked rice, barely enough to last the journey, so any delays meant that they ran out of food and the possibility of delays were numerous. They began with the boatmen in India refusing to take them across the Palk Straits without bribes, then in Ceylon the rivers in flood could hold them up for days and even when the "waters had subsided so that strong men and good swimmers" could cross they had to wait for "their weaker companions, the women and children". "Sour boiled rice, jungle roots, half cooked or eaten raw, and bad weather soon began to tell". Those who fell ill then began to lag behind and were "necessarily abandoned to die a lingering

[37] Memorial of the Planters, 19 December 1846, PRO CO 54/235, TNA.

[38] Tennent to the Secretary of State, 21 April 1847, TNA.

death from bowel complaint or starvation unless their sufferings are sooner terminated by their being devoured by jackals".

Furthermore, as Elliot pointed out, echoing the earlier accounts, "the seeds of illness are laid in those who immediately escape", and being unable to work, "they wander about until picked up by the police and taken to the pauper hospitals", hence the "frightful high mortality which our hospital returns show". Until a steamer service from India to Ceylon was fully established he suggested that a system of three ambulance bullock carts be established along the route in the charge of a man who would receive a basic training in administering medicine and who could offer food. "How many a poor creature would a single dose of medicine or a meal enable to reach the far-off estate or to keep up with his friends" or a "drink of water prevent a poor creature going to a mud-hole and with the noxious draft taking in the seeds of lingering illness and death". The government apparently approved this service at a cost of £18.70 a month.[39]

"The stalemate" between government and planter, Soma Hewa has argued, "contributed to a great deal of suffering among the immigrant labourers persisted throughout the late nineteenth and early twentieth centuries".[40] However, whilst there is no doubt that the health of the Indian labourer continued to be poor and that both sides were reluctant to make the necessary commitment towards ending their suffering, in the longer term it became increasingly difficult for the government to ignore the threat posed by the wandering sick and dying, and the conditions on the estates. Moreover, by the 1860s there was third actor emerging—the civil medical service.

A "disgrace to any civilised community": The Colonial Government and the Kandy Friend-in-Need Society Hospital

Thus, in the late 1850s the government came under increasing pressure to expand its hospital provision. The principal hospital in the

[39] Elliot to Colonial Secretary, 14 September 1858, Record Group (henceforth RG) 6/ 2461, Sri Lanka National Archives (henceforth SLNA); Minute, 15 September 1858, RG 6/ 2461, SLNA.

[40] Soma Hewa, *Colonialism, Tropical Disease and Imperial Medicine: Rockefeller Philanthropy in Sri Lanka* (Lanham: University Press of America, 1995), 46.

Central Province, where the coffee estates were concentrated, was still the charitable Kandy Friend-in-Need Society Hospital. In 1860 this voluntary hospital was taken over by the government to become the second major civil hospital of the island. This episode provides a further example of the conflict of interests between government and planter and illustrates the developing role of the newly created civil medical department.

According to Dr Charsley (PCMO in 1859) the Kandy Hospital had been founded in 1839 and until 1847 was supported by £500 worth of annual public subscriptions. The depression in the coffee industry of that year led to a drastic decline in its finances and in 1848 it had had to reduce admissions from an average of forty a month to only three or four. Such a sharp reduction in the service forced the government to make a direct annual subsidy to the Society of £350 on the condition that the hospital admitted all the sick who were sent. In 1858 this subsidy was increased to £900. In addition the government paid the £250 a year salary of the Assistant Colonial Surgeon in charge of the hospital and a further £40 towards the Society's Charitable Fund. This made an annual total of £1200. [41] At the same time Dr Charsley pointed out, the total of private subscriptions had fallen to £200. [42] Such a sizeable outlay by the government to an institution over which it had only limited control could not continue for long.

The impetus for a complete government takeover appears to have come from a member of the newly created civil medical department. Until 1859 the hospital had been under the charge of an Assistant Surgeon who occupied a somewhat ambiguous position in that he was responsible neither to the government who paid his salary nor to the hospital management committee of the Friend-in-Need Society who technically employed him. [43] In 1859 the Gover-

[41] Dr W. P. Charsley to the J. Bailey, Assistant Colonial Secretary, 5 September 1859, PRO CO 54/351, TNA.

[42] J. Bailey to Rev. G. W. Sprott,, Honorary Secretary of the Kandy Friend-in-Need Society, 18 January 1860, PRO CO 54/351, TNA.

[43] The Committee at the time was composed of the Government Agent of Kandy as President, a Major Bird as Vice-President, the Commandant of Kandy, the District Judge, the Police Magistrate, the Chief Kandyan,

nor, H. G. Ward, appointed Dr J. Johnston as District Medical Officer in the newly formed civil medical administration. As a result of what he had seen at the hospital Dr Johnston complained personally to the Governor that the colony was maintaining "the most horrible and loathsome of establishments" and suggest that the Governor visit to see the situation for himself. This the Governor did in June of that year. As his despatch to the Secretary of State explained, "I went instantly to see the place though in a state of health . . . which precluded me from entering the wards, without danger".[44] As the Colonial Secretary relayed to the Friend-in-Need Society, the Governor's personal observation impelled him to condemn the "Kandy Cooly Hospital" as a "disgrace to any civilised community: a mass of filth, and ordure, and vermin, and uncleanliness of every kind".[45]

The report commissioned from Dr Johnston in August supported this assertion. The hospital consisted of two buildings. One was intended as a surgical and one as a medical hospital. As the so-called surgical hospital had no privy (patients had to relieve themselves in the grounds around it, very close to the Medical Officer's house), it was used for the few convalescent patients who could walk to the medical ward when necessary. The result on Dr Johnston's inspection was that only five patients occupied the surgical hospital while seventy-eight crowded into the medical hospital. In addition the medical hospital's new female ward was half filled with stores so that women, even in the last stages of dysentery, were mixed in with the men in the remaining two wards. Some patients occupied the verandahs but most were crammed into the wards with doors and windows shut at night so that "hospital gangrene spread from sore to sore". As Dr Johnston related, "The sight of the beds and floors in the morning was very disgusting, and during the day the

---

Sinhalese and Tamil Mudaliyars (indigenous leaders), two Burghers, four clergymen, both the bankers of Kandy and the Chairman and Secretary of the Planters' Association. *Meeting of the Subscribers to the Kandy Friend-in-Need Society,* 6 February 1860, PRO CO 54/351, TNA.

44 H. G. Ward to the Duke of Newcastle, 5 March 1860, PRO CO 54/351, TNA.

45 J. Bailey to the Rev. G. W. Sprott, Secretary of the Friend-in-Need Society, 5 December 1859, PRO CO 54/351, TNA.

stench from the cases of gangrenous sores and, the cases of bowel complaint, was intolerable". When he asked for the back windows to be opened he was told that they "were always kept shut, to prevent the ingress of a *more unwholesome* atmosphere from the back verandah, where the worst cases of bowel complaint were kept". The back verandah, he said, was too disgusting to describe and had for some time been termed the "charnel house". Wards and patients were dirty, there was no discipline, no clothes to replace soiled ones, only a few mattresses and blankets "saturated with every kind of abomination", and in the small cemetery about forty yards behind the hospital, where 573 bodies had been buried in the previous year, "the surface of the ground was strewed with human bones". [46]

The Committee naturally defended itself from charges of mismanagement by claiming that the situation was beyond its control owing to the numbers of sick and dying labourers needing hospital care (115 patients housed in a building ideally meant for 20), and that its repeated requests for help from the government had met no response. [47] Feelings ran so high that for a time the dispute caused a major breach in the colonial elite. The Committee virtually accused the Governor of lying about what he saw and the Governor countered with accusations of "extreme impropriety". [48] An emollient statement from the Society in February 1860 expressing the wish that the medical department would takeover the hospital and a public apology from the Governor at the opening of the Katugastotte bridge ceremony, which was reported in the press, saved the situation. [49] The hospital was formerly surrendered to the govern-

[46] Dr J. Johnston, *Confidential Report on the Hospitals of the Kandy Friend-in-Need Society,* 15 August 1859, PRO CO 54/531, TNA.

[47] G. W. Sprott to L. Bailey, 20 December 1859, PRO CO 54/351, TNA.

[48] G. W. Sprott to L. Bailey, 20 December 1859, TNA; L. Bailey to G. W. Sprott, 18 January 1860, PRO CO 54/351, TNA.

[49] *The Statement of the Committee,* 11 February 1860, PRO CO 54/351,TNA; H. Ward to the Secretary of State, 5 March 1860, TNA. This despatch included a press cutting for the 1 or 2 March (it's not clear from which paper) entitled *Kandy Friend-in-Need Society Hospital* in which the Governor expressed regret that in "condemning a system he had done injustice to the hard working members of the committee".

ment on 2 March 1860. The government undertook to provide sufficient accommodation, medical attendance and medicines for the maximum average number of patients of the last five years, and the planters, as they were supposed to but frequently did not, would pay for all cases sent to the hospital. If this arrangement failed to work then the government would have to consider the possibility of a general assessment on the planting community to finance the medical care of their labour force.[50]

This episode has been covered in some detail for a number of reasons. First, it provides some idea of conditions within a mid-nineteenth-century colonial hospital. Secondly, it illustrates the process by which the government was drawn into taking responsibility for the medical needs of the broader population. The Governor felt impelled to act as a "duty of vital importance to the colony", and because to allow "so great a scandal" to continue would bring great discredit on it.[51] Thirdly, the creation of a civil medical department established a body of expertise, represented here by Dr Johnston, which had to exert itself in order to establish its credibility and its utility. At the Colonial Office (CO), Sir Henry Ward's actions were commended; "it seems to be the cardinal duty of the Governor of an island, inhabited by an inferior race, and destitute of the checks which exist in such a country as ours to exhibit a detestation of abuses. In such a community the example of the Head of the Society stands in the place of public opinion".[52] This observation on the nature of colonial governance at the Colonial Office leads naturally to a consideration of the role of the Imperial government.

The Imperial Government and Hospital Inspection

In 1867 a system of inspection and reporting on each hospital was instigated in Ceylon with the PCMO acquiring the additional powers of being the Inspector General of Hospitals. This development was the result of an Imperial government initiative. In January 1863

50 H. G. Ward, *Minute,* 5 March 1860, PRO CO 54/351, TNA.

51 H. Ward to Secretary of State, 3 March 1860, PRO CO 54/ 351, TNA; J. Bailey to G. W. Sprott, 5 December 1859, TNA.

52 Minute, 27 April 1860 (signature unreadable), PRO CO 54/351, TNA.

the Secretary of State had sent a circular despatch to all colonial Governors seeking detailed information on the state of all their hospitals. The precipitating event for this circular, it was stated in the resulting report, had been the exposure of the "evils and defects" of the public hospitals and the "cruelties and abuses" in the lunatic asylum of Jamaica.[53] As the Secretary of State pointed out in his follow-up despatch in 1864, in the United Kingdom the majority of hospitals "owed their existence to the bounty and philanthropy of private persons" and thus, the "beneficent spirit in which they originated has attended them continually". Consequently, there was a constant interest in their "progressive improvement of structure, arrangements, management and supervision". In the colonies however, the hospitals were founded and supported from public funds, and, echoing the comment of the CO official above, their "well-being" was dependent on the "Executive and Legislative authorities". The replies from the Governors, the despatch asserted, revealed that the state of their hospitals was "widely and deplorably different from what would be considered in this country to be consistent with humanity itself".[54]

H.G. Ward had eventually conceded in relation to the Kandy hospital that it was the system not the individuals which had been at fault. So too did the Secretary of State acknowledge that the state of colonial hospitals could not be attributed to "wilful and deliberate neglect" but to "a want of adequate knowledge of what such institutions ought to be, and of the methods by which improvements are to be brought about".[55] Part III of the Report therefore contained recommendations to remedy this. It was self-evident, the authors wrote, that the "object desired in the treatment of the diseased . . . are that the greatest proportion of patients should be cured and in the shortest possible time". Taking for granted that sufficient funds would be made available by governments, the way to improve-

[53] Circular Despatch, Report on Colonial Hospitals and Lunatic Asylums, 6 April 1864, 1, PRO CO 854/7, TNA.

[54] Secretary of State to the colonial Governors, 6 April 1864, PRO CO 854/7, TNA.

[55] H. G. Ward, *Minute,* 5 March 1860, TNA; Secretary of State to the colonial Governors, 6 April 1864, TNA.

ment was first to ensure that the sanitary conditions in hospitals and asylums were regulated. The "class for whom such institutions are intended", it was asserted, "have a strong claim to be treated according to conditions which scientific experience has found to be indispensable".[56] Secondly, management should be in the hands of those "who have necessary knowledge and are in a position to give necessary attendance and can be made responsible for to some other superior power".[57]

In order to effect these first two recommendations there was a further recommendation for a system of inspection of all hospitals and asylums and a "regular and better system of reports". Such reports would fulfil various functions. Making those in charge of the hospitals report on "the workings of the system" in a way which could not be "too many or too minute", would mean that "the official has to justify his actions" to the inspectors of hospitals.[58] Secondly, based on the information in these individual reports annual or bi-annual summaries would be distributed throughout all the colonies as a "valuable system of comparison, advice and suggestions". Thirdly, the reports would facilitate statistical analysis for scientific purposes.[59] The official inspection of hospitals by either a Board of Inspectors, or if this was not practical an individual, should also be supplemented by having a system of hospital visitors who should make their own observation.[60] The report concluded that:

> There is no excuse for any preventable excess in the rates of mortality or the duration of treatment, and if the institutions of mercy do not conform so far as reasonably practicable to those conditions under which alone their patients have a fair chance of recovery, it must be a question . . . whether they ought to exist at all.

The implementation of this practice in Ceylon, thus, meant that each MO in charge of a hospital was accountable to the PCMO

56 Circular Despatch, Report, 6 April 1864, Paragraph 49, 13, TNA.

57 Ibid., Paragraph 50, 13, TNA.

58 Ibid., Paragraphs 51, 17.

59 Ibid., Paragraphs 51, 18.

60 Ibid., Note III, Appointment, Powers and Duties of Inspectors.

and the Governor for the success or failure of their hospital when measured against the above criteria. It also meant that the PCMO was similarly accountable to the Imperial government for the overall performance of all hospitals in the colony. Failure to conform to the required standards thus presented a possible threat to their professionalism, status and even their livelihoods. The hospital returns of Ceylon's hospitals exposed their high mortality rates and brought into question the utility of these institutions and the expertise of those who ran them. These reports provided hard evidence in the stalemate between government and planter over the issue of what should be done and who should pay for the medical care of the immigrant labourer.

The Government, the Medical Department, the Planter and the Mortality of the Immigrant Labourer

The first health care requirement placed on the planter by law was in one short section of Ordinance No. 11, 1865 which established their duty to provide for treatment of the sick worker, either on the estate or if necessary by removal to hospital.[61] From the late 1860s however, there was increasing pressure on the government for more intervention, especially from members of the medical profession. One notable example was the controversial 1869 report on the immigrant hospital at Gampola by the Assistant Colonial Surgeon in charge, Dr W. G. Van Dort.[62] Dr Van Dort was a young Burgher doctor and his report aimed to shift the responsibility for the high mortality rates in his hospital to the planters, and to the labourers themselves. The principal diseases from which the worker suffered and subsequently died in the hospital were dysentery, diarrhoea (83 admissions in 1868, for example, of whom 31 died),

[61] Ordinance No. 11 1865, *Ordinance to Consolidate the Law Relating to Servants, Labourers, and Journeymen Artificers under Contracts for Hire and Services*, Section 27, PRO CO 56/9, TNA.

[62] Dr Van Dort rose to prominence in the profession and the colony. He was President of the Ceylon Branch of the British Medical Association, 1900–1903 and was the Burgher representative on the Legislative Council. Uragoda, *History of Medicine,* 137–38.

and anasarca and asthenia (143 admissions and 40 deaths), these last two conditions being a direct result of the bowel complaints. Basing his conclusion on the figures of immigration and emigration taken from Ferguson's Ceylon Directory, Dr Van Dort claimed the general death rate for all labourers was "nearly 1 in 4".

However, rather than ascribing these complaints to the conditions under which these men and women lived and laboured he concentrated his analysis on the character and habits of the Tamil worker. With regard to their character, they were "inoffensive, patient, docile, indisposed for exertion". Although with "great powers of endurance" they were also "unprincipled" and "untruthful". Moreover their "immoderate indulgence of gross and sensual appetites", "want of cleanly habits", "improvident and careless disposition", "apathy and indolence", rendered them "easy prey to disease".[63]

The report was circulated to Government Agents (GAs) and members of the Planting community for comment. The GAs tended to concentrate on disputing the overall mortality figures arguing that they were based on insufficient statistical information, and that many Tamils settled permanently in the island and thus did not appear in the emigration figures. E. N. Atherton the AGA for Mannar, for example, who had general supervision of the Immigration Service, claimed that the mortality rate, certainly for the previous five years, was 1 in every 647. He argued that Dr Van Dort was inaccurately extrapolating his figures from the mortality rates of those who entered Gampola Hospital.[64]

The Planters similarly disputed the figures but they also took objection to Dr Van Dort's comments on the "habits" of their workforce. H. Byrde the Secretary to the Planters' Association rejected his observations on the workers as "throughout exaggerated, and in some respects, wholly incorrect". The mortality at the Gampola hospital could be accounted for by the "great and . . . insuperable

[63] Correspondence on the Condition of Malabar Coolies in Ceylon, 1869–1870, PRO CO 54/475, TNA; Dr W. G. Van Dort, Report on the Gampola Civil Hospital (not dated).

[64] Malabar Coolies in Ceylon, 1869–1870, E. N. Atherton, AGA, Mannar, 24 December 1869, PRO CO 54/475, TNA.

objection" which the Tamils had to entering a hospital which meant they only did so when their case was desperate.[65] Mr J. Shipton, who was in charge of the Gampola Hospital for many years and claimed a twenty-year experience of the conditions on the coffee estates, similarly condemned the comments as "gross exaggerations" if not "quite untrue". The "poor diseased degraded wretch" portrayed by Dr Van Dort, he argued, bore little resemblance to the "fine healthy, contented, and orderly set of coolies that form the bulk of the labouring population of Ceylon".[66] Peter Moir with topical awareness averred that Dr Van Dort's comments on the physique of the Tamil "would enchant a Darwinian".[67] Perhaps R. B. Tytler's sarcastic reference to Dr Van Dort as "the medical youth who has aired his English and his professional attainments" came close to understanding the motivation of the government surgeon.[68] Appointed to the medical service of the colonising government, a position which necessarily carried some status and prestige for him, he found himself in a hospital which in his own words was deficient in a number of respects—the locality, the sanitary arrangements, the overcrowding, the unsatisfactory buildings—and in which his patients died at an alarming rate. The need to justify himself to his masters both in Ceylon and in London must have been a pressing imperative.[69]

This correspondence was an opening salvo in a renewed debate between planter and government on the question of what should be done, and by whom, for the sick immigrant labourer. Furthermore, it took place against the background of the newly instituted scrutiny of hospital performance by the Imperial government. The high rates of mortality exposed by the colony's hospital returns was sufficient to raise negative comments at the Colonial Office and led to urgent requests for an explanation. As Dr Charsley (PCMO)

65 Malabar Coolies in Ceylon, 1869–1870, H. Byrde (not dated), TNA.

66 Ibid., J. Shipton, Kandy, 30 October 1869, PRO CO 54/475, TNA.

67 Ibid., P. Moir, Matale, 10 November 1869, TNA.

68 Ibid., R. B. Tytler, Pallekelly, 29 October 1869, TNA.

69 Ibid., Dr W. G. Van Dort, Report on the Gampola Civil Hospital (not dated), TNA.

asserted in his reply to the CO in June 1870, "the whole despatch seems to cast serious reflections on the conduct of the hospitals generally for which I feel myself responsible". His defence rested in part on some rather dubious, in the eyes of the CO officials at least, claims about how to count the figures. But, more importantly, the "fatal state of things [was] in no respect due to any fault of the department" but was "dependent on conditions and circumstances over which neither the government nor the medical officers can exercise control". For one thing, he pointed out, Ceylon possessed no "workhouses, nor almshouses, nor infirmaries to which the sick poor can resort, but all at the moment seek the government civil hospitals in which to terminate their existence". And for another, there was the "objection of the Tamil cooly and I may add all other classes of natives to enter a government civil hospital until the last necessity compels them".[70]

In May 1871 the Planters' Association passed a resolution calling upon the government to adopt a system of outdoor medical relief at government hospitals as a way of solving the problem of providing treatment for the workers who refused to go into hospital.[71] The resolution's somewhat disingenuous claim that this would entail no extra expense for the government was vehemently rejected by Dr Charsley who saw the whole plan as a ruse by planters to get free medical treatment for their workers. There followed an acrimonious correspondence through the colonial secretariat between Dr Charsley and H. Byrde, the Secretary of the Planters' Association. Byrde condemned the PCMO's "presumptions" on the planters' motives as "unjust and incorrect"; hardly the way he said to "increase the practical utility of his department".[72] Dr Charsley retaliated with the claim that the Ceylon government had already extended its "beneficence to a degree unheard of in other places" where Indian immigration had been permitted, and reiterated his charges of neglect

[70] W. P. Charsley to H. Irving, 2 June 1870, PRO CO 54/478, TNA.

[71] Correspondence Relating to the Medical Treatment of Coolies, H. Bryde, Secretary of the Planters' Association, to Henry Irving, Colonial Secretary, 18 May 1871, PRO CO 54/478, TNA.

[72] Correspondence Relating to the Medical Treatment of Coolies, H. Byrde to H. Irving, 22 July 1871, PRO CO 54/478, TNA.

against the planters. Their excuse that the labourers refused to enter hospitals was odd, he noted, given that so many appeared willing to die in them. Ironically also this reluctance seemed to have "become so intensified of late" that the money received from planters for the treatment of their workers in the Kandy hospital, for example, had declined from £25 to £30 a month just a few years ago to a mere £2 16s in July 1870. His solution was a radical one: "Planters must be compelled to build district cooly hospitals, to provide them with all medical requirements".[73]

Despite the slight rebuke administered to Byrde by the Colonial Secretary that "hospitals are part of the necessary machinery of a civilised Government", the government was not yet ready for Dr Charsley's district hospital proposal. However, with pressure coming also from the Imperial Government on "the propriety of making better provision" for the immigrant labourers it had to do something consequently it proposed a more limited and jointly funded (government and planter) scheme.[74] The Planters' Association reaction to this was to appoint a select committee to consider both the government's plan and Dr Charsley's proposal.

The Planters' Select Committee circularised 735 owners and managers of estates to ask for their views on both these proposals. Of the 279 replies received (admittedly a limited response), 176 were in favour of the government scheme, 58 said they were already providing that kind of medical assistance and 45 thought no scheme at all was required.[75] Among the last category was R. B. Tytler who called upon his fellow planters not to be "mealy-mouthed" but to "manfully speak out in plain Anglo-Saxon common sense: Let us, and our coolies, alone". His objections rested both on the mere suggestion of government interference in planters' affairs but also

[73] Medical Treatment of Coolies, W. P. Charsley to H. Irving, 28 August 1871, TNA.

[74] Lord Kimberley to the Governor, 16 August 1870, PRO CO 54/457, TNA; Medical Treatment of Coolies, H. Irving to H. Byrde, 31 October 1871, PRO CO 54/478, TNA.

[75] Medical Treatment of Coolies, Analysis of the Replies received to Committee's Circular, 6 June 1872, PRO CO 54/478, TNA.

of course on the taxation that it would entail.[76] In contrast some planters not only supported the government's scheme but also favoured Dr Charsley's proposal. Stewart Jolly from the Mausagala Estate, for example, considered it "highly desirable" to have a district hospital not more than 12–15 miles distant and J. G. Toussaint of the Beredewelle Estate thought there should be hospital within 10 miles of each estate. Though neither of them explored the question of who would provide the finance.[77]

The level of support was considered sufficient to enable the government to legislate for its scheme in Ordinance No. 14, 1872. By the ordinance groups of estates elected a District Medical Committee, under the chairmanship of the GA, which would then be responsible for making the necessary medical arrangements for their district, and for the assessment and collection of the estates' contributions towards its funding.[78] As the Governor explained to the Secretary of State, he was convinced that the already existing hospitals were a "great success", but they were not enough, the ordinance would ensure that on each estate or group of estates a "small cottage or hut" was established to "which the sick may be removed where their diet may be under control and where they may enjoy some of the appliances of a hospital, however simple, as regards cleanliness and ventilation". He likened the planters' opposition to the compulsory element of this scheme with that of the Irish landowners' to the Medical Charities Bill of Ireland. They had similarly contended, he argued, that the "labouring poor would be better cared for by private supervision than by public" but the Bill had become law and as a past Chairman of a Poor Law Union he "could speak with authority as to the signal benefit which state medical relief had conferred on Ireland".[79]

During the next two years the ordinance was gradually introduced into the coffee districts; but as early as the mid-1870s it was

76 Medical Treatment of Coolies, R. B. Tytler to H. Byrde, 15 February 1872, TNA.

77 Ibid., Stewart Jolly, TNA: J. G. Toussaint, Replies 67, 68, TNA.

78 Ordinance no. 14 1872, *An Ordinance for the Medical Wants of the Coffee Districts*, PRO CO 56/10, TNA.

79 Governor to Lord Kimberley, 9 July 1872, PRO CO 54/477, TNA.

already apparent that the ordinance, relying as it did largely on the voluntary cooperation of the planters, was—as predicted by Herbert at the CO in 1872—a "clumsy" compromise.[80] For one thing, Dr Charsley's confident assertion in his 1872 medical report that the ordinance would reduce mortality rates in hospitals was soon proved to be optimistic.[81] The death rates continued to be unacceptably high, and to provoke comment at the CO. In 1875 Dr Kynsey (PCMO) was again justifying them by the fact that estate labourers were being sent to the government hospitals "at such a stage that recovery is impossible". The "present arrangements", he argued, were "defective" and in "urgent need of reformation".

In March 1875 the Medical Inspector of the coffee districts, Dr Coghill, was asked to report on the workings of the 1872 ordinance.[82] He found a good deal of variation in implementation. While most had already appointed a district surgeon, the hospitals had not all materialised. The Kelebokka District Hospital, for example, had been up and running for some time and the dispensary system of out-relief was already extensive. The hospital consisted of three wards, a dispensary, small kitchen but no latrine and it required "equipment supplies very much to make a suitable hospital".[83] In the Hunasgiriya district, on the other hand, a European MO had been engaged and a bungalow rented for him but the hospital was no further on than the drawing up of plans and the selecting of a site. In the meantime the District Committee was using an old store as a hospital.[84] In the Rangalla and Nitre Cave district where Dr Coghill reported there had been strong opposition to the ordinance, great difficulty had been experienced in finding a suit-

80 Minute, Herbert, 26 November 1872, PRO CO 54/478, TNA.

81 *Annual Medical Report, 1872*, PRO CO 54/494, TNA.

82 Sessional Paper XIII, Correspondence Relating to the Medical Wants Ordinance, G. O' Brien to J. D. M. Coghill, 3 March 1875, PRO CO 57/67, TNA.

83 J. D. M. Coghill to Colonial Secretary, 3 April 1875, Paragraph 22, PRO CO 57/67, TNA.

84 J. D. M. Coghill to Colonial Secretary, Paragraph, 23, TNA.

able site for a hospital and the MO was dispensing drugs to the sick from his own house.[85]

There was thus considerable deviation from the prescribed arrangements. In addition, virtually no estates had set aside quarters on the 'cooly lines' for sick workers as laid down in Section 21 of the Act, and this could not easily be rectified. With "a few exceptions", Dr Coghill noted, "no existing cooly lines are capable of being converted into sick lines". Indeed he felt that to establish sick quarters adjacent to healthy workers would be unsuitable instead he recommended that estates of over 50 acres should be compelled by the government to set up separate sick quarters. These "cottage hospitals", as he termed them, would be very "advantageous" as the sick worker would receive treatment "at their own door and amongst their friends".[86] His report also highlighted a further problem. He pointed out that there were large numbers of Sinhalese labourers and artisans who "were absolutely unprovided with medical aid, although particularly, liable to severe injuries received whilst following their calling", and there was a "large bazaar population similarly circumstanced". The government should, he argued, give a "grant-in-aid" in support of the district scheme and public labourers should have access to the district hospitals.[87] Dr Coghill was in effect already recommending a substantial extension of the district hospital scheme.[88]

The Planters likewise were, for different reasons, unhappy with the workings of the ordinance. In a resolution to the government in July 1877 they complained that it was, from their viewpoint as rate-payers, "costly and vexatious" and moreover a "source of increased disease and death among Indian labourers". In response,

[85] Ibid., Paragraph 24, TNA.

[86] Ibid., Paragraphs 2–4, TNA.

[87] Ibid., Paragraphs 11–12, TNA.

[88] The term 'hospital' in this context might be a misnomer. The 'hospital' at Kelebokka, for example, was built of brick pillars with wattle and daub walls, white washed with a shingle roof. It held a maximum of four patients at any one time and had no blankets, mats, pillows, stool buckets, bed-pans, urinals etc. Annexure C, Diary of the Medical Inspector of the Coffee Districts, J. D. M. Coghill, 3 March 1875, PRO CO 57/67, TNA.

the government set up a Commission composed of planters and officials to look into the possibility of an improved scheme.[89] They interviewed eighty-two witnesses among them members of the planting and mercantile communities, and the medical profession. Drs Kynsey (PCMO), Coghill (Medical Inspector), Tothill (District Surgeon, Maskeliya) and Arthur (District Surgeon, Dimbulla) all submitted schemes to the Commission favouring the transfer of all responsibilities to the civil medical department, with some kind of assessment from the Planters to provide funding.[90]

The full extent of the problem faced by the government and the medical services was outlined by Dr Kynsey in his proposal. In 12 Government Civil Hospitals in 1876 the percentage death rate for Malabar coolies was 20.9 but for all other races it was 6.73. In 13 out of 20 district hospitals which had sent in returns the death rate was a horrifying 42.5 per cent; a situation which he said caused "much anxiety to the medical officers in charge".[91] He gave fourteen reasons for this state of affairs which included the state of ill-health of the Indians before they even left their home country, the rigours of the journey, changes in food and climate, lack of proper clothing, the insanitary conditions of many estates and impure water supplies. These things were exacerbated by some of the habits of the workers themselves. The last on his list was the "defective working of the Medical Wants Ordinance". As he saw it there were only two ways to provide for the medical care of the workers. The first was to have an entirely voluntary system run by the planters supplemented by government inspection. The second, which he favoured was for a government scheme run by the civil medical department and but funded by the planters. Under this scheme medical aid would be given by indigenous medical assistants trained in the Medical College at Colombo but supervised by medical men with European qualifications who could speak Tamil. Sick workers would be

89 Sessional Paper V, *Medical Aid Commission Report, 1879*, vi., PRO CO 57/78, TNA. The Report was signed by F. B. Templar, F. R. Saunders, W. D. Gibbon and A. T. Carslake.

90 Sessional Paper V, *Medical Aid Commission Report, 1879*, ix., TNA.

91 Ibid., Proposed Schemes, Dr Kynsey, Section VII and VIII, 179. The returns for the hospitals at Kelebokka and Humasgiriya had been eaten by rats.

treated on the estates where possible or if not in a small district hospital. It might also be necessary in the future, he argued, to have two large central hospitals in the planting district at Dimbulla and Hapatule.[92]

Despite the fact that the majority of the planters opposed any transfer of the scheme to the medical department the government acted on the lines of Dr Kynsey's suggestions.[93] Ordinance, No. 17 1880 *An Ordinance to provide for the Medical Wants of the Immigrant Labourers in Certain Planting Districts* grouped estates into districts under the charge of an MO appointed and directed by the PCMO. The district MO would be assisted by one or two medical assistants, and each district would have a hospital with one or more dispensaries. In other words there was to be a substantial extension of the government's hospital provision. The part of the ordinance which provoked howls of protest from the planters was the means of financing it. An export duty on all coffee, tea, cocoa and cinchona, would be imposed and the proceeds placed into a special Medical Aid Fund for the expenses of the scheme.[94] The battle between planter and government over this financial exaction lasted for the next two years and culminated in a petition from the Planters to Queen Victoria in February 1882.

This petition reiterated the customary grievances of the planters: that the 1865 Ordinance was sufficient; that it was the government's failure to provide hospitals as the coffee districts had expanded which had created the problem; that to expect them to pay for a more extensive health-care system was unjust, especially when the coffee districts were increasingly populated by Sinhalese and permanently settled Tamils; and that it was, therefore, the government's responsibility to pay for this out of the general revenue.[95] This petition had the opposite of the desired effect. The planters' objections

[92] Dr W. R. Kynsey, 17 April 1879, PRO, CO 57/78, TNA.

[93] Medical Aid Commission Report, 1879, vii., TNA.

[94] Ordinance No.17 1880, *An Ordinance to Provide for the Medical Wants of Immigrant Labourers in Certain Planting District,* PRO CO, TNA.

[95] Petition to Her Most Glorious Majesty Victoria, included in the despatch of February 1882, PRO CO 54/537, TNA, and signed by the Chairmen of the Planters' Association and the Ceylon Chamber of Commerce.

were unequivocally rejected by CO officialdom: "the expense was too great to throw upon government", and moreover their attitude was totally unacceptable. The threats in the petition that they would refuse to cooperate with the new ordinance and that they would reduce wages if they had to pay the tax, horrified officials at the CO. As Sir Charles Lucas averred, "it is a serious matter when a class of English, for whom a great deal has been done by the government . . . openly declare that they will do their best to defy the law".[96] The Secretary of State rejected the planters' petition.

The 1882 Ordinance remained the basis of the medical wants system until the government passed further legislation in 1912.[97] The fact that it lasted for three decades did not mean that the matter was settled and that improvement necessarily resulted. The matter rumbled on through to the next century for two principal reasons. These were, as stated by the Governor, Sir Arthur Hamilton Gordon as early as 1884, 'the high death rate in the district hospitals and the enormous cost of the medical aid rendered'.[98] Improvements to the scheme were periodically attempted. For example, an attempt by the colonial government in 1890 to make the planters pay more of the costs through an additional export tax faltered in the face of their opposition.[99] The 1893 review of the scheme found that the death rate in the district hospitals in the years 1883–91 had averaged 20.87 per cent, double the rate in other hospitals. To ensure earlier treatment and thus hopefully lower death rates, additional estate dispensaries were established in the 1890s.[100] However, no substantive changes were made to the scheme until 1912.

[96] Minute, Charles Lucas, 5 April 1882, PRO CO 54/537, TNA.

[97] Ordinance No. 9, 1882, *An Ordinance to Amend the Medical Wants Ordinance 1880, and to Repeal the Amendment Ordinance of 1881,* PRO CO 56/11, TNA; Ordinance No. 9, 1912 *Medical Wants Ordinance,* PRO CO 56/17, TNA.

[98] Hamilton Gordon to Secretary of State, 9 July 1884, PRO CO 54/554, TNA.

[99] See Medical Wants Ordinance 1890, PRO CO 54/590, TNA.

[100] Sir Arthur Havelock to the Secretary of State, 5 November 1893, PRO CO 54/610, TNA.

Conclusion

By 1890 there were various kinds of hospitals operating in the colony some totally and some only partially funded by the government. There were civil hospitals, specialist hospitals like the Leper and Lunatic Asylums and the De Soysa Lying-in Home, and immigrant, field and parangi hospitals. All these were totally funded government institutions and open to all. In addition there were the Medical Aid Hospitals funded by the government and the planting industry, at this stage for the use of the estate workers. These hospitals provided free medical care although planters were expected to, but often did not, pay a per diem fee for the treatment of their workers. The distribution of all these hospitals throughout the island was not even but reflected both the indigenous and European population distribution, and the routes and patterns of settlement of the immigrant workers. Table 1.3 illustrates this distribution by province.

TABLE 1.3 Distribution of hospitals by type and province, 1890

Province	Government Civil Hospital	District Hospital	Parangi Hospital	Field Hospital[101]
Western	6	-	-	-
Central	5	5	-	-
Eastern	3	-	-	-
Uva	1	2	-	3
Northern	3	-	-	-
Southern	4	-	-	-
North-Western	4	-	-	1
Sabaragamuwa	2	3	2	-

Source: Ceylon Blue Book of Statistics 1890, PRO CO 50/101, TNA.

This chapter cannot explore all the precipitating factors which explain this pattern, but as has been seen the high death rates and ill-health of the Indian worker was pivotal to the extension of hospital provision. From the onset of Indian immigration in the 1840s

[101] Field Hospitals were set up to treat government workers on public building works. The immigrant hospitals are subsumed within the numbers for government civil hospitals

basically laissez-faire colonial state was drawn reluctantly and incrementally into committing more government resources for building hospitals and providing the medical expertise to run them. Firstly, the presence of large numbers of workers needing hospital care put pressure on the rudimentary existing provision initially intended solely for the indigenous population. These hospitals had to be improved to deal with the crisis. The government takeover of the Kandy Friend-in-Need Society Hospital illustrates this process. Secondly, the presence of the sick, the dying and the dead on the roads and in the streets of the colony's towns presented a visible need requiring a response from the authorities. To begin with, hospitals were constructed along the routes used by the migrant workers. It was soon apparent that this in itself was insufficient. The migrants were not immune to sickness once they had reached their destination; treatment and care had to be provided in the plantation areas and it was soon clear that the employers were not willing to take that responsibility voluntarily. The resulting legislation between 1872 and 1882 created a framework for the further expansion of hospitals to the more rural and remote parts of the colony.

This process of government intervention provides an insight into the development of nineteenth-century colonial society and state in Ceylon. The two obvious players in deciding the ways and means of providing medical care for the Indian labourer were the employers—the planters—and the colonial government. The impasse between these groups was, however, mitigated and even manipulated by two other interested parties who had their own agenda. At the metropolitan centre the imperial government adopted a more interventionist role after the imperial hospital survey of 1863. From 1867 the colonial government was subject to a review of its capacity to deal with a problem that was crucial to the economic development of the island and therefore of critical importance to the imperial government. The hospitals were found to be wanting and remedial action was expected. The colonial government was therefore under pressure to adopt a more interventionist and expansive role.

The other no less significant interested party was the government medical service. The practitioners of the colonial medical service were under pressure to justify and defend their professional performance to both the imperial and the colonial government. They, therefore, increasingly put pressure on the government to increase its commitments arguing that only by legislating for, and funding increased hospital provision would the situation improve. Dr Johnston's intervention in Kandy in 1859–60 offered an early example of this. The role of the PCMOs in the development of medical wants legislation further illustrates its salience. A further significant factor in Ceylon was that from 1870 the Colombo Medical School was turning out indigenous practitioners who sought the financial security, career opportunities and professional status that employment in the government service offered. This could only be achieved in a medical service which was not restricted to caring for the coloniser but covered the entire population whether settled or migrant. The desire to provide 'native doctors' for the 'natives' was a primary motivating factor in the establishment of the Colombo School and it was its graduates who eventually worked in the district hospitals and served the remoter and more rural areas. Ultimately the expansion of the medical service over the entire island staffed with locally trained doctors resulted in a unique situation. The Ceylon colonial medical service was by the turn of the century fast developing into an indigenous service where Europeans were in the minority.

However, the self-interest of the medical profession was supplemented by a more nebulous ethos which impacted on the nature of Ceylon's colonial society. Harold Perkin has claimed that a significant influence in the formation of nineteenth-century English society was the development of the professional ideal. Doctors, he argued, along with other professionals, belonged to "a distinct class" and though "not altogether immune from market forces" their incomes were not the direct "result of bargaining in the market". The professions were characterised by "expert, esoteric service demanding integrity in the purveyor and trust in the client and the community". Thus "emancipated", professionals could be "the philosophers of society", and postulate the vision of an ideal society in which economic interests were sublimated and the ideals of the other classes were transformed from "mere apologetics for self-interest into moral theories of society".[102] As David Marquand has more recently argued doctors, like lawyers and civil servants contributed to the development of a "public service ethic" and the evolution of what can be termed the "public interest". This public interest is "inherently contestable, both in the sense that agreement can never be final, and in the sense that it is defined through conflict and the resolution of conflict".[103] In other words in the contest between the various interested parties—the planters, the colonial administration, the imperial government and the medical profession—over the medical care of the Indian immigrant worker some notion of a public interest began to evolve in Ceylon to place it on a trajectory not totally dissimilar from that of the colonial masters. In the period under discussion these processes were as yet in their infancy. Their main impact came later but a framework had been established both for the specific case of hospital provision, the subject of this paper and for the wider commitment to the welfare of the population of the colony evidenced by the preventive and curative services which developed in the twentieth century.

[102] Harold Perkin, *Origins of Modern English Society* (London and New York: Ark Paperbacks, 1986), 257–61.

[103] David Marquand, "The Public Domain is a Gift of History. Now It Is at Risk", *New Statesman*, 19 January 2004, 25–28.

2

For God, Emperor and Science: Competing Visions of the Hospital in Manchuria, 1885–1931

Robert John Perrins

Introduction

Located at the junction of a number of major rail-lines, and within 100-kilometres of both the Japanese-run steel mills in Anshan and the great colliery at Fushun, the Manchurian railway town of Mukden witnessed tremendous growth during the first three decades of the last century.[1] In addition to thousands of Chinese who migrated to the city from the surrounding rural counties, tens of thousands more journeyed to Mukden from as far away as the neighbouring provinces of Hebei and Shandong in order to find employment in the town's new factories and businesses. In the decades following the Russo-Japanese War, thousands of Japanese also settled in Mukden's railway concession zone, and in the Kwantung Leased Territory (*Kantôshu*) to the south, where they hoped to build brighter

The author would like to acknowledge the support of Associated Medical Services, and specifically the Hannah Institute for the History of Medicine's Grant-in-Aid programme, that provided the financial support and made this research possible.

[1] Throughout this paper I have used the name Mukden when discussing the history of the city now known as Shenyang, the capital of Liaoning Province in the People's Republic of China. During the late nineteenth and early twentieth centuries, the city was referred to by several other titles, including: Shengjing or Fengtian (Fengtien) by the Chinese, and Hôten by the Japanese. I have also used the term 'Manchuria' throughout this chapter to denote the region of China that comprised the Republican provinces of Heilongjiang, Jilin and Fengtian (now Liaoning).

futures for themselves in Japan's newest overseas possessions.[2] By the early 1920s, Mukden was not only home to the headquarters of the Manchurian warlord, Zhang Zuolin,[3] but also an important administrative centre for the Japanese-controlled South Manchuria Railway Company, commonly referred to as Mantetsu,[4] and a military base for an elite battalion of the Kwantung Army (*Kantôgun*) that was garrisoned in southern Manchuria to protect the Japanese railway and attached lands.[5] In the years immediately following the First World War, the city boasted a population of more than a quarter of a million persons, and had emerged as the key political, military and industrial centre in central Manchuria.

Manchuria was one of the most contested borderlands in Asia during the late nineteenth and early twentieth centuries.[6] As the Qing dynasty collapsed, only to be replaced by a weak Chinese Re-

[2] Adachi Kinnosuke, *Manchuria a Survey* (New York: Robert M. McBride & Company, 1925), 129–30; and Owen Lattimore, *Manchuria: Cradle of Conflict* (New York: The Macmillan Company, 1935), 209–21, and 262–63.

[3] On the Zhang Zuolin's rise to power and the establishment of his headquarters in Mukden, see Gavan McCormack, *Chang Tso-lin in Northeast China, 1911–1928: China, Japan, and the Manchurian Idea* (Stanford: Stanford University Press, 1977), 15–33.

[4] Mantetsu is an abbreviation of the full Japanese name of the railway company, *Minami Manshû tetsudô kabushiki kaisha*. For an introduction to the history of this enormous colonial enterprise in English, see Ramon H. Myers, "Japanese Imperialism in Manchuria: The South Manchuria Railway Company, 1906–1933", in *The Japanese Informal Empire in China, 1895–1937*, ed. Peter Duus, Ramon H. Myers and Mark R. Peattie (Princeton: Princeton University Press, 1989), 101–32; and Yoshihisa Tak Matsusaka, *The Making of Japanese Manchuria, 1904–1932* (Cambridge, MA: Harvard University Asia Center, 2001).

[5] On the history of the founding of the Kwantung Army and its early role as a garrison force in southern Manchuria, see Carl Walter Young, *Japanese Jurisdiction in the South Manchuria Railway Areas* (Baltimore: The Johns Hopkins Press, 1931), 261–315; and Alvin D. Coox, "The Kwantung Army Dimension", in Duus et al., *The Japanese Informal Empire in China,* 395–98.

[6] I have borrowed the phrase 'contested borderland' from Pransenjit Duara, who uses it to describe Manchuria in his latest study, *Sovereignty and Authenticity: Manchukuo and the East Asian Modern* (New York: Rowman and Littlefield Publishers, 2003), 41–86.

public, a number of outside parties became interested in establishing a presence in the region. While imperialist dreamers in both St.Petersburg and Tokyo cast their eyes on Manchuria as a vast warehouse of natural resources, scores of Western missionaries saw the frontier as an untapped reservoir of souls that required saving. While much of this international rivalry was played out on the battlefield or through diplomatic manoeuvrings, the medical sphere was also an important arena of competition between the various foreign interests.[7]

The residents of Mukden faced a variety of pressures during the early twentieth century including widespread social and economic disruptions caused by the Boxer Uprising of 1900, the Russo-Japanese War (1904–1905), and the numerous military campaigns launched by the local warlord, Zhang Zuolin, in the 1920s. In addition to the dangers brought on by warfare, the local population also faced regular threats at the microbial level. During the first three decades of the last century Mukden's residents were plagued by endemic diseases such as tuberculosis, scarlet fever, and a plethora of intestinal-track ailments that resulted from poor sanitation. The region of central Manchuria, in which the city was located, was also struck by several epidemics during this period, including outbreaks of pneumonic plague (1910–11, 1920–21), bubonic plague (1928–30) and cholera (1919 and 1926).

In the city of Mukden, practitioners of traditional Chinese medicine and owners of local apothecaries confronted new challengers to their professional status and livelihoods in the late nineteenth and early twentieth centuries. European missionary doctors, as well as Japanese and Western-trained Chinese physicians who practised 'modern' medicine, worked to establish both themselves and their form of medical treatments among the local population. Despite their different visions of Manchuria's future, agents of Japanese colonialism and the local community of foreign missionaries did share a common belief in the importance of Western, scientific medicine as a tool for bringing 'modernity' to the region and its inhabitants.

[7] See Carl F. Nathan, *Plague Prevention and Politics in Manchuria, 1910–1931* (Cambridge, MA: East Asian Research Centre, Harvard University, 1967), 1–6, and 74–78.

A central component in the medical strategies of both foreign interests was the construction of hospitals.

By the late 1920s, two large teaching hospitals were competing to serve the residents of Mukden: a three hundred-bed missionary hospital established in 1885 by Dugald Christie and run by the Mission Board of the United Presbyterian Church of Scotland,[8] and a second, even larger facility opened in 1915 by the South Manchuria Railway Company to serve both its employees and local residents. In the early twentieth century, these two hospitals, along with the Peking Union Hospital and the Mantetsu Hospital in the Manchurian port city of Dairen[9] were the largest hospitals in northern China. Each of the hospitals in Mukden boasted Western-styled operating theatres and pharmacies, as well as an assortment of imported medical machinery such as X-ray machines and assorted laboratory equipment.[10]

Diseases of all types were major social and economic concerns for colonial rulers including the Japanese in Taiwan, Korea and Manchuria. Throughout Manchuria's cities and along the region's

[8] In 1900, the United Presbyterian Church of Scotland merged with the majority of congregations of the Scottish Free Church to form the United Free Church of Scotland. See H. H. Tsai, "Dugald Christie, CMG, FRCS, FRCP Edin: Scottish Medical Pioneer in Manchuria, 1883–1923", *Scottish Medical Journal* 34, no. 2, 1989, 443–44; and Austin Fulton, *Through Earthquake, Wind and Fire: Church and Missions in Manchuria, 1867–1950: The Work of the United Presbyterian Church, the United Free Church of Scotland, the Church of Scotland and the Presbyterian Church of Ireland with the Chinese Church in Manchuria* (Edinburgh: Saint Andrew's Press, 1967), viii, 27–37, and 285–93.

[9] On the history of the Mantetsu hospital in Dairen, see Robert Perrins, "Doctors, Disease and Development: Engineering Colonial Public Health in Southern Manchuria, 1905–1931", in *Building a Modern Nation: Science, Technology and Medicine in Japan*, ed. Morris Low (London: Palgrave Macmillan, 2005), 103–33.

[10] See China Medical Commission (henceforth CMC) of the Rockefeller Foundation, *Medicine in China* (New York: Rockefeller Foundation, 1914), 20–21; John Z. Bowers and Akiko K. Bowers, "Japanese Medicine in Manchuria: The South Manchuria Medical College", *Clio Medica* 12, no. 1, 1977, 5; and Liu Zhongming, *Fengtian Yike Daxue (Liaoning Yi Xueyuan) jianshi* [A Brief History of the Mukden Shenyang Medical College] (Shenyang: Fengtian Yike Daxue, 1992), 49.

rail-lines, the Japanese authorities adopted a variety of provisions that aimed not only to control and cure disease, but also to demonstrate the modernity of post-Meiji Japan and its ability to govern and develop a colony.[11] Efforts related to the improvement of public hygiene and sanitation, the quarantining of new arrivals at the colony's ports, and the creation of modern hospitals such as the Mantetsu facility in Mukden, all stemmed, in part, from the necessities of governing a colony. Such efforts, however, also developed as part of the belief in a greater vision that would see its eventual fruition with the creation of the puppet state of Manzhouguo in the 1930s.[12] Japanese colonial administrators in Manchuria justified their activities using the notions of science and progress; ideas that had recently played central roles in the transformation of Japanese society in the Home Islands during the Meiji period.[13] The Japanese civilian and military governors of the Manchurian territories, following the guidelines and vision of the first Mantetsu President and former Civilian Governor of Taiwan, Gotô Shinpei, believed in a rational and scientific approach to colonial administration.[14] They

[11] For a more detailed discussion of Japanese perceptions of how their activities in the colonies were elements of a broader 'civilizing mission,' see Marius B. Jansen, "Japanese Imperialism: Late Meiji Perspectives", in *The Japanese Colonial Empire, 1895–1945*, ed. Ramon H. Myers and Mark R. Peattie (Princeton: Princeton University Press, 1984), 61–79.

[12] Recent works on the history of Japanese colonial activities in Manchuria, and the creation of Manzhouguo in the 1930s include Louise Young, *Japan's Total Empire: Manchuria and the Culture of Wartime Imperialism* (Berkeley: University of California Press, 1998); Rana Mitter, *The Manchurian Myth: Nationalism, Resistance, and Collaboration in Modern China* (Berkeley: University of California Press, 2000); and Matsusaka, *Making of Japanese Manchuria*.

[13] Bill Sewell, "Public Health Concerns in a Manchurian Treaty Port" (Paper presented at the conference, "Foreign Fevers and Colonial Cures: Disease and Medicine in the British, French and Japanese Empires", Acadia University, Canada, 23 August 2003), 4–5.

[14] For an introduction to the colonial, and particularly medical ideas of Gotô Shinpei and how they were implemented in the Japanese colonies of Taiwan, Manchuria and Korea see Liu Shiyung, "Medical Reform in Colonial Taiwan" (PhD diss., University of Pittsburgh, 2000), 65–81; Bowers and Bowers, "Japanese Medicine in Manchuria", 4–6; and Barbara Brooks, "Colonial Power and Public Health in Japanese-held Korea" (Paper

saw themselves as pioneers who were developing Manchuria in a manner similar to the way in which one would conduct a laboratory experiment.

Japanese governors in Manchuria were not alone in their attempts to create modern medical facilities in China in the early twentieth century. The government of Jiang Jieshi's (Chiang Kai-shek's) nationalists also attempted "to build a modern healthcare system in the context of national reconstruction,"[15] during the 1920s. The nationalists worked at formulating policies, establishing agencies, and initiating programmes that aimed at rebuilding China. An important component in this work was the creation of hospitals. In Manchuria, the Chinese-run North Manchuria Plague Prevention Service, under the leadership of Dr Wu Liande, established seven hospitals during the 1910s and early 1920s to deal with outbreaks of plague and other epidemic diseases.[16] These hospitals in the cities and towns of Haerbin (Harbin), Sanseng, Lahasusu, Daheiho, Manzhouli, Niuzhuang (Newchwang), and Andong, served as emergency quarantine and treatment facilities during times of crisis, but "in the lulls between epidemics . . . were thrown open as a general medical service for Northern Manchuria."[17] Unfortunately for the residents of Mukden, no Plague Prevention Service hospital was established in their city.

During the late nineteenth and early twentieth centuries, Western colonial powers were also active in China where they worked to establish policies and programmes related to public health. The British, in the treaty ports of Shanghai and Hong Kong, worked to bring their brand of medical modernity to China, establishing

---

presented at the Association for Asian Studies Meeting, Washington, D.C., 5 April 2002), 2.

15 Ka-che Yip, *Health and National Reconstruction in Nationalist China: The Development of Modern Health Services, 1928–1937* (Ann Arbor: Association for Asian Studies, 1995), 5.

16 Wu Liande (Wu Lien-teh), ed., *Manchurian Plague Prevention Service: Memorial Volume, 1912–1932* (Shanghai: National Quarantine Service, 1934), 3–4, and 397–408; and Wu Liande, "How I Built Hospitals in China", *National Medical Journal of China* 10, no. 2, 1924, 265–77.

17 Nathan, *Plague Prevention and Politics in Manchuria*, 55.

quarantine regulations, public hospitals, municipal sanitation codes, and medical schools.[18] The most active Western participants in the development of hospitals and the provision of medical treatment in China during this period, however, were not the metropolitan governments or their official representatives. Rather, it was the growing contingent of foreign missionaries who had the greatest impact on the early development of modern healthcare facilities in the 'Middle Kingdom.'

Although traditional accounts of the history of Christian missionaries in China often begin with the work of the Jesuit fathers Matteo Ricci and Adam Schall von Bell at the Ming and Qing courts in the seventeenth century,[19] it was really the latter half of the nineteenth century, following the 'Great Awakening' amongst evangelical Protestants and the establishment of foreign residency rights granted under the terms of the treaties that ended the Opium Wars, that witnessed the growth of the foreign missionary presence throughout China.[20] Almost sixty major foreign missionary boards sent missionaries to China during the last two decades of the nineteenth and the first half of the twentieth centuries.[21] While the activities and scope of many of these organisations were limited

[18] See Kerrie MacPherson, *A Wilderness of Marshes: The Origins of Public Health in Shanghai, 1843–1893* (Hong Kong: Oxford University Press, 1987); and Elizabeth Sinn, *Power and Charity: The Early History of the Tung Wah Hospital* (Hong Kong: Oxford University Press, 1989), 1–4, and 184–208.

[19] For example, see Kenneth Scott Latourette, *A History of Christian Missions in China* (New York: The Macmillan Company, 1929).

[20] Jonathan Spence, *To Change China: Western Advisers in China, 1620–1960* (New York: Penguin Books, 1980), 129–30; John Z. Bowers, *Western Medicine in a Chinese Palace: Peking Union Medical College, 1917–1951* (Philadelphia: Josiah Macy, Jr. Foundation, 1972), 17–18; Alvyn J. Austin, *Saving China: Canadian Missionaries in the Middle Kingdom, 1888–1959* (Toronto: University of Toronto Press, 1986), 3–20; and Karen Minden, *Bamboo Stone: The Evolution of a Chinese Medical Elite* (Toronto: University of Toronto Press, 1994), 13–16.

[21] For a fairly comprehensive list of the foreign mission boards who were engaged in sending missionaries to the China field, see Dan Cui, *The Cultural Contribution of British Protestant Missionaries and British-American Cooperation to China's National Development During the 1920s* (New York: University Press of America, 1998), xi–xii.

to establishing isolated churches, schools or stations (sometimes equipped with a small dispensary and/or clinic) in Chinese towns and villages, some of the larger mission boards oversaw extensive ventures that included the construction and staffing of entire colleges and modern, Western-styled hospitals.[22]

By the early 1900s, medical missionaries throughout Asia had emerged as the leading force in the effort to spread the Christian faith. Rosemary Fitzgerald, in an essay that explores missionary medicine in colonial India, writes:

> At the beginning of the twentieth century, many mission-minded Christians were convinced that 'clinical Christianity', as missionary medicine was sometimes known, provided the most impressive and persuasive means of presenting the gospel message to the peoples of other cultures and faiths. Medical agents were assigned a vanguard place in the missionary army; their work was believed to constitute "one of the most powerful forces for spreading a knowledge of Christianity."[23]

Although Fitzgerald is examining the history of medical missionaries in colonial South Asia, the consensus amongst historians exploring the missionary enterprise in modern China is strikingly similar.

In his study of the China Inland Missions, Alvyn Austin argues that by the turn of the twentieth century, the proponents and practitioners of 'clinical Christianity' in the China-field had not only concluded that medical work was the most effective way of gaining acceptance in the foreign land, but also that missionary medicine had become a legitimate goal in and of itself. He writes:

> The construction of hospitals as modern as those in the home countries, symbolized the new place of medical work in mission policy. The change

[22] Kwang-Ching Liu, "Early Christian Colleges in China", *Journal of Asian Studies* 20, no. 1, 1960, 71–73; and Michelle Renshaw, *Accommodating the Chinese: The American Hospital in China, 1880–1920* (New York: Routledge, 2005), 45–117.

[23] Rosemary Fitzgerald, "'Clinical Christianity': The Emergence of Medical Work as a Missionary Strategy in Colonial India, 1800–1914", in *Health, Medicine and Empire: Perspectives on Colonial India*, ed. Biswamoy Pati and Mark Harrison (New Delhi: Orient Longman, 2001), 89.

in purpose came so gradually as to be almost imperceptible. Medical work was no longer to be a mere means to an evangelistic end. It was in itself to be a living expression of the Christian Gospel and must, therefore, maintain the highest standards. [24]

The founder of the United Presbyterian Church of Scotland's Mission in Mukden, the physician Dugald Christie, was a firm believer in this approach to mission work, and in fact took the argument one step further in an address that he gave at a 1907 conference in Shanghai celebrating the centenary of the arrival of the first Protestant missionary in China. He concluded his address with the lines:

> Let us realize that by healing a man we are letting in a ray of Divine Light on the darkness of his surroundings, even if he takes absolutely no interest in the Divine message. Let us seek to let the heathen and hostile world read more plainly in our Christianity, the same Gospel as it finds in the Gospels. Let the whole work of Medical Missions be lifted to this higher plane, as a necessary and fundamental part of missions, not a mere aid to them. Let this be our practical aim, and so shall we hasten the time we are all longing for, when the whole world shall stretch out its hands to God. [25]

Christie's vision that medical work was a 'necessary and fundamental' component of missionary activity was in some sense similar to the Japanese administrator, Gotô Shinpei's belief that medical reforms and the improvement of public health were central priorities in the development of a successful colonial policy. While both views agreed on the importance of medical work in places such as Manchuria, there were important differences between the two visions. The competition between Christie's and Gotô's philosophies regarding both clinical work and medical education was played out in Mukden's two largest hospitals and medical colleges during the early decades of the twentieth century.

[24] Austin, *Saving China*, 167.

[25] The text of Christie's 1907 address can be found in Dugald Christie and Iza Inglis Christie, *Thirty Years in Moukden, 1883–1913: Being the Experiences and Recollections of Dugald Christie* (London: Constable & Company, 1914), 216–22.

Dugald Christie and the Mukden Missionary Hospital and Medical College

Born in Glencoe in 1855, Dugald Christie had a difficult childhood. His father died while Dugald was still an infant, and his mother passed away when he was only eleven years old. Christie was then raised by his devotedly religious elder sister Jessie until the age of fifteen when he began an apprenticeship in a Glasgow drapery shop. Christie was later encouraged to pursue a university education in order to become a missionary, and eventually Dugald wrote Edinburgh University's entrance examination and was successful in gaining admission to the school's medical programme in the autumn of 1877.[26]

Christie completed his medical education in four years, graduating in July 1881. He was then appointed by the directors of the Edinburgh Medical Missionary Society as the resident physician at the Cowgate Dispensary and Clinic located in the city's slums. While serving at Cowgate, Christie considered his plans for the future, and after contemplating, pursuing missionary work in either India or Africa, was approached by the Mission Board of the United Presbyterian Church to head their new mission in the Manchurian capital of Mukden. As it was expected that a missionary would travel with a spouse, Christie's blossoming relationship with Elizabeth Hastie Smith, whom he had met at his parish church, was finalised with a quickly-arranged marriage in August 1882. The newly married Christies, along with Dugald's close friend James Webster and his wife, set off on their journey to Manchuria that September.

Before they could begin their missionary work in Mukden, however, Christie and Webster spent the winter of 1883 in the Manchurian port of Yingkou where they worked on learning some Chinese and gaining advice on how to establish a mission station from the Reverends John Ross and John Macintyre who headed the United Presbyterian Church of Scotland's mission in south-western

[26] Iza Inglis Christie, *Dugald Christie of Manchuria, Pioneer and Medical Missionary: The Story of a Life with a Purpose* (London: James Clarke & Company, 1932), 9–24.

Manchuria.[27] In early May 1883, the Christies and Websters set off on the 200-kilometre journey inland to Mukden.[28]

The Scottish missionaries faced a difficult task when they arrived in the walled-city that had served as the first capital of the Manchus in the early 1600s. The local population was openly hostile to the newcomers. Rumours circulated that Christie and Webster were possibly the vanguard of a planned British invasion, and that the young Scottish doctor was working with local Catholic priests and nuns who it was claimed were "anxious to obtain children's hearts and eyes, and were willing to give large sums for them."[29] Despite being confronted by an extremely suspicious local population, Christie was determined to fulfil his calling and decided that the best way to overcome resistance to the presence of the Scottish mission, as well as its religious message, was to begin to offer medical services as soon as possible.

After providing irregular medical care in the parlour of his house, Christie finally opened the first hospital in Mukden to offer Western medical treatments in the spring of 1885. This hospital was little more than a small shack that was located behind the missionaries' residence, offering room for only a dozen patients at a time.[30] In addition to supplying basic Western pharmaceuticals, the Scottish doctor performed regular surgeries at the clinic.[31] Two procedures in particular, cataract surgeries and amputations, so impressed the local Chinese population that Christie at last found acceptance for himself, his hospital, and the Presbyterian mission. Dozens, and on some days even hundreds, of Chinese visited the missionary hos-

[27] On the history of John Ross's role in establishing the Scottish Presbyterian mission in Yingkou, see James Horne Morrison, *The Scottish Churches' Work Abroad* (Edinburgh: T. & T. Clark, 1927), 162.

[28] Liu, *Fengtian Yike Daxue*, 5 and 48.

[29] On the Chinese suspicions surrounding the activities of the Catholic missions, see Daniel T. Robertson, *The Story of Our Mission, Manchuria* (Edinburgh: Foreign Mission Committee, United Free Church of Scotland, 1913), 102.

[30] "Dr Christie, Founder of Mukden Hospital and Medical College of Church of Scotland, Passes Away", *Manchuria Daily News*, 8 December 1936.

[31] Christie and Christie, *Thirty Years in Moukden*, 40–41.

pital not to seek treatment for themselves, but to watch the foreign doctor perform surgical operations. In the fall of 1885, Christie performed cataract surgeries on two prominent members of the local community, a merchant who had been blind for several years, and a school teacher from a neighbouring village who had lost his livelihood due to his recent blindness. Both surgeries were successful, and when Christie asked the merchant to state how many fingers he was holding up, only minutes after the operation was completed, the crowd was impressed when the formerly blind man replied correctly. By the mid-1880s the success of Dugald Christie's open-air surgeries had paved the way for his acceptance into the local community.

The original hospital building soon proved to be an unsuitable location for a medical clinic. In the summer of 1885, only months after the hospital was opened, one of its mud walls collapsed during a flood. In the spring of 1887, Christie negotiated the purchase of a suitable piece of land in the south-eastern district of Mukden near a small stream called 'Small River', or Xiao He, by the locals. This land had been formerly owned by a Chinese mandarin official named Sun who had recently been reassigned to another province, and who had decided to offer his compound to the Scottish missionaries who were now establishing themselves as respected members of the community. Christie and Webster relocated their own residences to this site and began construction of a new chapel and hospital. Completed in late 1887, the new mission hospital was a tremendous improvement over the previous incarnation, having a waiting room that could hold 150 people, and two separate patient wards that could accommodate 50 men and 15 women.

During Christie's first six years in Mukden he continued to pursue the practice of what scholars now refer to as 'clinical Christianity,' that is, providing medical treatment in order to gain the necessary degrees of social and cultural acceptance that were required before proselytising could be expected to have any chance of success. Christie, like earlier foreign missionaries, quickly became aware of the fact that if one wanted to be taken seriously in China, providing free medical care to the poor and members of the merchant class was not enough. One had to cultivate the local *literati* and officials. Recounting his medical activities during this period, Christie remarked in 1914:

> At the outset, a doctor has the great advantage that he may have an opportunity of relieving bodily suffering, and thus gain an entrance [to Chinese society]. The maintenance of a friendly footing afterwards, and the extension of acquaintance among these classes, will depend largely on the extent to which he himself cultivates [the] 'rules of propriety.' Our relation with the officials was a most vital matter thirty years ago, as the common people were greatly influenced by the attitude taken up by them regarding us and our work.[32]

In this regard, Christie was particularly successful. Not only did he garner an important level of official support for his mission by manufacturing a set of dentures for Mukden's Manchu governor (who was embarrassed to appear before the Qing emperor in Beijing having lost two of his front teeth) but he also cultivated a number of important political relationships during these early years by providing a variety of medical services to other prominent members of the governor's court and local mandarins.

In the early autumn of 1888, Christie was ordered to return to Scotland with his wife Elizabeth and their three small children. Not only had the exhausted Dugald contracted a fever, however, but his wife was also suffering from a mysterious illness, and by the time the Christies reached Scotland, Elizabeth was beyond treatment and died shortly after arriving at the family home in Bothwell. For the next three years, Dugald toured his homeland giving talks to Presbyterian congregations extolling the value of missionary medicine and particularly the work of the hospital that he had founded in Mukden. In the autumn of 1891, having completed the training required for his ordination by the Presbytery of Edinburgh, as well as a number of additional medical courses at his alma mater in anaesthesia and new surgery techniques, Christie left his three young children in the care of his sister Jessie's family and returned to Manchuria.

During the 1890s the mission hospital in Mukden continued to grow. By 1894 several new buildings had been completed, and in

[32] Christie and Christie, *Thirty Years in Moukden*, 26.

that year a total of more than five hundred in-patients were provided with care, in addition to over twenty thousand out-patients and a thousand surgeries.[33] Christie was assisted during this period by four female doctors, Mary Campbell Horner, Katherine Kirk Paton, Isabella Aitken and Ethel Louie Starmer, who were sent to Manchuria by the mission board of the United Free Presbyterian Church of Scotland between 1894 and 1899.[34] The arrival of these new physicians was fortuitous as Christie would require additional trained hands to treat not only thousands of additional civilian patients, but also Chinese soldiers who were wounded in battle during the first Sino-Japanese War of 1894–95.

During the conflict, Christie brought his new wife married for two years, Eliza, as well as his friends the Websters and Dr Mary Horner, to what he hoped was the relative safety of the treaty port of Yingkou. The mission hospital in Mukden, meanwhile, was placed in the hands of eight trusted Chinese assistants whom Christie had been training as medical assistants since his return to Manchuria in 1892. One of these assistants, Wang Yachin, who had proven himself as both the top student in the class of eight, and who had a long experience working at the mission's hospital, was placed in charge and instructed to keep the clinic open if at all possible for the duration of the hostilities and to provide basic medical services even in the absence of the foreign staff.[35] Christie's acceptance of Western female physicians, as well as his confidence in the abilities of the Chinese medical assistants whom he was training, made his vision of missionary medical work in hospitals fairly unique in Asia during the late nineteenth century.[36]

[33] See H. H. Tsai, "Scottish Women Medical Pioneers: Manchuria 1894–1912", *Scottish Medical Journal* 37, 1992, 56; and Christie, *Dugald Christie of Manchuria*, 66–68.

[34] Tsai, "Scottish Women Medical Pioneers", 56.

[35] Liu, *Fengtian Yike Daxue*, 50–51; and Christie, *Dugald Christie of Manchuria*, 76–77.

[36] Christie's confidence in the abilities of Chinese assistants was echoed in the attitudes of some, but not many, other foreign missions in China in the late nineteenth century. For similar missionary attitudes in the China Inland Mission in Sichuan Province, see Austin, *Saving China*, 176–82.

In Yingkou, Christie helped to establish one of the first branches of the Red Cross in China. He worked with seven other missionary doctors and the local medical officer employed by the Imperial Chinese Maritime Customs Service, Dr C. de Burgh Daly, in the new Red Cross hospital in Yingkou providing emergency service to the besieged citizens of the city as well as to thousands of wounded Chinese soldiers.[37]

When the war finally ended, the foreign missionaries returned to Mukden in July 1895 after being absent from the city and their hospital for almost a year. Within weeks of the missionaries' return, word was received that both Christie and Dr de Burgh Daly had been awarded a special commendation, the Imperial Order of the Double Dragon, from the Qing ruler, Emperor Guangxu, for their medical services during the conflict.[38] Honours aside, Christie's medical mission received another boost during this period as his hospital was the recipient of a large financial grant from the executive committee of the Chinese Red Cross Society's headquarters in Shanghai. This body had raised a great deal of money during the war, and after all expenses were paid for the work conducted by its representatives in Mukden and Yingkou, the decision was made to transfer most of the remaining monies to Christie so that he could expand his medical work in Manchuria. With this windfall, Christie purchased a large tract of land adjacent to the existing hospital site, and ordered the construction of a new women's hospital and the purchase of additional medical equipment from Europe and North America. After a decade and a half of turbulent growth, the future of the Mukden hospital appeared bright in the late 1890s.

In 1900, however, yet another crisis confronted Christie and the staff at the Mukden mission hospital—the arrival of supporters of the Boxer movement in central Manchuria. In the spring of 1900, the number of peasants and itinerant labourers who comprised the majority of the movement's supporters had exploded into the tens of thousands, and large contingents of Boxers entered Beijing and the northern treaty port of Tianjin where they harassed and killed

[37] Christie and Christie, *Thirty Years in Moukden*, 91–108.

[38] "Dr Dugald Christie", *Manchuria Daily News*, 8 April 1926.

foreigners and Chinese Christian coverts, or sometimes those who simply possessed foreign objects like watches or boxes of matches. By early June Boxers were seen in increasing numbers on the streets of Mukden and rumours began to circulate that a large rebel force was approaching the city with the intention of slaughtering all of its foreign residents and their Chinese supporters. In his memoirs, Christie vividly recounted the growing unrest of this period.

> Placards were posted on the walls and passed from hand to hand, telling of the evil doings of foreigners to China, including the poisoning of wells and the killing of little children. . . . On Wednesday the 20th [of June], vile posters were put up everywhere with horrible charges against foreigners, and all the loyal people of China were called on to rise up and sweep them out of the land. The 24th was fixed for the burning of the buildings, and rewards were promised to all who helped.[39]

After first receiving rather cold assurances from the Governor-General that the situation was under control and then being told by a former mandarin who was a close friend of Christie that they "should leave without any delay,"[40] the decision was made on Friday, 22 June 1900, to evacuate all but three members of the foreign community from Mukden to the port of Yingkou.

Dugald Christie and two others, Dr Thomas Young and the Reverend T. C. Fulton, remained in the city. On Sunday, 24 June the date given as the commencement of the destruction of all foreign buildings, the three remaining foreign missionaries in Mukden attended service at the chapel of the Scottish mission. Although several Chinese members of the congregation proclaimed their willingness to die for their new faith, the majority of patients in the mission's hospital were not so enthusiastic about the prospects of martyrdom. Following the service, Christie received a final telegram from the British consul in Yingkou ordering the three missionaries to leave at once. After gathering a few possessions and closing the chapel and hospital doors, Christie and his companions slipped out of Mukden early Monday morning. The following Saturday he received a

[39] Fulton, *Through Earthquake, Wind and* Fire, 35; and Christie and Christie, *Thirty Years in Moukden*, 136.

[40] Ibid., 137.

telegram from Mr Wei, one of the hospital's Chinese assistants. The message read:

> About four o'clock today the church was burned, and the hospitals and houses are burning. It is not known whether the Pastor [Liu, a Chinese convert] is dead or alive, nor how many Christians have been killed. [41]

This message was followed by a final telegraph two hours later, stating that the "Men's and women's hospitals, dwelling houses, Bible Society buildings, church and chapels have all been burned to ashes by the Boxers." [42] Almost two decades of work on the part of Christie and his staff had just gone up in smoke.

From Yingkou, the foreign missionaries travelled to Japan and eventually Christie decided to send his family to Scotland in early September, and then return alone to Manchuria. On 9 November 1900 Christie finally returned to the site of his mission where he viewed a complete destruction of the hospital compound. After visiting all of the surviving Chinese members of his medical staff and the local congregation that he could locate, Christie immediately set about rebuilding the mission's hospital. By 1903 a new, expanded women's hospital had been built and the men's hospital was scheduled to be reopened in 1904. [43] This event, however, was delayed by the outbreak of yet another war in Manchuria, this one between Russia and Japan. This conflict was the first modern war of the twentieth century and witnessed tremendous number of battlefield fatalities in both armies, as well as hundreds of thousands of casualties who required medical treatment. [44]

While Christie left the mission hospital, now largely confined to work in the new women's ward, in the care of female missionary doctors who had joined his staff in the 1890s, he escorted his

41 Ibid., 139.

42 Ibid., 140.

43 Ibid., 163.

44 For a recent account of Western military observers' accounts of the medical side of the conflict, see Claire Herrick, "'The Conquest of the Silent Foe': British and American Military Medical Reform Rhetoric and the Russo-Japanese War", in *Medicine and Modern Warfare*, ed. Roger Cooter, Mark Harrison and Steve Sturdy (Amsterdam: Rodopi, 1999), 99–131.

wife and four children to the safety of the Port of Tianjin where he left them for the duration of the war. Christie then returned to Mukden where he was summoned by the province's Chinese Governor-General who requested that the missionary establish and head a relief committee to deal with the growing medical and refugee emergency. Together with the Reverend J. W. Inglis (his wife's father) and two Chinese officials appointed by the Governor-General, Christie approached the Chinese Red Cross and Refugee Aid Society for Assistance. This agency, with whom Christie had worked a decade earlier, authorised the Scottish doctor to draw upon whatever funds were required in order to meet the emerging crisis. Christie commandeered the largest Buddhist temple in Mukden, along with a number of theatres, inns, warehouses, and even the grounds of the mission compound that had been destroyed during the Boxer Uprising, in order to house the thousands of Chinese refugees who were flooding into the city. In a temporary hospital that now flew a Red Cross flag from its roof timbers, Christie worked with another Scottish missionary doctor, W. A. Young, to treat not only thousands of Chinese civilian patients, but also hundreds of wounded Japanese and Russian soldiers who were transported to the clinic during the Japanese siege of Mukden in the winter of 1905.[45] When the war ended, the status of Christie, his fellow missionary doctors, and their mission hospital was assured. Again Christie received high honours, this time in the form of military decorations and financial grants for his hospital from both the Russian and Japanese governments, as well as a gold pocket watch from the Russian Tsar, a letter of thanks from President Yuan Shikai of the Chinese Republic, and most importantly the patronage of the highest-ranking Chinese official in all of Manchuria, the Viceroy Xu Shichang.[46]

Although Christie's vision of medical missionary work was successful, the series of crises of the 1890s and early 1900s also demonstrated to the Scottish doctor that it was not enough to simply perform modern, Western-styled medicine for the good of all who

[45] Christie, *Dugald Christie of Manchuria*, 98–99.

[46] Ibid., 101–3.

required his services and his small staff of foreign physicians. There simply would never be enough foreign doctors available to help everyone who needed medical care. Between 1905 and 1910, Christie's vision of 'clinical Christianity' was modified, as he shifted focus from serving the Chinese to educating them. In 1909, Viceroy Xu presented Christie and the United Free Church of Scotland's Mukden mission with a large property just to the east of the hospital compound as well as funds for the construction of a modern medical school under Christie's leadership.[47] With local finances secured, Christie decided to return to Scotland for a brief furlough in order to convince his mission board to support the new college both theoretically as well as financially, and to recruit a second male medical missionary to work in the hospital and as a teaching professor in the planned medical college. When he landed in Scotland in October 1909, Christie had four thousand pamphlets printed, outlining his vision of the new medical college. Dugald knew his audience well. "The object of the college," read the pamphlet:

> is to give young men a thorough training in the knowledge and practice of medicine and surgery, and to prepare as many of them as possible for Medical Missionary work. It will be essentially a missionary institution, run on Christian principles, permeated by Christian influence. . . . It is proposed to draw up a plan for the entire building, and to erect at once as much as our funds allow. We shall not go into debt.[48]

Christie's appeal to his supervising mission board was successful in that its members approved of the idea of the college, but could not provide all of the funds that were required for such a major new venture. Dugald estimated that £4,000 would be needed to construct the college in addition to the salary of at least one additional doctor and a small annual sum for operating expenses. Christie turned to the people of Scotland for support and printed five thousand letters of appeal that were circulated in church congregations and meeting halls. In his letter, Christie wrote:

[47] Liu, *Fengtian Yike Daxue*, 7 and 43.

[48] Christie and Christie, *Thirty Years in Moukden*, 232.

> There are two methods of starting a medical college. One is to gather a substantial sum of money, erect a large building, equip it thoroughly, provide a staff of professors, and then begin to seek for students. The other is to begin in a humble way, providing accommodation for as many as are certain, and extending as the work develops. We propose to adopt the latter course.[49]

Throughout the fall and winter of 1909, donations began to arrive at Christie's Edinburgh address. Following an article on the proposed medical missionary college in the United Free Church's official magazine in March 1910, however, there was a flood of letters. Through the example of his missionary work and letter of appeal, Christie had successfully transformed the limited evangelical vision of not just his mission board, but that of much of the membership of the United Free Church's Scottish congregations into one that was far more ambitious than the 'clinical Christianity' of the late nineteenth century. The new vision was one that viewed the purpose of the Manchurian mission as spreading the Christian faith through the work of foreign doctors, as well as one that believed in educating Chinese physicians to eventually assume control of the mission's medical activities on their own. Christie returned to Mukden in September 1910 with a total of almost £5,000, and a promise that two young male doctors would be despatched within weeks to join him in the Manchurian mission.[50]

The plan to construct the new medical college did not mean that Christie abandoned the mission's hospital. In fact, during the years immediately following the conclusion of the Russo-Japanese War, the hospital witnessed its greatest period of growth. Between 1906 and the spring of 1907 a new hospital complex was constructed on the banks of the 'Little River'. The hospital was a large, two-storey building comprising a large waiting room, two wards able to accommodate 110 patients, a modern operating theatre and dispensary, and several staff offices. The opening of the new facility was a major social and political event in Mukden, with dozens of local Chinese

[49] Christie, *Dugald Christie of Manchuria*, 124.

[50] Moukden Medical College (henceforth MMC) Board of Management, *The Moukden Medical College: Report and Annual Statement, for the Year 1919* (Edinburgh: Darien Press, 1920), 3–4.

officials, members of the foreign consular community from Yingkou, Japanese military officers from the town's railway garrison, and two Buddhist monks in attendance. Following the evening banquet, a fireworks display was provided by members of the local Chinese merchant guilds who wished to recognise the work Christie had performed for the town's residents during the past quarter century. Over fifty thousand people assembled on the banks of the 'Little River,' to celebrate the opening of the city's largest public hospital.

These celebrations were perhaps premature, as yet another medical emergency befell the people of Mukden three years later—the arrival of pneumonic plague. The Manchurian plague epidemic in the winter of 1910–11 marks a major turning point in the modern medical history of the region. Again, Christie's services were called upon by the local Chinese authorities, this time in co-operation with Russian railway officials and doctors headquartered to the north in the city of Harbin, and Japanese military and railway health officers stationed in southern Manchuria. This massive medical response to the crisis was co-ordinated by the Western-educated Chinese physician Wu Liande.[51] In Mukden, Christie worked as a member of the city's Plague Prevention Bureau (*Fangyi zongju*), the leadership of which also included the chief and deputy-chief of police, the director of the fledgling Fengian Provincial Hospital, and the heads of the provincial Chinese government's Commission of the Interior (*Mingzheng si*) and the Commission of Foreign Affairs (*Jiaoshe si*).[52] After initial reports of the first plague case being found near Mukden's main railway station on 2 January 1911, followed three days later by several other cases being found within the city's walls, Mukden's Plague Prevention Bureau ordered the city closed to railway traffic from the north.[53] For the next few weeks, Christie, working along with two other British doctors, A. R. Young and Arthur Jackson, as well as local police officers, attempted

[51] On the career of Wu Liande, see Wu Liande (Wu Lien-teh), *Plague Fighter: The Autobiography of a Modern Chinese Physician* (Cambridge: W. Heffer & Sons, 1959).

[52] See Carol Benedict, *Bubonic Plague in Nineteenth-Century China* (Stanford: Stanford University Press, 1996), 156–63.

[53] Christie and Christie, *Thirty Years in Moukden*, 234–37.

to locate and treat carriers of the disease. While Christie divided his time between the mission hospital and the municipal anti-plague headquarters in the provincial Viceroy Xiliang's [54] compound, Jackson volunteered to work at Mukden's main railway station where he was to inspect all incoming passengers and provide medical care to the sick.

Jackson had only just arrived in the city, the previous November, after being sent by the United Free Church of Scotland's mission board to be the first of the two additional doctors requested by Christie in 1909 to staff the new hospital and medical college. Arthur Jackson had received his medical training at Cambridge, and had also taken additional diploma training in tropical medicine at the new school in London. On 14 January 1911, the last train, before Christie and the Chinese Governor ordered the suspension of all rail service, left Mukden's railway station headed north towards Harbin. It was stopped at a medical check-point by Russian and Chinese medical officers after several hours, and at this time it was discovered that two of the Chinese labourers in one of the railcars had died of plague. The train was ordered to return to Mukden. Jackson was alone on duty when the train pulled into the central station, and he began to inspect all 470 passengers for signs of infection. Even though no others appeared to be ill, Jackson could not let them leave the station to mingle with the city's population. With no official quarantine facilities available, Jackson commandeered several inns near the station and began a vigil. He did not have long to wait, as several died that night, and by the next day dozens were showing symptoms of the plague. For the next nine days Jackson tended to the sick, and refused to allow any other physician to take his place. On Tuesday, 24 January, the last of the itinerant labourers from the 'plague train' were transferred to the city's emergency hospital. Although his efforts to prevent the plague from spreading to Mukden's population were successful, Jackson would not survive the epidemic. He had contracted the disease while treating one of the Chinese sufferers, and died early the next evening. He was bur-

[54] On late Qing reforms of police sanitation work carried out by Governor Xiliang and his predecessors, see Benedict, *Bubonic Plague*, 156–57.

ied the following Saturday 2 kilometres outside of the city's walls in a piece of land donated by the Governor-General of the Three Eastern Provinces, Xiliang. Christie's medical mission had its first martyr.[55]

In the two decades that followed the 1910–11 plague epidemic, the Scottish Presbyterian Mission Hospital in Mukden grew dramatically. By 1913, it had a staff of thirteen physicians, nurses and dispensary clerk, and had emerged as one of the most famous medical missionary enterprises in all of China.[56] This recognition was the result of not only Christie's efforts to deliver medical treatment to the people of Manchuria, but also because of the emotional and spiritual appeal of the example of Arthur Jackson's ultimate sacrifice. Jackson's story was retold in a popular work by the missionary writer Alfred Costain, in his book, *The Life of Dr Arthur Jackson of Manchuria* (1911), a book that was a best-seller throughout Britain, and particularly in Scotland, in the years before First World War. Jackson's tale was often repeated in the annual reports of the Mukden medical college and hospital, as well as in missionary literature published by the United Free Church of Scotland.[57] By his untimely death, Arthur Jackson was indirectly responsible for guaranteeing the Manchurian mission the funding that it required to continue and to expand its medical work. The hospital and college suffered temporary staff shortages during the Great War as four of its six doctors returned to Europe to serve in a variety of capacities, but overall the two decades that followed the great Manchurian plague epidemic were the calmest the mission had known.

[55] For more detailed discussions of Jackson's efforts during the plague outbreak, see Alfred J. Costain, *The Life of Dr. Arthur Jackson of Manchuria* (London: Hodder and Stoughton, 1911), 127–43; and Christie and Christie, *Thirty Years in Moukden*, 237–40.

[56] Christie, *Dugald Christie of Manchuria*, 161.

[57] For examples of Arthur Jackson as the missionary exemplar, see William Watson's Preface to Costain, *The Life of Dr. Arthur Jackson*, 7–9; as well as Costain's own account, particularly pages 68, and 142–43; Morrison, *The Scottish Churches' Work Abroad*, 177; Christie, *Dugald Christie of Manchuria*, 134; the MMC Board of Management, *The Mukden Medical College, Report for the Year 1919*, 4; and Robertson, *Story of Our Mission*, 107.

In 1923, Dugald Christie announced his retirement, and together with his wife Eliza left Manchuria to return to Scotland. Christie left behind a legacy of dedication to serving the people of Manchuria by offering his own medical services, and by founding three institutions that were manifestations of his vision of 'clinical Christianity'—the men's and women's hospitals of the United Free Church of Scotland's mission and the Mukden Medical College. As in the past, Christie had secured a powerful local patron for these institutions by the early 1920s, this time the local Manchurian warlord, Zhang Zuolin. Christie frequently visited Marshall Zhang at his headquarters in Mukden, where the two men talked of politics, world events and the future of China. During the early 1920s, Zhang presented Christie's hospital and college with generous bequests of land for an athletic field, thousands of pounds in financing, as well as gifts in the form of valuable medical equipment. With the funding from Marshall Zhang, as well as grants from the China Medical Board of the Rockefeller Foundation and the Foreign Mission Committee of the United Free Church, the Mukden hospital embarked on a major expansion drive in the early 1920s. A new patient ward was completed, as were new nurses' residences and a new central medical building. [58] When constructing these new hospital facilities, the 1920 report of the Mukden Medical College noted:

> [A] special effort was made to make [them] a model in equipment and all arrangements, and to have the nursing, sanitation, and cleanliness, equal to that in a home hospital. . . . It is not intended that this [new] ward should be an exception, and all the doctors and nurses, and no doubt all patients too, long for the time when every ward in the Hospital shall be as well equipped and provided for. [59]

The vision of missionary medicine that Dugald Christie left in Mukden was now much more demanding than it had been four decades earlier as the basic care that he had first provided in the mis-

[58] MMC Board of Management, *The Mukden Medical College,Report for the Year 1919*, 4–5; and Board of Management, *The Moukden Medical College: Report for 1918, Ninth Annual Statement* (Edinburgh: Darien Press, 1919), 15.

[59] Board of Management, *The Mukden Medical College: Report for 1920, Eleventh Annual Statement* (Edinburgh: Darien Press, 1921), 23.

sion's early primitive hospitals was no longer seen as good enough. For the Mukden hospital and its associated medical college, now both under the management of Dr William A. Young, to be truly successful as medical and educational facilities, and as 'showcases' of both the mission's Christian faith and Western science, they had to be as modern and well-equipped as possible.[60] By the late 1920s, the Mukden Medical College and hospital boasted modern operating rooms, patient wards, classrooms, library, a foreign teaching staff of almost twenty, and an enrolment of almost eighty Chinese medical students and was a far cry from the mud-walled shack where Christie had performed his first surgeries forty years earlier.

Gotô Shinpei and the Japanese Hospital and Medical College in Mukden

As Dugald Christie was the guiding force in the history of the Scottish missionary medical presence in Mukden, Gotô Shinpei played a similar, albeit less direct role, in the development of Japanese public health policies and medical facilities in the city.[61] Born in 1857, Gotô hailed from an impoverished samurai family. Due to his family's financial difficulties Gotô was forced to go to work as a minor assistant in the local prefectural government at the age of thirteen. There Gotô found a mentor and sponsor in Yasûba Ichihira, Iwate's magistrate. Yasûba provided the funds to send his young assistant to Fukushima in western Japan, where Gotô completed his primary

[60] On the growing perceived importance in the vision of the foreign missionaries in Manchuria of building modern, well-equipped, scientific hospitals and colleges, see CMC of the Rockefeller Foundation, *Medicine in China*, 18.

[61] For an introduction to the career and medical ideas of Gotô Shinpei, see Kitaoka Shin'ichi, *Gotô Shinpei: Gaikô to bijon* [Gotô Shinpei: A Vision of International Politics] (Tokyo: Chûô Koronsha, 1988); Tsurumi Tasukuho, *Gotô Shinpei* (Tokyo: Kubisô shoten, 1985); Edward I. Chen, "Gotô Shinpei: Japan's Colonial Administrator in Taiwan; A Critical Re-examination", *The American Asian Review* 13, no. 1, 1995, 29–59; Ruth Rogaski, *Hygienic Modernity: Meanings of Health and Disease in Treaty-Port China* (Berkeley: University of California Press, 2004), 153–54; and Liu, "Medical Reform in Colonial Taiwan", 65–80.

education as well as medical school studies, graduating from the new Sukagawa Medical College in 1876.

Armed with a medical degree, Gotô then began his residency training in Aichiken prefecture where his sponsor Yasûba had recently been posted as chief magistrate. In Aichiken, Gotô's training benefited from his relationship with two new medical colleagues. The first was Shiba Ryôkai, a military physician in the local hospital who taught the young Gotô to read German and introduced him to the concepts of military medicine and hygiene. The second was the Austrian doctor Albrecht von Roretz who instilled in the resident a belief in the importance of public health and sanitary medicine. When Saigô Takamori launched his rebellion against the Meiji government in 1877, Gotô went to Osaka in order to serve at a military hospital. Here he worked under Ishiguro Tadanori, the founder of modern military medicine in Japan, and made important personal connections with many members of the fledgling Meiji government's medicine and public health bureaucracy—connections that would prove to be extremely valuable in his later career. [62]

After serving in Osaka during the Saigô insurrection, Gotô returned to Aichiken where he was elevated to the positions of deputy chief of the prefectural hospital and principal of its small medical college. During the next several years, Gotô transformed Achiken's college into a medical school modelled on the German system. The curriculum adopted German-styled courses and emphasised the importance of new medical diagnostic instruments and laboratory science. [63] During this time Gotô also developed a new-found belief in the importance of public health. After only a year in his new post, Gotô was able to convince magistrate Yasûba to establish a sanitary police system in the prefecture in order to improve public health.

In 1882, Gotô moved to the city of Nagoya where he was appointed to be a technical investigator for the national government's sanitation board. During his time in central Japan, Gotô continued to refine his medical thinking. In his extensive sanitation reports,

[62] See Liu, "Medical Reform in Colonial Taiwan", 68–69.

[63] On the central role of the German model of medical science and education in Meiji Japan, see John Z. Bowers, *When the Twain Meet: The Rise of Western Medicine in Japan* (Baltimore: Johns Hopkins University Press, 1980).

Gotô included not only basic statistics on disease morbidity and mortality rates, but also detailed analysis of the local environment, customs, geography, and economy. This work marked the beginning of Gotô's emphasis on 'biological principals' (*seibutsugaku no genri*), a concept that would be more fully developed during his tenure as Chief Civil Administrator of Taiwan in the late 1890s and then a decade later in Manchuria when he headed the South Manchuria Railway Company.[64] These 'biological principals' reflected the widespread belief in Meiji Japan in the value of rational, scientific governance as well as certain traits associated with the biological determinism that lay at the core of the ideas of Herbert Spencer and late nineteenth-century social Darwinism—a philosophy that had had a great impact on many Meiji intellectuals.[65]

In 1890, Gotô received an opportunity to continue his post-graduate studies in Germany where he completed a thesis on the development of medical police and public health administration in Japan. Gotô's experiences and training in Europe affected his vision of modern medicine, further enhancing his belief in the importance of state involvement in sanitation and public health. When he returned to Japan, Gotô was appointed to head the Home Ministry's Medical Bureau where he worked to expand the Meiji government's medical bureaucracy as well as to establish an integrated national hospital system. Before these plans could be fully realised, however, Gotô was appointed to work with General Kodama Gentarô as the chief of the Army's Quarantine Office. After serving as the Chief Inspector of Military Hygiene during the Sino-Japanese War of 1894–95, Gotô followed General Kodama, his newest mentor and sponsor, to Taiwan where the General had just been appointed to serve as the colony's first Governor General. Kodama asked Gotô to join his new administration as the Chief Civilian Administrator (*Minsei Chokan*).[66]

In Taiwan, Gotô, writes Bill Sewell, "turned his attention to colonial development, overseeing railway construction, economic

64 See Liu, "Medical Reform in Colonial Taiwan", 70–71, and 76–80.

65 Rogaski, *Hygienic Modernity*, 153.

66 Bowers and Bowers, "Japanese Medicine in Manchuria", 4.

growth, and urban planning, all while keeping his administration in the black."[67] A central component in Gotô's efforts to develop Taiwan as a model colony using rational scientific principles was the development of a comprehensive public health programme. Medical reforms and the drafting of public health ordinances assumed high priority in Gotô's administration as the colonial administration attempted to use the rhetoric of bringing civilisation and modernity to Taiwan.[68] In 1901, Gotô delivered a speech at a conference of public physicians in Taiwan outlining the centrality of medical issues in Japan's colonial efforts. He claimed:

> If we take a look at colonial policies in other countries, we find that there is not a country which does not use religion to facilitate its rule. In other words, the aid is to increase the regime's popularity by resolving mental confusion for, and providing spiritual comfort to, the colonised. However, the native religion in our country has not fully developed. But physical diseases, like mental confusion, are also a human weakness, which provides a space [in which the regime can alleviate people's pains in order to] enhance approval in the popular mind. That's why we adopted the system of public physicians. . . . Physicians will function in our colony the way missionaries did in other colonies.[69]

In some sense, therefore, Gotô's form of 'clinical colonialism' can be viewed as a secular version of the 'clinical Christianity' practised by Dugald Christie and other western medical missionaries in the late nineteenth and early twentieth centuries. After serving for ten years in Taiwan, Gotô was elevated to the rank of Baron, and appointed the first President of the South Manchuria Railway Company. He would now have the opportunity to supervise the economic and industrial development of Japan's newest overseas possession, as well as "to integrate other Asians into the empire through [Japan's] enlightened policies of leadership."[70]

[67] Sewell, "Public Health Concerns", 10.

[68] Ming-cheng Lo, *Doctors Within Borders: Profession, Ethnicity, and Modernity in Colonial Taiwan* (Berkeley: University of California Press, 2002), 35–43.

[69] Lo, *Doctors Within Borders*, 40.

[70] Sewell, "Public Health Concerns", 10.

As the Mantetsu President, Gotô wielded a great deal of power in Manchuria. While the defence of the territory was charged to the newly formed Kwantung Army, Gotô was granted a great deal of freedom to develop the colony's economy and social policies.[71] As the vehicle for delivering Gotô's vision of colonial rule, the Mantetsu giant was responsible for administering the region's railway and harbour facilities; running its largest factories, coal mines, and experimental farms; assisting in the governing of cities; and providing educational and medical facilities.[72] By the time Gotô left Manchuria in 1908 to assume the presidency of the Japanese Railway Board and the post of Minister of Communications in the national government in Tokyo, Mantetsu was supervising a growing array of medical institutions in southern Manchuria, including a two hundred-bed hospital in the port of Dairen, as well as smaller hospitals and clinics in most of the towns and cities along its raillines.[73] By the mid-1910s, the number of hospitals had grown to eighteen with facilities located in all the major cities in Manchuria, the largest ones being found in Dairen, Andong, Yingkou, Anshan, Fushun, Changchun, and Mukden.[74]

[71] Joshua A. Fogel, trans., *Life Along the South Manchurian Railway: The Memoirs of Itô Takeo* (Armonk, NY: M. E. Sharpe, 1988), 7–9.

[72] Myers, "Japanese Imperialism in Manchuria", 105–09; the South Manchuria Railway (henceforth SMR) Company, *Educational Activities of the South Manchuria Railway Company* (Dairen: South Manchuria Railway Company, 1937); and the Sanitary Office of the South Manchuria Railway Company, *A Glimpse of Public Hygiene in South Manchuria* (Dairen: SMR Sanitary Office, October 1925).

[73] Wang Bingzhong, trans., and ed., *Manzhou kaifa sishinian shi* [A Forty-year History of the Development of Manchuria] (Shenyang: Dongbei lunxian sishinian shi Liaoning bianxie zu yi, 1987), 1: 485–86, and 490–92; and Manshikai [Manchurian History Society], ed., *Manshû kaihatsu yonjûnen shi* [A Forty-year History of Manchuria's Development] (Tokyo: Manshikai, 1964), 1: 137–39.

[74] SMR, *A Glimpse of Public Hygiene in South Manchuria*, 4–5; South Manchuria Railway Company, *Report on Progress in Manchuria* (Dairen: South Manchuria Railway Company, 1929 ed.), 165–66; and Tsurumi Mitsuzo, "Public Hygiene in Manchuria and Mongolia", *Light of Manchuria: The Monthly Organ of the Manchuria Enlightening Society,* 6 February 1921, 5–10.

After the railway hospital in Dairen, the second largest Japanese-run medical facility in colonial Manchuria was the Mantetsu hospital established in Mukden in April 1907.[75] Initially, this facility was housed in a number of abandoned buildings that had been used by the Russian Army's medical corps during the war with Japan. On 23 October 1908, the Mantetsu administration made the decision to construct a new, modern hospital in the growing Japanese concession zone that was located just over a kilometre west of the walled Chinese city. Construction of this facility began that autumn, but the pace of building was quite slow as the company's main efforts were focussed on developing the basic infrastructure in the Japanese concession by laying new roads, electric tram lines, and a modern sewage system.[76] By the summer of 1909, however, a four-storey main hospital building had been completed. During its first year of operation, the new Mantetsu hospital in Mukden treated a total of more than twenty-three thousand patients. It must be noted, however, that the overwhelming majority of patients who received treatment in this modern hospital were Japanese employees of the Mantetsu giant. Only 1,925 of the hospital's patients were Chinese, compared to more than 21,500 Japanese who received treatment.[77]

During the great plague epidemic in the winter of 1910–11, the staff at the new western-styled hospital left the responsibility for the majority of care of the city's population in the hands of the local Plague Prevention Bureau.[78] While Dugald Christie and his

[75] "South Manchuria Medical College: Tenth Anniversary Celebrated", *The Light of Manchuria: The Monthly Organ of the Manchuria Enlightening Society*, 15, 1 November 1921, 49–50.

[76] On the construction of the Japanese railway town in Mukden, see Kinnosuke, *Manchuria a Survey*, 129–34; and Arthur R. Wellington, *Hygiene and Public Health in Japan, Chosen [Korea] and Manchuria: Report of Conditions Met with During the Tour of the League of Nations Interchange of Health Officers* (Kuala Lumpur: Federated Malay States Government Printing Office, 1927), 50.

[77] SMR, *A Glimpse of Public Hygiene in South Manchuria*, 48.

[78] Ishimoto Rikizo, *Nan Man Igakudô jûnen shi* [Ten-year History of the South Manchuria Medical College] (Hôten: Nan Man Insatsusha, 1922), 1–4; and "Manchuria Medical College Takes Honorable Place in Innumerable Contributions Made by SMR towards Development of Manchuria", *Manchuria Daily News*, 22 December 1934.

fellow missionary doctors worked with the town's Chinese police to control the spread of plague, doctors at the Mantetsu hospital focussed their efforts on manning quarantine inspection posts along the numerous rail-lines that radiated out from Mukden.[79] When the plague epidemic finally subsided, Mantetsu's Governors re-evaluated their medical strategies and decided to expand their company's involvement in supervising and indeed improving public health in Manchuria. The central component in this new, more dynamic, vision was the establishment of a medical college attached to the company's hospital.

This is not to say that the Mantetsu managers had not already accomplished a great deal during the first six years of the company's existence. In addition to constructing the new modern hospitals in Dairen and Mukden, the company had also built water reservoirs and sewers in a number of cities, and established regulations for the quarantining of passengers arriving by both rail and sea.[80] The Mantetsu hygiene staff had also assisted the Kwantung Government (*Kantôchô*) in the Japanese leasehold in southern Manchuria in drafting dozens of public health ordinances that aimed to improve 'public hygiene' in the colony.[81] The medical crisis of 1910–1911, however, clearly demonstrated that more needed to be done. Not only had the plague outbreak seriously threatened the economy of

[79] It should be noted that Christie's medical efforts in Manchuria were widely respected by the Japanese, not only in Manchuria, but also in the Home Islands during the colonial period. Two popular translations of his memoirs were published in Japan where they were widely read. See Yanaihara Tadao, trans., *Hôten sanjûnen* [Thirty Years in Mukden] (Tokyo: Iwanami shoten, 1938); and Etô Toshio, trans., *Manshû siekatsu sanjûnen: Hôten no seija 'Kurisuti' no omoide* [Thirty Years Living in Manchuria: Reminiscences of Saint 'Christie' of Mukden] (Tokyo: Dai Ajia kensetsusha, 1937).

[80] Kantô-kyoku (The Kwantung Bureau), *Kantô-kyoku shisei sanjûnen shi* [A Thirty-Year History of the Guandong Bureau] (Tokyo: Toppan insatsu kabushiki kaisha, 1936), 61–78; Gu Mingyi et al., *Riben qinzhan Luda sishinian shi* [A Forty-year History of Japan's Occupation of Lushun and Dalian] (Shenyang: Liaoning renmin chubanshe, 1991), 39–42, and 68–77; and Kwantung Government, *The Kwantung Government: Its Functions and Works* (Dairen: Manchuria Daily News, 1929 ed.), 16–21.

[81] Kwantung Government, *The Kwantung Government* (1929 ed.), 72–74.

the region, but there was also a growing recognition that major investments needed to be made in further developing both modern medical facilities and medical education in the colony as part of Japan's 'civilising mission' in Manchuria. Remembering this time of crisis almost two decades later, a Mantetsu staff writer claimed:

> It was vitally important to diffuse sanitary and medical knowledge and skill in Manchuria and Mongolia in order to promote the general welfare. The dreaded pneumonic plague, which broke out in the winter of 1910–11 and swept over Mongolia and Manchuria claiming 50,000 victims, attracted the eyes of the whole medical world to these regions, and resulted in the assembly of the International Plague Conference at Mukden at the end of the visitation. A medical college was contemplated by the South Manchuria Railway Company, chiefly in order to train Chinese physicians, and this finally came into existence in June, 1911 at Mukden, being named the South Manchuria Medical College.[82]

Although never publicly stated, another possible motivation for both continuing the expansion of the Mukden hospital and establishing the associated medical college was the need to compete with the medical facilities operated by Dugald Christie and the United Free Church of Scotland for the title of 'messenger of modern civilisation'.[83]

On 20 May 1911, senior Mantetsu administrators submitted a request to the National Hygiene Office in Tokyo for permission to establish a medical school in Manchuria. Given that the plague outbreak had ended only weeks earlier, the request was quickly approved by Tokyo, and on 7 June General Ôshima Yoshimasa, the Governor-General (*Kantô totoko*) of the Kwantung Leasehold and commander of the Kwantung Army, announced the plans for the construction of a major expansion to the railway hospital in Mukden

[82] SMR Company, *Report on Progress in Manchuria* (1929 ed.), 167.

[83] A similar speculative conclusion regarding the possible 'competitive stimulus' role of missionary enterprises has recently been drawn by Barbara Brooks in her examination of the history of hospitals and medical colleges in colonial Korea where the Japanese had to compete with the famous Presbyterian Severance Hospital and Medical School in Seoul. See Brooks, "Colonial Power and Public Health", 3.

that would house the new South Manchurian Medical College.[84] Construction began that summer on a parcel of land adjacent to the hospital. The campus of the Mantetsu medical showcase facility when it was completed in 1914 would occupy the entire southern quadrant of the 'great plaza' in the Japanese concession zone.

As construction continued on the new medical college, the railway hospital in Mukden continued to grow. The hospital in Mukden now dwarfed the Scottish mission hospital across town. By the mid-1910s, it boasted nine medical divisions, including a comprehensive clinic, surgery, paediatrics, ophthalmology, gynaecology and obstetrics, dentistry, dermatology, rhino-laryngo-otology, and public health.[85] Stocked with the latest medical, pharmaceutical and laboratory equipment and supplies, the Mukden Railway Hospital treated hundreds of out-patients daily, and had beds for almost four hundred more in its in-patient wards. By the late 1910s, the hospital required an enormous number of people to operate its facilities and treat more than 100,000 patients it serviced annually. Its staff now included 56 physicians, 6 pharmacists, 6 technicians, 15 clerks, and more than 100 midwives and nurses.[86]

Not all residents of Mukden and its environs, however, were to benefit from the facilities that could be found in the new hospital. The grand Mantetsu hospital and medical college had been constructed, despite propaganda claims to the contrary, primarily for the treatment of the territory's sizable Japanese community. However, even within this group not all would have access to the hospital's 'medical wonders'. Although its spokesmen often bemoaned the financial sacrifice that Mantetsu was forced to endure in providing health care facilities in the colony, the company, through the fees charged in facilities such as the hospital at Mukden generated sizable revenues throughout the colonial period.[87] Daily room fees

[84] *Manchuria Daily News*, 22 December 1934; SMR Company, *Report on Progress in Manchuria* (1929 ed.), 167; and Ishimoto, *Nan Man Igakudô jûnen shi*, 1.

[85] Manshikai, ed., *Manshû kaihatsu yonjûnen shi*, 1: 158; *The Light of Manchuria*, November 1921, 49–50; and Ishimoto, *Nan Man Igakudô jûnen shi*, 5–18.

[86] *The Light of Manchuria*, February 1921, 6.

[87] "SMR Hospitals: What Sacrifice is Paid for Their Maintenance", *Manchuria Daily News: Monthly Supplement*, 1 July 1923, 15.

in the new hospital ranged from over ten yen for a bed in one of the four first-class rooms, down to a figure between one and two yen for one of the 276 beds in the third-class ward. Even the lower fee was not trivial as the average weekly salary for even a skilled Japanese worker in the railway town was only a few yen.

While Japanese labourers faced a financial hurdle while seeking treatment in the new hospital, the situation was far worse for members of Mukden's Chinese community. Chinese employees of Mantetsu were permitted to seek basic treatment at the hospital, although they were placed in a segregated 'special third-class' ward.[88] Hundreds of thousands of other Chinese residents in the railway town, however, were never allowed to step into the edifice to colonial modernity. Several smaller clinics and hospitals were built to treat Mukden's Chinese majority, but these facilities could not offer the level of care provided by the staff and equipment at the main hospital. In their efforts to construct a 'healthy colony', the Japanese Governors were also constructing barriers not only between diseases and people, but also between rulers and the ruled.

The institution that theoretically was supposed to bridge the colonial divide between the Japanese rulers and the Chinese 'ruled,' was the South Manchurian Medical College in Mukden. The stated aims of the college were:

> To turn out good doctors of fine character who [would] be capable of contributing to the advance of medical relief and public hygiene in China; [and] secondly to prosecute the study of medical science to keep abreast with the western elders and to elevate this college to a place of high repute among its kind in China. The primary object of founding the college consists in laying the foundation of Sino-Japanese co-existence and co-prosperity.[89]

When the college opened in October 1911, however, all 20 members of the first class of students admitted were Japanese.[90]

[88] SMR, *A Glimpse of Public Hygiene in South Manchuria*, 49; and Wang, *Manzhou kaifa sishinian shi*, 1: 486.

[89] Wellington, *Hygiene and Public Health in Japan, Chosen [Korea] and Manchuria*, 51.

[90] Ishimoto, *Nan Man Igakudô jûnen shi*, 37.

This situation did gradually change throughout the next decade as more Chinese students gained admission, and by 1921 the college had graduated a total of 185 doctors with the title *Igakushi* ('medical graduate'), 130 of whom were Japanese, and the remaining 55 Chinese.[91]

Under the supervision of its first director, Dr Kanai Kenji, formerly the superintendent of the Mantetsu Hospital in Dairen, the South Manchurian Medical College in Mukden became one of the leading medical schools in not just China or the Japanese empire, but even one that was highly thought of in Japan itself. The entrance examinations were rigorous, and often only 10 per cent of those who wrote them were able to secure admission.[92] In addition, all students had to demonstrate proficiency in both written and spoken Japanese and Chinese as part of the college's stated purpose of bringing the two cultures together in harmony. The school's curriculum followed the guidelines dictated for all 'medical colleges' by the Japanese Ministry of Education. All students were required to take German classes for all four years of the programme, in addition to the standard medical classes in chemistry, anatomy, physiology, pathology, pharmacology, surgery, hygiene, ophthalmology, obstetrics, psychiatry, dermatology and bacteriology. Japanese students were also required to take additional courses in the Chinese language, while Chinese students were to continue their study of Japanese. This language work, it was hoped, was to serve as a "linguistic bridge [between] the young students of different nationalities [who] are brought into mutual contact personally and spiritually."[93]

What made the Mantetsu medical institutions in Mukden unique in not only Manchuria, but also the colonial empire, was not its attempt to create a co-operative spirit between the two nationalities in the colony. Rather it was the volume of high calibre research that

[91] Wellington, *Hygiene and Public Health in Japan, Chosen [Korea] and Manchuria*, 51.

[92] *Manchuria Daily News*, 14 September 1914; and SMR, *A Glimpse of Public Hygiene in South Manchuria*, 32.

[93] Wellington, *Hygiene and Public Health in Japan, Chosen [Korea] and Manchuria*, 50.

was carried out by the college's twenty-three professors and dozens of the associated hospital's doctors. The research work conducted by this cohort of physicians involved the fields of bacteriology, physiology, surgical technique, public health, and virology. These men formed the core of the South Manchurian Medical Association and oversaw the publication of one of the leading Japanese-language medical journals in the early twentieth century, the *Nanman Igakukai Zasshi* (South Manchurian Medical Association Journal). Established in 1912, this journal merged in 1923 with another published by the Mantetsu Hospital in Dairen and became the *Manshû Igaku Zasshi* (Manchurian Medical Journal). During its more than three decades of existence, this journal was one of the premier medical research publications in East Asia, and its quarterly editions were often more than four hundred pages in length.[94] In recognition of both the quality of the college's research output, and the education of its students, the Japanese Education Ministry upgraded the institution's status to that of an imperial university with a faculty of medicine (*Nanman Igaku Semmon-bu*) in May 1922. By the late 1920s, the Mantetsu hospital and medical university in Mukden had emerged as institutional showcases of modernity and scientific expertise that Japanese administrators believed symbolised their 'enlightened colonial rule.' The only problem was that the show was not open to everyone.

Conclusion: Legacies and Shifting Chinese Views of the Past

Today, one of the largest and most prestigious medical schools in the People's Republic of China (PRC) is the China Medical University (*Zhongguo Yike Daxue*) located in the capital of Liaoning Province, Shenyang—the city that was formerly better known in the West as Mukden. The school's campus is an extensive complex housing more than thirteen thousand students and more than 1,100 teaching staff in 18 colleges, 130 research departments, a centre for Japanese-language training, a rural health college, 18 research laborato-

[94] See Bowers and Bowers, "Japanese Medicine in Manchuria", 12.

ries, and one of the largest medical research libraries in the PRC.[95] The website for this university contains a short description of the institution's glorious and decidedly revolutionary history, noting that it was formerly the Chinese Workers' and Peasant's Red Army Medical School (*Zhongguo Gong Nong Hongjun Yi Xuexiao*) founded in the southern province of Jiangxi in 1931, and that following the Long March of 1934–35, the school was renamed the China Medical University by Mao Zedong and the Central Committee of the Chinese Communist Party. Only in a single sentence at the end of the historical biography of the school is mention made that the institution's origins in Shenyang were the Scottish missionary Mukden Medical College, and the Manchuria Medical University established by the South Manchuria Railway Company.[96]

Such use of ideological blinkers when discussing the pre-1949 past is not an uncommon approach in Chinese scholarship. In their study of the Manchurian city of Harbin, Soren Clausen and Stig Thogersen cite the Chinese historian Yu Ciyun who described the attitude amongst his colleagues regarding the history of the colonial period of the region as:

> Because of the influence of "leftist" ideology it has always been felt that [this period] was "false" [or "puppet," *wei*], so there was no need to write about it. Why glorify the colonial puppet regime by writing its historical records? "We don't recognise it at all!"[97]

[95] China Medical University (henceforth CMU), Information Center, "China Medical University: Survey," Shenyang, 2003. http://www.cmu.edu.cn/overview/overview.htm (accessed 1 August 2004).

[96] CMU, "China Medical University", 2003. http://www.cmu.edu.cn/overview/overview.htm (accesed 1 August 2004). Although the correct date of 1911 is cited as the founding of the Manchurian Medical University by the Japanese-run South Manchuria Railway Company, the website mistakenly claims that the missionary college was founded in 1882, when in fact it was opened three decades later in 1912. The earlier date probably refers to the date when Dugald Christie began to practise medicine in Shenyang (Mukden).

[97] Soren Clausen and Stig Thogersen, *The Making of a Chinese City: History and Historiography in Harbin* (Armonk, NY: M. E. Sharpe, 1995), 122.

While the majority of Chinese historiography has tended to write off entirely Manchuria's pre-1949 past as a false story, this is not the case in the work by all historians. During the late 1980s and 1990s there was a surge in interest in local-level history throughout the north-eastern provinces as some Chinese scholars attempted to reclaim their region's colonial past.[98] The administrations of several cities organised teams of researchers to compile municipal gazetteers that charted Manchuria's history from literally the dawn of geological time through to the period of the post-Mao reforms. As part of this broader movement, the municipal government of Shenyang oversaw the publication of a seventeen-volume series that documented the city's past, one volume of which examined the topics of culture, the news media, the publishing industry, sports, and public health. Although this volume, edited by the historian Meng Jie, continues the tradition of largely ignoring the history of Japanese activities in the city, it does contain detailed descriptions of the medical and education work conducted by the Scottish missionaries in the late nineteenth and early twentieth centuries. Dugald Christie, referred to by his 'Chinese name' Ke Duge, is cited as being the first 'modern' (*jindai*) doctor in Shenyang, and his pioneering efforts to establish the Scottish missionary hospital are hailed as benefiting the people of the city.[99]

Liu Zhongming's history of the city's medical college goes even further in its praise of Christie and his fellow missionaries. On the founding of the hospital and attached college, Liu writes:

> The initiation and development of the hospital and the college were chiefly due to the vision, endeavour and wisdom of a young Scottish doctor, whose name was Dugald Christie, a graduate of Edinburgh University, in 1881. . . . In 1883, he came to Mukden (Shenyang) on a cart pulled by a cow, spending fully eight days for the journey. Through his devotion, hard work and medical skill, he built a hospital to start and be-

[98] Clausen and Thogersen, *The Making of a Chinese City*, 3–4, 48–50, 122, and 202–6.

[99] Meng Jie et al., eds., *Shenyang shi zhi: Wenhua, xinwen, chuban, weisheng, tiyu, wenwu* [History of the City of Shenyang: Culture, News, Publishing, Public Health, Sports, and Cultural Relics] (Shenyang: Shenyang chubanshe, 1990) 13: 199–200, and 244.

gan to enrol apprentices in the late nineteenth century; a regular medical school was established in 1912.[100]

Liu's praise of Christie's efforts and the work of the missionary college is followed by detailed lists of the college's alumni from the entering class of 1912 through to the last graduates in 1951. This list contains the names of all 682 Chinese physicians, 329 nurses, 78 pharmacists, and 40 laboratory technicians who were trained at the college and notes the institutions where many went on to practice their profession.[101] After noting the tens of thousands of Chinese who were treated at the Scottish mission's hospital, Liu concludes that the "Mukden Hospital, in its existence from 1884 to 1948, rendered efficient medical services of the people of the three north-eastern provinces and gained a very good reputation for its therapeutic care to the sick and injured at all times."[102]

Not only is Liu's work representative of the shift in local historical scholarship in Manchuria, but it also reflects the broader reassessment in the People's Republic of China, the past educational and medical work conducted by foreign missionaries. In her study of Western medical missionaries in Sichuan Province, Karen Minden notes that in the 1980s Chinese historians began to re-examine the roles that foreign missionaries had played in China's educational history and modernisation. She notes that, "[i]t has been increasingly acknowledged that [the] missionary-run schools were an essential conduit for the introduction of modern methods of education and research into China."[103] As China opens to the world it is perhaps only natural that the early social and educational work conducted by Western missionaries is now viewed with a certain nostalgia and that figures such as Dugald Christie are now seen as 'heroes' (*yingxiong*) in a manner similar to past officially-sanctioned portrayals of foreign friends (*guowai youren*) such as the revolutionary martyr Dr Norman Bethune.

[100] Liu, *Fengtian Yike Daxue*, 5–6.

[101] Ibid., 58–78.

[102] Ibid., 50.

[103] Karen Minden, *Bamboo Stone*, 19.

If the history of foreign missionaries is now viewed through the lenses of 'rose-coloured glasses,' has there been a similar reappraisal in the PRC of the medical and public health work conducted by the Japanese during the colonial period? The simple answer to this question is no. The activities of the Japanese colonial authorities and the Mantetsu giant continue to be portrayed by Chinese historians as the products of 'colonial oppression' (*zhimin yapo*) and the work of an 'imperialist power' (*diguozhuyi lieqing*). Such assessments are harshest for the post-1931 period. While Manchuria's colonial history is no longer necessarily a 'false' past that is best left ignored, Chinese scholars continue to rely on simplistic interpretations of the period that highlight the worst excesses of Japanese rule, such as the activities of Unit 731, the infamous bacteriological warfare division of the Kwantung Army, or the exploitative conditions in Japanese-run coal mines and factories.[104] While these are important topics, the histories of which clearly demonstrate both the war crimes committed by certain elements in the Japanese military as well as the terrible conditions under which many Chinese lived during the Japanese occupation, there are many issues which get painted over when one employs such broad brush strokes.

Recent scholarship on the history of medicine in the Japanese colonies of Taiwan and Korea has provided more nuanced interpretations of the past that demonstrate the need for new topics of enquiry—topics that should also now be pursued as part of a reconsideration of Manchuria's colonial history. By examining official colonial public health policies and medical programmes along with the roles played by Taiwanese, Korean and Chinese physicians who were educated by and who worked under the Japanese, as well as private Japanese and missionary doctors, the picture of medicine

[104] Examples of this rather 'black and white' version of Manchuria's colonial history include: Jie Xueshi, *Wei Manzhouguo shi* [History of the False Manzhouguo] (Beijing: Renmin chubanshe, 1995); Chang Cheng et al., *Xiandai Dongbei shi* [The History of the Contemporary Northeast] (Haerbin: Heilongjiang jiaoyu chubanshe, 1986); and Tan Yi, ed., *'Jiu Yiba' kangzhan shi* [A History of the War of Resistance] (Shenyang: Liaoning renmin chubanshe, 1991).

within the Japanese empire has become more complicated.[105] In the colonial world, "doctors [may have] served as agents of modern civilisation,"[106] but it must be remembered that there existed competing, or at least evolving, visions of what constituted 'modern civilisation' even amongst members of this profession. This chapter has explored the two dominant foreign visions of both the hospital and Western medicine as vehicles for bringing 'civilisation' to Manchuria that were at play in the railway town of Mukden during the early twentieth century. The missionary vision, personified in the life and work of Dugald Christie, believed in modern, Western scientific medicine, but it also maintained at its core a spiritual and evangelical component. The 'clinical Christianity' of Christie and the United Free Church of Scotland's Mukden mission, however, did evolve during the late nineteenth and early twentieth centuries, and by the 1920s there was a growing sense that medical and educational work in China was not only God's work, but also a service to be commended in and of itself. On the other side of the coin stood the 'clinical colonialism' of Gotô Shinpei and the company that he forged in his image, Mantetsu. In this competing vision, modern science and medicine were also valued, but were to be employed in the service of creating a strong, 'healthy' colony for the benefit of Japan. Even here, however, one must be careful not to construct an overly simplistic picture of the past. Although the overwhelming majority of both patients treated in the Mantetsu hospitals and physicians trained in the Manchurian Medical College were Japanese, hundreds of thousands of Chinese also received medical care and hundreds of Chinese doctors, who would later assume leadership roles in the post-war period, were educated during the early colonial period. The mixed legacies of the colonial period continue to resonate decades after the liberation of Manchuria.

[105] See Brooks, "Colonial Power and Public Health", 16–17; Ming-cheng Lo, "Between Ethnicity and Modernity: Taiwanese Medical Students and Doctors under Japan's *Kôminka* Campaign, 1937–1945", *Positions* 10, no. 2, 2002, 285–332.

[106] Lo, *Doctors Within Borders*, 39.

3

Obstetrics and Obstruction: Maternity Provision in Madras, 1840–1852

Seán Lang

Introduction

In the course of the 1840s the Government of Madras found its attention repeatedly being drawn to the issue of maternal care for Indian women.[1] It began in 1840 when a group of nine British surgeons formed themselves into a committee to revive their earlier attempt to set up a Lying-in Hospital in the city.[2] They approached the Governor-in-Council for his support, and he in turn approached the Government of India.[3] Calcutta expressed some doubt whether the proposal would work, but agreed that the hospital might go ahead with the Government of Madras undertak-

I acknowledge with gratitude the advice and encouragement I received while undertaking the research for this paper from Professor Mark Harrison, Professor Sir Christopher Bayly, Professor Barbara Ramusack, Dr Rosemary Fitzgerald and Professor Sarah Hodges. Dr Margaret Jones was very patient in helping prepare the manuscript. I am also grateful for the research grant I received from the Wellcome Trust and the invaluable and unfailing help of the staff at the Oriental and India Office Collection in the British Library.

1 For the background to Madras's maternity policy, see Seán Lang, "Drop the Demon Dai: State Maternity Policy in Madras Presidency, 1840–1875", *Social History of Medicine* 18, no. 3, 2005, 357–78; Sarah Hodges, "Women in Madras Presidency Health Policy, 1840–1890" (unpublished paper, University of Wisconsin, 1992).

2 *Madras Public Consultations*, 4 August 1840, no. 77, Oriental and India Office Collections P/247/53, British Library (henceforth OIOC, BL).

3 *Madras Public Consultations*, 15 March 1841, no. 12, OIOC P/24/59, BL; Government of India (henceforth GOI) *Public Consultations* 17 February 1841, nos. 6–7, OIOC P/186/97, BL.

ing to subsidise its costs.[4] Suitably encouraged, the committee set about finding a site. After some tricky negotiations with the elders of St Andrew's Scottish Church, they obtained a site adjacent to the church and close to the River Cooum.[5] The hospital finally opened its doors in 1844 and, although its riverside site left it vulnerable to frequent flooding, the hospital quickly developed a very favourable reputation.[6] The Governor meanwhile was discovering to his dismay that the hospital was going to cost far more to run than he had realised; in 1847 government bowed to the inevitable and took the hospital over formally.[7] Although officially called simply the Madras Lying-in Hospital, it was often known as the Government Lying-in Hospital and it was subject to the same regime of inspection and accountability as any other government medical institution.

This hospital was not to be the Madras Government's only encounter with Indian maternity in the 1840s and 1850s. Within a year of the government's takeover of the hospital, a second Lying-in Hospital was opened in Madras, this time an independent venture under the supervision of a Dr John Scott recently arrived from Ceylon.[8] Scott was a private surgeon and his hospital was administered by an independent committee. However, since it proved impossible to finance the hospital entirely from private subscription, Scott applied for and got a monthly government subsidy; in return, the hospital was to be subject to inspection by the government medical authorities.[9]

By the end of the 1840s, therefore, the Government of Madras found itself responsible, directly or indirectly, for two Lying-in Hospitals, both of them engaged, or planning to engage, in midwife training. The evidence suggests that the Madras Government took its responsibilities in this field seriously. To understand the signifi-

[4] Ibid., no. 7.

[5] *Madras Public Consultations*, 15 February 1842, no. 11, OIOC P/247/68, BL.

[6] For details of the problems of the riverside site, see J. L. Ranking, *Report upon the Lying-in Hospital and Dispensary for Women and Children* (Madras, 1869).

[7] Ranking, *Report upon the Lying-in Hospital and Dispensary*.

[8] *Bombay Times*, 7 October–1 November 1848.

[9] *Madras Despatches*, 14 January 1852, 230, OIOC E/4/976, BL.

cance of this it is important to put it into its broader context. State medical policy in India has generally been understood as having been determined largely by the needs of the European population which, in the 1840s and 1850s, was largely engaged in the military or in the civil service.[10] Moves to develop women's medicine, and especially care in childbirth, have usually been dated to the second half of the nineteenth century and ascribed in the first instance to missionary societies, which did indeed make a tentative start in the field in the late 1850s.[11] By the 1880s the missionaries were joined by a number of voluntary organisations, such as the Bombay-based Medical Women for India Fund and the Countess of Dufferin's Fund.[12] State involvement has been characterised as reluctant and penny-pinching, trailing behind the efforts of the religious and voluntary agencies;[13] a major British provincial government in India

[10] David Arnold, "Medical Priorities and Practices in Nineteenth-Century British India", *South Asia Research* 5, no. 2, 1985, 167–83; Radhika Ramasubban, "Imperial Health in British India, 1857–1900", in *Disease, Medicine and Empire: Perspectives on Western Medicine and the Experience of European Expansion*, ed. Roy MacLeod and Martin Lewis (London and New York: Routledge, 1988).

[11] Rosemary Fitzgerald, "A 'Peculiar and Exceptional Measure': The Call for Women Medical Missionaries for India in the Later Nineteenth Century", in *Missionary Encounter: Sources and Issues*, ed. Robert A. Bickers and Rosemary Seton (Richmond: Curzon Press, 1996); Rosemary Fitzgerald, "'Clinical Christianity': The Emergence of Medical Work as a Missionary Strategy in Colonial India, 1800–1914", in *Health, Medicine and Empire: Perspectives on Colonial India*, ed. Biswamoy Pati and Mark Harrison (New Delhi: Orient Longman, 2001); Margaret Balfour and Ruth Young, *The Work of Medical Women in India* (London: Oxford University Press, 1929).

[12] For Bombay, see Mridula Ramanna, *Western Medicine and Public Health in Colonial Bombay, 1845–1895* (London: Sangam Books, 2002). For the Countess of Dufferin's Fund, see Maneesha Lal, "The Politics of Gender and Medicine in Colonial India: The Countess of Dufferin's Fund, 1885–1888", *Bulletin of the History of Medicine* 68, no. 1, 1994, 29–66; Seán Lang, "Saving India Through Its Women", *History Today* 55, no. 9, 2005, 46–51.

[13] David Arnold, *Colonising the Body: State Medicine and Epidemic Disease in Nineteenth-Century India* (Berkeley: University of California Press, 1993), 254; Balfour and Young, *Work of Medical Women in India*, 13–14. See also Geraldine Forbes, "Managing Midwifery in India", in *Contesting Colonial Hegemony: State and Society in Africa and India*, ed. Dagmar Engels and Shula

taking such an active interest in the issue of maternity provision so early in the century appears to challenge this received wisdom. This study will show that, as well as the undoubted humanitarian concern of the doctors for the lives and well-being of the Indian women they treated, the development of maternity services in Madras also owed much to political in-fighting and manoeuvring at the highest level of government.

Establishing the Government Hospital

From the start, the main factor which drove nineteenth-century European interest and involvement in Indian maternity was concern at the very high death rate among parturient women and the need "to lessen so fearful a loss of life".[14] There were no accurate records, but the general consensus was that the rate was extremely high, and that the main cause lay in the unsanitary conditions in which women gave birth and in "the amount of mischief done by native midwives" known as *dais.*[15] Tetanus, for example, from the practice of cutting the cord with a sharpened piece of shell or bamboo smeared in dung, was a major killer in traditional Indian child-

---

Marks (London and New York: I. B. Tauris, 1994); Dagmar Engels, "The Politics of Childbirth: British and Bengali Women in Contest, 1890–1930", in *Society and Ideology: Essays in South Asian History Presented to Professor K. A. Ballhatchet*, ed. Peter Robb (Delhi: Oxford University Press, 1994); Supriya Guha, "'The Best Swadeshi': Reproductive Health in Bengal, 1840–1890", in Reproductive Health in India: History, Politics, Controversies, ed. Sarah Hodges (New Delhi: Orient Longman, 2006); Anshu Malhotra, "Of Dais and Midwives: 'Middle Class' Interventions in the Management of Reproductive Health in Colonial Punjab", in Hodges, *Reproductive Health in India.* For a positive reassessment of the colonial state's role in female health, see Margaret Jones, "Infant and Maternal Health Services in Ceylon, 1900–1946: Imperialism or Welfare?" *Social History of Medicine* 15, no. 2, 263–89.

14 *Madras Public Consultations*, 6 August 1844, no. 29, OIOC P/248/14 BL.

15 Norman Chevers, *A Commentary on the Disease of India* (London: J. & A. Churchill, 1886), 748. For the continuing uncertainty surrounding maternal mortality statistics in India, see *Census of India*, 1911, India: Report, vol. 1, part 1, 218–19; A. Lakshmanaswamy Mudaliar, *Maternity and Child Welfare* (Madras: Everyman's, 1922), 6.

birth, as indeed it still is.[16] European doctors wrote gruesome accounts of the violent treatment meted out to mothers and children by untrained dais, and much of the work undertaken by the government hospital consisted in trying to save the life of mothers taken out of the hands of the dai by concerned friends and relatives.[17]

The Government Lying-in Hospital's prospectus emphasised the high levels of maternal mortality resulting from the "barbarous" practices of the dai and appealed to "the best feelings of those who have witnessed the sufferings of their fellow creatures, which might be obviated by the introduction of European treatment and practice".[18] This was not mere rhetoric; appealing for funds to "the charitable feelings of the community of Madras" meant involving the whole community, European and Indian, in a public renunciation of the dai and all she stood for, and in a vote of confidence in the superiority of European medical science.[19] As if to emphasise their personal commitment to the issue, the founding surgeons were offering their services to the hospital free of charge.[20] They were conscious that they were following the lead set by Calcutta, where in 1840 a Lying-in Hospital had opened in connection with the Medical College. The Madras hospital committee pointed to

[16] Mridula Bandyopadhyay and Stewart MacPherson, *Women and Health: Tradition and Culture in Rural India* (Aldershot: Ashgate, 1998), 15–21; Roger Jeffery, Patricia Jeffery and Andrew Lyon, "Only Cord-Cutters? Midwifery and Childbirth in Rural North India", *Social Action* 34, no. 3, 1984, 229–50.

[17] Accounts of rough treatment by dais are common in European medical literature in India throughout the nineteenth century. In 1829 *The Lancet* described the dai's methods as "the most rough and inhuman conceivable" (*The Lancet*, 12 September 1829, 758); Superintending Surgeon F. Godfrey claimed that dais' "present meddling practice can in many instances be termed (saving intent) little better than murderous", *Madras Public Consultations*, 21 July 1849, 1, 658, OIOC P/248/53, BL.

[18] *Madras Public Consultations*, 26 January 1841, no. 17, 272, OIOC P/247/58, BL.

[19] Ibid.

[20] Ibid., 273, BL. Working free of charge in charitable hospitals was not in itself unusual: Scott did so at the Black Town Lying-in Hospital and so did the surgeons at the Calcutta Lying-in Hospital. Nevertheless, it was regarded as a significant measure of personal commitment.

the Calcutta scheme in their own prospectus, stressing that the Bengal Government had undertaken to finance the operating costs of the hospital if its building could be erected from public subscriptions; they hoped that their own government would take a similarly generous line.[21] The Madras Government in its turn pointed out to the Government of India that it was merely asking "that the same assistance which has been given to a similar institution at Calcutta may be extended to that proposed to be established at this Presidency".[22] For Madras, always sensitive to issues of hierarchy and authority, it was a question of political equity; if the Government of India did not allow it to establish a Lying-in Hospital when it had given Calcutta the go-ahead, it would be taken as a sign that Madras was being treated as a second-rank presidency. By the same token, having a Lying-in Hospital when Calcutta also had one meant that Madras was maintaining its importance within the political and social structure of British India as a whole.

Like the Madras proposal, the Calcutta hospital's prospectus, a copy of which appears in the Madras Government's proceedings, spoke of "the great mortality among lower orders of the female population during parturition" but it noted that "it chiefly affects the females of the Christian and Jewish religions".[23] Like the Madras surgeons, the Calcutta surgeons were also offering their services gratuitously; unlike Madras, the Calcutta hospital was to be closely tied to the local medical college. It was to provide training opportunities for midwives and for male medical students, thereby enabling the college to establish a Chair of Midwifery. The pupil midwives were to be taught by a European matron under the general direction of the Professor of Midwifery. Calcutta was conscious that it was following standard European practice: the matron was to "conduct the instruction of the pupils on the system followed at the great Lying-in Hospitals of Paris, London and Dublin."[24]

[21] Ibid., 272, BL.

[22] Ibid., 275, BL.

[23] Ibid., 268, BL.

[24] Ibid.

Madras's approach was significantly different. Its Lying-in Hospital was, at least initially, to be kept separate from the local medical school. The Government Medical Board was concerned about the need to encourage women to come into the hospital and noted in 1847 that opening the hospital to medical students "would have the effect of preventing Native Females from resorting to the Hospital as freely as they have heretofore".[25] Rather than training medical students it was intended that the hospital should be geared to the training of midwives.[26] The plan, which was to become characteristic of Madras's approach to midwifery, was to train up a body of midwives in Western practice who would receive a certificate "which will be a guarantee that they are sufficiently educated to give their assistance to the community at large, whether at the Presidency, or, outstations".[27] Although the prospectus did not specify whether or not they should be Indian, the reference to working in "the community at large" would suggest that at least some of them would be; when the midwifery school was launched in 1854 the Madras Government insisted that half its intake should be Indian.[28] From the start that the hospital's midwives were to be the conduit for spreading the hospital's influence in the city and beyond.

Saving Indian Women

The first attempts to establish a Lying-in Hospital in Madras came within a few years of Bentinck's famous outlawing of *sati* in 1829.[29]

[25] *Madras Public Consultations*, 28 May 1847, no. 48, 1,963, OIOC P/248/37, BL.

[26] *Madras Public Consultations*, 4 August 1840, no. 77, OIOC P/247/53, BL; *Madras Public Consultations*, 1 August 1854, no. 65, OIOC P/249/30, BL.

[27] *Madras Public Consultations*, 4 August 1840, no. 77, OIOC P/247/53, BL

[28] *Madras Public Consultations*, 1 August 1854, no. 55, OIOC P/249/30, BL.

[29] The hospital prospectus stated that, "The members of the Medical profession at the Presidency have for Several years past considered the establishment of a Lying-in Hospital of the greatest importance and the endeavours of a few were some time back exerted to effect this desirable object which was partially accomplished, but abandoned for want of the means of supporting it" (*Madras Public Consultations*, 4 August 1840, BL). I have not been able to trace any other record of this earlier scheme. It seems likely, from the

It has long been recognised that *sati* provided a very potent set of imagery for the British imaginative construction of the Indian woman: meek, oppressed, and in desperate need of rescue from the pernicious effects of her own culture.[30] The British liked to see themselves in the chivalrous role of rescuer of the Indian damsel in distress, and those who were not able literally to pluck widows from funeral pyres adopted the same mental picture in relation to other aspects of Indian womanhood. In 1835, for example, the Court of Directors directed the magistrates in Rajahmundry and North Arcot in Madras Presidency to investigate the apparently high number of female suicides recorded by the local coroners: 140 in one year in North Arcot, 109 in six months in Rajahmundry.[31] The Rajahmundry magistrates, while finding that the figure had been inflated, nevertheless attributed female suicides to "the degrading and often cruel treatment to which especially the younger women are exposed in their families."[32] The usual culprit was held to be the woman's in-laws, especially her mother-in-law; significantly, it was her mother-in-law who invariably exercised control over her daughter-in-law's labour.[33]

---

wording here, that it dates from the early 1830s at the latest, which would place it contemporaneously with the abolition of *sati*.

30 C. A. Bayly, *Indian Society and the Making of the British Empire* (Cambridge: Cambridge University Press, 1993), 122; Lata Mani, "Contentious Traditions: The Debate on Sati in Colonial India", in *Recasting Women: Essays in Colonial History*, ed. Kumkum Sangari and Sudesh Vaid (New Delhi: Kali for Women, 1989), 90–118.

31 Report Relative to the Prevalency of Suicides in Rajahmundry and North Arcot, *Board's Collections* 61215, vol. 1539, 1835–36, OIOC F/4/1539, BL. I am grateful to Professor C. A. Bayly for bringing this information to my attention.

32 *Board's Collections* 61215, BL.

33 Ghulam Murshid, *Reluctant Debutante: Response of Bengali Women to Modernisation, 1849–1905* (Rajshahi: Rajshahi University, 1983); Dr Adityanjee, "Suicide Attempts and Suicides in India: Cross-Cultural Aspects", *International Journal of Social Psychiatry* 32, no. 2, 1986, 64–73; Carol Vlassoff, "The Status of Women in Rural India: A Village Study", *Social Action* 32, October–December, 1982, 380–407. While this paper was being composed, on 9 September 2004, the BBC Radio 4 programme "You and Yours" carried a report on the high levels of suicide among British Asian women brought about by family pressures.

Two of the North Arcot suicides were of women in labour, apparently seeking release from the pains of childbirth. The most common cause of suicide listed among the female cases was stomach pains, which can probably be explained in terms of uterine disease; the surgeon Norman Chevers found it the most common cause of suicide among Indian women.[34] Actual cases of suicide by mothers in labour were understandably rare but the link between childbirth and death, including suicide, was very close.[35] Improving the conditions of childbirth would address a whole raft of issues which were increasingly exercising the reform-minded British by the 1840s: suicide; child marriage, which meant that some primiparae women were still in puberty; female seclusion, more common in the south among Muslims than among Hindus but which still denied many women access to male doctors; and female infanticide, in which the dai often played a central role.

The Hospital and the State

Government was intimately connected with the Lying-in Hospital from the outset. The founding surgeons were Government Medical Officers and their meetings were held at the offices of the Government Medical Board; the land on which the hospital was built was government land originally ceded to the Scottish kirk and now resumed by government; the building was designed and built by government engineers and, although the initial financing came from private subscriptions, it was clear to the surgeons that government would have to pick up the tab for the day-to-day running of the hospital.[36] No sooner had the hospital opened its doors in 1844

[34] Chevers, *Diseases of India*, 712.

[35] The Government Maternity Hospital did record a successful suicide attempt by a woman in labour in 1881. See A. M. Branfoot, "Annual Report of the Madras Lying-in Hospital for 1881", in *Annual Report on the Civil Hospitals and Dispensaries in the Madras Presidency for the Year 1881* (Madras, 1882).

[36] *Madras Public Consultations*, 26 January 1841, no. 17, BL; *Madras Public Consultations*, 1 March 1842, nos. 11–12, OIOC P/247/68, BL; *Madras Public Consultations*, 4 April 1843, nos. 56–57, OIOC P/248/4, BL; *Madras Public Consultations*, 23 May 1843, no. 36, OIOC P/248/5, BL.

than it was importuning the government for a roadway up to the entrance;[37] it was exasperation at the seemingly endless requests for equipment, staff and extra capacity that drove the Madras Government to take over the running of the hospital in 1847.

For the hospital, the change of status meant constant application to the Governor-in-Council for authorisation to make any alteration to the fabric of the building or to its staffing. All expenditure had to be submitted for approval, which was usually, though not always, forthcoming; in 1850, for example, the Governor-in-Council declined to sanction indents for balances and clocks for the Lying-in Hospital and for Dr Scott's hospital, "not considering them necessary for either of the institutions";[38] in 1852 the government rather grudgingly sanctioned new *punkahs* for new wards, noting that "they doubt the necessity of a Punkah in the Native confinement ward of the Lying-in Hospital."[39] Above all, as a state institution, the hospital had to show itself, in the parlance of the day, "useful", which meant, essentially, providing the state with value for money. From the tone of the hospital's reports to government and from government concern about the number of women passing through the hospital's doors it is clear that the Lying-in Hospital was expected to maintain a high turnover of patients and a low mortality rate, while all the time keeping expenditure down. On the whole the hospital met these expectations. The hospital's high patient turnover obliged the government, immediately on taking the hospital over in 1847, to build two new wings, and the first major round of repairs was needed in 1850.[40] Soon the hospital was pressing strongly for accommodation for the resident apothecary; accommodation would also soon be needed for the expanding midwifery school.[41] In 1854, with patients having to be housed in specially-bought tents in the hospital grounds, the government finally authorised the building of

37 *Madras Public Consultations*, 24 September 1844, nos. 24–25, OIOC P/248/15, BL; *Madras Despatches*, 14 January 1852, 673–74, OIOC E/4/966, BL.

38 *Madras Public Consultations*, 29 October 1850, nos. 27–28, OIOC P/248/63, BL.

39 *Madras Public Consultations*, 23 November 1852, no. 3, OIOC P/249/10, BL.

40 *Madras Public Consultations*, 31 January 1850, nos. 42–43, OIOC P/248/58, BL.

41 *Madras Public Consultations*, 1 August 1854, no. 65, OIOC P/249/30, BL.

an upper storey.[42] The Madras Lying-in Hospital now constituted a major area of state financial responsibility.

TABLE 3.1 Admissions to the Madras Lying-in Hospital, 1845–51

1845	*1846*	*1847*	*1848*	*1849*	*1850*	*1851*
67	104	116	161	216	311	407

Source: Reports of the Madras Lying-in Hospital, *Madras Public Consultations*, 1845–52, OIOC.

In return for this financial outlay, the government expected regular reports on the hospital's work, and these reports show a steady increase in the number of women resorting to it (tables 1 and 2). Women were classified by the racial and religious groupings usual in British official documentation: Europeans; those of mixed race (variously designated as Eurasians or Indo-Britons); Hindus, Muslims (normally rendered as Mussulmans); and Pariahs, who constituted by far the largest group. Difficult deliveries, especially where they resulted in maternal or infant deaths, were written up in detail, and the reports were addressed, through the Government Medical Board, to the Governor-in-Council. From the detailed comments made on them it does seem that the reports were read; we can perhaps say that these reports brought some of the reality of difficult labour or death in childbirth directly to the attention of the Governor and his Council, so that they knew in some detail exactly what they were financing.

TABLE 3.2 Indian and European Admissions to the Madras Lying-in Hospital, 1845–49

	1845	1846	1847	1848	1849
Europeans	No information	19	29	31	30
Indians	No information	85	87	130	186
Total	67	104	116	161	216

Source: Reports of the Madras Lying-in Hospital, *Madras Public Consultations*, 1845–50. OIOC.

[42] *Madras Public Consultations*, 14 November 1854, nos. 104–105, OIOC P/249/33, BL.

The Hospital and Its Women

How good was the care on offer in the government hospital? Since most women only resorted to it in desperate circumstances the hospital was bound to have a high death rate, and it did. The hospital's reports stress that most deaths occurred in cases where a dai delivery had gone badly wrong and the woman was so badly ill that there was little the hospital could do.[43] Similar points were made about the use of instruments. The 1849 report pointed out that all the instrumental deliveries were of patients brought in after having spent long periods in labour under a dai, and that "Not one occurred amongst the patients in Hospital"; this reference to in-patients as opposed to emergency cases would seem to indicate that even by 1849 some women were choosing to deliver within the hospital rather than by traditional means.[44]

Working out why women might have chosen to deliver in the hospital rather than going through a traditional birth is not easy. The hospital certainly offered a marked contrast to the traditional experience of the Indian birthing chamber, though there were many ways in which women were able to mitigate the effects of the "Western" environment. Friends and relatives, sometimes including husbands, seem to have accompanied the women into the hospital, often making it almost as crowded as the traditional birthing chamber. Importantly, instead of dieting the women the hospital paid them a daily sum (*batta*) with which their friends could buy food to cook on the premises.[45] The general effect was to make the hospital experience much closer to what the women would have been familiar with at home.

[43] *Madras Public Consultations*, 23 July 1850, no. 15, *Annual Report of the Lying-in Hospital from 1st January to 31st December*, 1849, 2, 372, OIOC P/248/61, BL; *Madras Public Consultations*, 31 March 1851, no. 15, OIOC P/248/66, BL.

[44] *Madras Public Consultations*, 23 July 1850, no. 15, BL.

[45] *Madras Public Consultations*, 20 April 1847, no. 25, OIOC P/248/37, BL; *Madras Public Consultations*, 8 February 1848, no. 5, OIOC P/247/43, BL.

The Black Town Lying-in Hospital

In the early 1850s maternity provision in Madras became unexpectedly the subject of political controversy. The trouble centred around the relationship between the independent hospital set up by Dr Scott to serve the poor quarters of Madras known as Black Town and the Superintending Surgeon to whom fell the task of inspecting the hospital on behalf of government, Dr Thomas Key.

Scott had made his name running a hospital for women and children in Colombo, and had been particularly commended for persuading a wide range of castes and classes to attend it. The *Bombay Times*, for example, noted that, "even Mussulman females took advantage of his skills, and submitted to the performance of operations".[46] On his arrival in Madras, even though the Government Lying-in Hospital had only opened four years earlier, Scott immediately set about the business of setting up a second Lying-in Hospital in the city. At first he settled on Triplicane as a suitable site, but the Government Medical Board objected that it was close to two existing government dispensaries, so Scott moved to Mount Road, the main thoroughfare through the European city. However, at the earnest invitation of "seventy two Respectable Native residents of Black Town" he soon moved again, this time to Armenian Street in the heart of Black Town.[47] The position of the two Lying-in Hospitals thus neatly encapsulated the two dominant philosophies of British rule: the state institution was situated in its own enclosure, separate from the Indian town, and invited Indian women to come into it; Scott's hospital adopted the more proactive approach of the missionary, independent of the state though dependent upon its goodwill, advancing into the heart of the indigenous community.

At first, Scott's scheme seems to have been generally well received. Leading figures in Madras society subscribed to Scott's hos-

[46] *Bombay Times*, 17 October–1 November 1848.

[47] Scott to Chief Secretary, Government of Fort St George (henceforth GFSG), 7 June 1848, GOI Home, 8 February 1850, no. 5, OIOC P/187/27, BL; Secretary, Madras Government Medical Board, to Chief Secretary, GFSG, 2 November 1848, GOI Home, 8 February 1850, no. 5, OIOC P/187/27, BL.

pital, including members of the Governor's Council.[48] The Governor himself, General Sir Henry Pottinger, subscribed to the tune of Rs 200 and donated Rs 100 more. Unlike the government hospital, which had declared that it would train Indian women as midwives but had not yet got round to doing so, Scott proposed to set about the task immediately. He even offered to train students at the Medical College, a request the college rather indignantly turned down.[49] Like the surgeons who set up the government hospital, however, Scott soon realised that he could not rely entirely upon private subscriptions for the daily running of the hospital, and he applied to the government for a grant. Government agreed to a monthly sum of Rs 200 to cover the costs of inexpensive medicines, but in return the hospital was to be subject to inspection by the presidency Superintending Surgeon.[50]

This deal brought Scott's independent charitable institution within the purview of government just like its state-run counterpart, and both hospitals therefore found themselves subject to the Benthamite efficiency drive which had been galvanising Indian administration since the 1830s. Immediately, the new arrangement provoked problems. The government disputed Scott's indents for expensive medicines and iron cots, reminding him that they had agreed to bear the cost of inexpensive medicines only.[51] The authorities at the Medical College clearly regarded Scott as something of an upstart and alleged that Scott's apothecary had been discharged from the Company's Medical Service for incompetence.[52] Never-

[48] *First Annual Report of the Black Town Lying-in Hospital and Dispensary for Diseases of Women and Children, 1848–49*, GOI Home, 8 February 1850, no. 5, OIOC P/187/27, BL; Third Annual Report to the Managing Committee of the Black Town Lying-in Hospital, 20 December 1851, *Madras Public Consultations*, 16 January 1852, no. 20, OIOC P/248/76, BL.

[49] G. Harding, Superintendent of Madras Medical School, to Superintending Surgeon, GOI Home, 8 February 1850, no. 5, OIOC P/187/27, BL.

[50] Chief Secretary, GFSG, to Secretary to Government of India, 18 December 1849, GOI Home, 8 February 1850, no. 5, OIOC P/187/27, BL.

[51] Secretary, Madras Medical Board, to Chief Secretary, GFSG, 31 May 1849, GOI Home, 8 February 1850, no. 5, OIOC P/187/27, BL.

[52] G. Harding, Superintendent of Madras Medical School, to Superintending Surgeon, GOI Home, 8 February 1850, no. 5, OIOC P/187/27, BL.

theless, Scott seems to have got on well with the Superintending Surgeon, J. Godfrey, who was a frequent visitor and who reported very favourably on what Scott was doing, especially in training native midwives, a task which Godfrey described as "a measure of great utility and also of humanity".[53] Godfrey considered the Black Town Hospital "of unquestionable utility" and Scott himself "a well educated and intelligent Practitioner—who appears to have devoted much attention to the study of Female complaints"; he even reported that the maligned apothecary "is considered to be remarkably steady and attentive and performs his duty in a very satisfactory manner."[54]

Scott's work was soon attracting official attention, not least because his statistical returns suggested that his hospital was treating anything up to twice as many patients as the government hospital and four times as many as the Lying-in Hospital in Calcutta. By 1851 this discrepancy was sufficiently marked for the Court of Directors, concerned as always about value for money and worried that the government hospital might be slacking, to direct the Madras government to look into the matter.[55] The Madras Government Medical Board declared itself "at a loss to understand how a contrast in disparagement of the Government Hospital could have been made" and suggested that the Court and the Madras Government might be forgetting that, whereas the government hospital was limited to confinement cases, Scott also dealt with cases of uterine disease.[56] However, a close analysis of the government hospital's statistical returns by the Hon. Daniel Eliott, a member of the Governor's Council, suggested that it was the government hospital itself that was at fault, for listing all its admissions as confinements, what-

[53] Secretary, Madras Medical Board, to Chief Secretary, GFSG, 8 November 1849, GOI Home, 8 February 1850, no. 5, OIOC P/187/27, BL.

[54] Secretary, Madras Medical Board, to Chief Secretary GFSG, 1 March 1851, *Madras Public Consultations*, 18 March 1851, no. 6, OIOC P/248/66, BL; Secretary, Madras Medical Board, to Chief Secretary, GFSG, 8 November 1849, GOI Home, 8 February 1850, no. 5, OIOC P/187/27, BL.

[55] GOI Home, 4 October 1850, no. 1, OIOC P/187/31, BL; *Madras Public Consultations*, 31 January 1851, no. 22, OIOC P/248/66, BL.

[56] Ibid.

ever the result of the labour; its figures were thus inflated and bore even worse comparison with Scott's. The Governor-in-Council accepted Eliott's analysis and asked the Medical Board to explain itself.[57] However, at this point the heat was taken off the government hospital by the intervention of the new Superintending Surgeon, Dr Thomas Key.

From the start, Key seems to have determined to expose Scott as a cheat and a fraud. He wrote to the Medical Board in March 1851:

> I may mention that I have all along suspected that the working of Doctor Scott's Institution was not faithfully reported and that both Government and the Public have been deceived as to the extent of his operations.[58]

He simply did not believe that Scott could be dealing with 70–90 out-patients each day between the hours of 6:00 and 8:00 in the morning, especially in view of Scott's own complaints that he did not enjoy anything like the resources and help available at the government hospital. Key inspected Scott's reports and found numerous inaccuracies, to the point that Key declared the hospital's reports "were calculated to mislead".[59] Specifically, Scott was in the habit of adding the figures for women still in hospital but undelivered at the end of the year to the totals both for the previous year, when they were admitted, and for the following year, when their babies were born: these women were therefore counted twice. Moreover, Key found evidence to substantiate the government hospital's claim that Scott was not distinguishing clearly between diseases of women, such as uterine diseases, and parturition cases. Scott's figures were therefore heavily inflated and, Key claimed, "both Government and the Public have been deceived".[60] Key further reported finding gaps in the hospital's nominal register, which in any case contained over two thousand male names, one Thomas Drysdale appearing in

57 Ibid., nos. 23–24.

58 Key to Secretary, Medical Board, 13 March 1851, *Madras Public Consultations*, 17 June 1851, no. 44, OIOC P/248/69, BL.

59 Ibid.

60 Key to Secretary, Medical Board 13 March 1851, BL.

the register twice, first as a patient and a few days later as the father of another patient. In effect, Key accused Scott of running a general hospital under the guise of a Lying-in institution and claiming government money under false pretences. To the military-minded British authorities in Madras there could be no more serious charge.

Scott defended himself as best he could, though he did not help himself by submitting his report very late and initially resisting the Medical Board's requests for sight of his record books.[61] He pointed to the support he had always received from Godfrey and criticised Key for "attempting to throw doubt on his predecessor's honesty or ability"; he also produced testimonials from Government Medical Officers, including Edward Balfour and Robert Cole, one of the founders of the Government Lying-in Hospital, backing up Godfrey's good opinions and stressing the importance of his hospital's work in uterine disease. Scott denied that the hospital had been treating adult males, pointing out that some of the Tamil names Key had picked out as male were applicable to either sex, and that the undoubted male names belonged to male children: his was a hospital for women and children; Thomas Drysdale, for example, was a child and bore the same name as his father, which explained the reference in the register. He even brought in Tamil language experts to rule on which names were male and which female. Where male names appeared next to female diseases, he explained, it was because there was not enough room on the forms to separate the different classes of patient. Scott accepted that adding "remaining" patients to the totals of both years was an error, though it was unintentional and Key had in any case told him it was unimportant; the gaps in the register had occurred when "domestic affliction" had kept him away from the hospital and his apothecary had been laid out by an accident.[62] Scott also attacked the basis of Key's criti-

61 *Madras Public Consultations*, 29 April 1851, no. 84, OIOC P/248/66, BL; Scott to Secretary, Medical Board 17 April 1851, *Madras Public Consultations*, 29 April 1851, no. 84, OIOC P/248/66, BL; Scott to Secretary, Black Town Hospital Committee, n.d., *Madras Public Consultations*, 17 June 1851, no. 44, OIOC P/248/69, BL.

62 Scott to Secretary, Medical Board, 29 March 1851, *Madras Public Consultations*, 17 June 1851, no. 44, OIOC P/248/69, BL.

cism, pointing out that his hospital was in a very different situation from the government hospital, which was "provided with every necessary, and with an efficient and well qualified staff", and was in no position to provide the sort of regular detailed statistical returns that were expected of government institutions. He also asserted that government had been aware of this when it had first granted the hospital its subsidy and that government expected no more of him than "care in the expenditure of the public money":

> The Government never expected that the institution should present a pattern of Hospital statistics; had such been their object, they would no doubt have afforded a sufficient staff for that purpose.[63]

Scott then turned his fire on Key. He pointed out that Key had not even visited the hospital before making his accusations: he had simply taken the hospital records away and kept them for a very long time. Since making his accusations, Scott claimed, Key had made one five-minute visit to the hospital, at six o'clock in the morning when the hospital opened for the day.[64] Clearly stung by this attack on his professionalism, Key defended himself vigorously. He had confined himself to inspecting the records, he said, simply to save Scott from an inquisitorial-style, on-the-spot inspection which would have appeared as "a species of espionage" and might have deterred patients from coming to the hospital: "and then", he added, "I should have been accused of injuring the Institution!"[65] There was no excuse for Scott's incompetence in record-keeping:

> I would simply ask what would become of the Commission and of the character at the same time of any Medical Officer of the Most HEIC's service who might be discovered thus dealing with his Hospital records?[66]

63 Scott to Secretary, Medical Board, 29 March 1851, 2515, BL.

64 Ibid., 2512–13, BL.

65 Key to Secretary, Medical Board, 3 April 1851, *Madras Public Consultations*, 17 June 1851, no. 44, OIOC P/248/69, BL.

66 Scott to Secretary, Medical Board, 29 March 1851, BL.

Given Scott's chaotic record-keeping, Key protested that he could hardly be blamed for not being able to distinguish between male and female names in Scott's registers. He disputed Scott's version of his visit, saying it had taken place at 6:40 a.m. and that he had stayed for fully twenty minutes, adding further that Scott knew the truth of the matter perfectly well.[67] He suggested that his predecessor, Godfrey, had failed in his duty by not checking up on Scott more rigorously. Meanwhile, if Scott wanted Key to inspect his hospital more regularly, then Key was happy to do so: and, indeed, within a year Scott was complaining that Key was never out of place:

> He has indeed "watched" the working of the Hospital; he has "watched" the registers with unswerving zeal, and superintended the Books of the out patients seeking eagerly though without success, for an occasion of complaint; but he has not "watched" the cases in the wards of the Hospital, he has not superintended either their nature or their management. . . . he has really stooped to this degrading office, and now accuses me of deliberately, by means of the Apothecaries, stating what I know to be untrue, by entering as patients the names of persons who never existed or at least never received relief from me; I cannot express in language sufficiently strong the indignation I feel in being treated in so unworthy a manner, by a professional brother and a Gentleman.[68]

Key was attempting to prove that Scott was negligently leaving serious cases to be dealt with by the apothecary, a charge that Scott denied but which required yet more detailed written justification of his procedures.[69]

All of this increasingly voluminous and acrimonious correspondence eventually made its way to the Governor's Council where Eliott noted the affair as "another of those unhappy Controversies with which the Government has been harassed, and distracted from more important subjects."[70] Nevertheless, the Governor and his Council

[67] Key to Secretary, Black Town Hospital Committee, 26 April 1851, *Madras Public Consultations*, 17 June 1851, no. 44, OIOC P/248/69, BL.

[68] Scott to Secretary, Black Town Hospital Committee, n.d., *Madras Public Consultations*, 16 January 1852, no. 20, OIOC P/248/76, BL.

[69] Ibid.

[70] Minute by Eliott, 16 May 1851, *Madras Public Consultations*, 17 June 1851, no. 44, OIOC P/248/69, BL.

recognised that behind the personal arguments there was an important issue at stake: was Scott's hospital a state institution, subject to state discipline, or was it not? In what relation did government stand to independent medical ventures to which it chose, or might choose in the future, to offer financial support? It was to be a recurring theme in the debates surrounding missionary medicine and the Countess of Dufferin's Fund; however, the Madras dispute also reflected a significant shift in the power relations within government itself.

The dispute centred essentially on two major issues: first, the question of authority and the relationship of an independent hospital to state supervision; second, the importance to government of the medical work undertaken at the Black Town Lying-in Hospital. Of the two questions, to Pottinger the first was always the more important and straightforward: Scott was in receipt of government money and was therefore subject to government authority in the person of the Superintending Surgeon. Key's complaint, aside from the irregularities in the records, was that Scott "deliberately, and without provocation, set aside my authority";[71] the Medical Board noted tersely that "Dr Scott is in no way under the authority of the Board, and . . . accedes to their requests or refuses compliance as he thinks proper".[72] Scott, however, simply did not accept that his hospital was answerable to the state. He declined to obey a general order requiring Public Dispensaries to submit weekly reports of sick, pointing out that "this institution is not a public dispensary in the sense in which the others are";[73] writing to his own hospital committee Scott made his feelings even clearer:

> The Government do not bear the relation to the Institution in Black Town, which they bear to the public dispensaries; they are merely large

[71] Key to Secretary, Medical Board, 5 July 1851, *Madras Public Consultations*, 19 August 1851, no. 33, OIOC P/248/70, BL.

[72] Secretary, Medical Board, to Secretary, GFSG, 24 April 1851, *Madras Public Consultations*, 17 June 1851, no. 44, OIOC P/248/69, BL.

[73] Scott to Key, 21 April 1851, *Madras Public Consultations*, 17 June 1851, no. 44, OIOC P/248/69, BL.

subscribers, and as such ought to have merely a considerable voice in the management of its affairs. [74]

While there was sympathy in government for certain specific points in Scott's defence, such as the issue of male names on the register, and no one disputed the medical value of his hospital's work, the Medical Board found his defence of his inaccurate statistical returns unconvincing, noting that, "Government and the Public have therefore been deceived as to the extent of its operations in no trifling degree." [75] For Pottinger the issue was a straightforward one of insubordination; he gave Key his full backing, condemned Godfrey, saying that if he had not gone home to England he would have been open to serious censure, and minuted on 12 May 1851 "that the support and countenance hitherto extended by Government to Dr Scott's Institution cannot be longer continued." [76]

It was at this point that political considerations intervened to save Scott. The provincial governments of Bombay and Madras had lost their independent power to legislate in 1833 by order of the Court of Directors in London, and their governing councils, which had consisted of the governor and three senior merchants, had been reformulated to consist of the Governor, the local Commander-in-Chief and two civilians. [77] In theory, in any dispute between the military and the civilians this could mean stalemate; in practice, since Governors usually preferred not to take sides, the arrangement could allow the civilians to outvote the military. Pottinger adopted a quiescent role as Governor: he generally deferred to the judgement of the civilians on his council, Eliott and the Hon. J. R. Thomas; Lord Dalhousie, the forceful Governor-General, even spoke of the "stagnation" prevalent in provincial government in Madras and

[74] Scott to Secretary, Black Town Hospital Committee, n.d., *Madras Public Consultations*, 16 January 1852, no. 20, OIOC P/248/76, BL.

[75] Secretary, Medical Board, to Secretary, GFSG, 24 April 1851, *Madras Public Consultations*, 17 June 1851, no. 44, OIOC P/248/69, BL.

[76] Minute by Pottinger, 12 May 1851, *Madras Public Consultations*, 17 June 1851, no. 44, OIOC P/248/69, BL..

[77] H. H. Dodwell, ed., *The Indian Empire, 1958–1918 and The Last Phase of British Sovereignty in India by R.R. Sethi*, The Cambridge History of India, vol. 6 (Cambridge: Cambridge University Press, 1964), 41.

Bombay.[78] However, Pottinger could be stirred into action, and the question of the proper relationship between government and the Black Town Lying-in Hospital achieved this, becoming, in effect, a field of manoeuvre between the military and civilian interests on the Governor's Council.

It was Eliott who took up the defence of Scott against the Superintending Surgeon. Where Pottinger had judged the issue purely in terms of the obedience Scott owed to a superior officer, Eliott, who had been away from Madras when the matter was first brought to the Governor's attention, adopted more of a lawyer's approach, scrutinising Scott's records and the correspondence between Scott and Key carefully and drawing reasoned conclusions from them. He consistently found that the evidence favoured Scott. Without defending Scott's statistical carelessness, he pointed out that the very scale of Scott's miscalculations militated against the idea that he had been seeking to defraud: "the error was palpable and open to detection on the most cursory inspection by anyone conversant with statements of the kind"; it was clearly the result of Scott's inexperience in statistics rather than any attempt to deceive. He pointed out that if Scott had really wanted to pass male patients off as females he would hardly have entered male names in the register; similarly, he would have invented names and dates rather than leaving gaps in the register.[79] Thomas agreed with Eliott's analysis, adding that Scott had nothing to gain from deceiving government since he "does not receive one farthing of emolument; his time and services are perfectly gratuitous".[80] However, the most significant aspect of Eliott's analysis was the way he turned the focus of criticism away from Scott to Key. He pointed out that the solution to the "male names" issue was so obvious that it had immediately occurred to him when he read of it; "it seems strange that it did not occur to the

78 George Pottinger, *Sir Henry Pottinger: First Governor of Hong Kong* (Stroud: Sutton Publishing, 1997), 159.

79 Minute by Eliott, 16 May 1851, *Madras Public Consultations*, 17 June 1851, no. 44, OIOC P/248/69, BL.

80 Minute by J. J. Thomas, 17 May 1851, *Madras Public Consultations*, 17 June 1851, no. 44, OIOC P/248/69, BL.

Superintending Surgeon".[81] He deprecated Key's attempt to criticise his predecessor when Godfrey was in England and unable to answer the accusations against him: a serious breach of professional etiquette. By his own admission, Eliott pointed out, Key had spent no more than twenty minutes in the hospital and had concentrated his attention not on the hospital's medical work but on its registers; as a result of his negligence, Eliott pointed out, government was uninformed as to the true value of the hospital it was supporting. Thomas noted that Key would be better employed following Godfrey's example, visiting the hospital regularly and lending a hand in the delivery room: "Till this is done", Thomas added, "I cannot attach much value to his [Key's] opinion".[82]

Pottinger's sympathies were strongly on Key's side and when Eliott was absent from Madras he gave rulings in favour of Key and against Scott, on straightforward lines of obedience to authority. However, on his return Eliott was always able to swing opinion back in Scott's favour. In government's formal resolution on the dispute, Scott was reprimanded for "blamable laxity and carelessness" in not keeping his records in order and he was told in no uncertain terms to mend his ways: at Thomas's suggestion, two Government Medical Officers chosen by the Black Town Hospital Committee were to sit on the hospital's committee to ensure this happened.[83] As a further concession to Scott, it was agreed that he should submit monthly returns instead of the weekly ones required of government hospitals, and the government grant to the hospital was to be continued.[84] Thus government was retreating from a previously-held position vis-à-vis an independent hospital. Key, on the other hand, was officially censured for having allowed his personal feelings to get in the way of his duty and basing his whole judgement on Scott's hospital on a single twenty-minute visit.[85] It was a significant victory for the civilians.

[81] Minute by Eliott, 16 May 1851, BL.

[82] Minute by J. J. Thomas, 17 May 1851, BL.

[83] Ibid., no. 57, BL.

[84] *Madras Public Consultations*, 19 August 1851, no. 36, OIOC P/248/70, BL.

[85] *Madras Public Consultations*, 17 June 1851, no. 57, OIOC P/248/69, BL.

Pottinger was deeply unhappy at this outcome, which had been forced on him by Eliott and Thomas; when Key subsequently came up with a detailed justification of his conduct Pottinger was quick to endorse it as "very satisfactory" and to direct that it should be sent to the Court of Directors and the Government of India "without further procrastination".[86] The reference to procrastination suggests that there had been some resistance within the offices of government to carry out the Governor's wishes. However, Eliott dissented from Pottinger's opinion, pointing out that Key had been in serious dereliction of his duty in not visiting the hospital more often, the more so since Scott was engaging in "a novel and interesting experiment" which government had wanted "to be watched with more than ordinary attention", a reference to Scott's work with uterine disease.[87] Pottinger backed down and withdrew his endorsement; Key's explanation was forwarded to Calcutta and to London without commentary from government. Pottinger's minute of 26 June 1851 stated that he deferred to the sentiments of the two civilians on the Council, although he maintained his own views on the matter. His minute also reveals the internal conflict which the issue had given rise to within the Madras administration:

> At least mine [his views in favour of Key] have been strengthened and confirmed by all I have seen further of this matter, and I particularly hold that the publication of a garbled portion of the Papers, including the Minutes of Consultation, is highly objectionable and has led to feelings of ill will which cannot fail to do harm and prevent the Public Service going on with that cordially [*sic*] which it ought always to do whatever differences of opinion may arise.[88]

Not surprisingly, Key felt his professional integrity had been called into question by the government's decision and he was infuriated that Scott had been left "under the impression that his defi-

[86] Minute by Pottinger, 19 July 1851, *Madras Public Consultations*, 15 August 1851, no. 16, OIOC P/248/70, BL.

[87] Minute by Eliott, 24 July 1851, *Madras Public Consultations*, 15 August 1851, no.17, OIOC P/248/70, BL.

[88] Minute by Pottinger, 26 July 1851, *Madras Public Consultations*, 15 August 1851, no.18, OIOC P/248/70, BL.

ance of authority was not deserving of reproof, and may be repeated, when it pleaseth him, with impunity".[89] Key particularly resented the proposal to appoint two Medical Officers to the hospital committee to whom he would have to report, since they would inevitably be junior to him; he took the matter directly to Pottinger, who told him to submit his complaint through the proper channel, via the Medical Board. The Board agreed that Key's position was anomalous and referred the matter to the Governor-in-Council. Key, who thought Scott had arrived at a very cosy situation whereby he could effectively choose his own inspectors, added that if the Black Town Hospital Committee wished to be relieved of his supervision altogether "I have not the slightest objection, but, on the contrary, will be thankful to be allowed to relinquish a charge which, in an honest and impartial endeavour to discharge my duty, has proved a very painful one".[90]

The question of the two Medical Officers appointed to the Black Town Committee raised a matter of basic military protocol and it roused Pottinger to outraged fury on Key's behalf, the more so as he had not spotted the anomaly when the proposal was first passed by his Council:

> It may so turn out that there will occur no difference of opinion [between Key and the two officers], but suppose it is otherwise what is the consequence? Why! That the Senior Executive Medical Officer at the Presidency is to be forced into an official controversy with those under him in rank and station. I must withhold my personal sanction from any such anomalous state of affairs.[91]

So incensed was he that he even declared that those Medical Officers who had written in support of Scott's work, and thereby, in Pottinger's eyes, impugned the judgement of the Superintending

[89] Key to Secretary, Medical Board, 5 July 1851, *Madras Public Consultations*, 19 August 1851, no. 33, OIOC P/248/70, BL.

[90] Key to Secretary, Medical Board, 11 May 1852, *Madras Public Consultations*, 6 July 1852, no. 62, OIOC P/249/6, BL; Secretary, Medical Board, to Secretary, GFSG, 27 May 1852, *Madras Public Consultations*, 6 July 1852, no. 62, OIOC P/249/6, BL.

[91] Minute by Pottinger, 30 May 1852, *Madras Public Consultations*, 6 July 1852, no. 63, OIOC P/249/6, BL.

Surgeon, had "laid themselves open to severe censure for a gross breach of official, and particularly military, etiquette".[92] In Eliott's absence from Madras it was left to J. F. Thomas to put the civilian answer to Pottinger's military case. Thomas stressed the medical value of Scott's work, pointed out that the two Medical Officers would be sitting on the hospital committee in their private capacity, and finally declared himself "unable to see the necessity of dealing with Dr Scott's Institution as a Public or Government Institution".[93] Pottinger took the opposite view:

> I have only to propose that so long as the Black Town Lying-in Hospital is supported in any degree by Government Funds it should be subject to all the Rules and Regulations of other Public Establishments, of a like nature.[94]

Thomas's most telling line of argument, and the one which finally won the argument, was the legal one closest to Pottinger's own position, namely that the arrangements Key complained of had been approved by the majority vote of the Governor's Council and, until such time as the Council voted to change them, they should be allowed to run.[95] Thomas saw no need to change the decision and he doubted that Eliott would either; and, he hinted, not even the Governor had the power to overturn a decision of his own Council:

> So far as I can see my way they [the Council's proceedings] could not be cancelled by a single voice—without admitting an illegal precedent I believe.[96]

The official resolution of the matter left the arguments themselves unresolved: in accordance with his wishes, Key was relieved of responsibility for inspecting the Black Town Hospital; instead

92 Minute by Pottinger, 30 May 1852, BL.

93 Minute by J. F. Thomas, 3 June 1852, *Madras Public Consultations*, 6 July 1852, no. 64, OIOC P/249/6, BL.

94 Minute by Pottinger, 30 May 1852, no. 63, BL.

95 Minute by Thomas, 3 June 1852, *Madras Public Consultations*, 6 July 1852, no. 64, OIOC P/249/6, BL.

96 Minute by Thomas, 25 June 1852, *Madras Public Consultations*, 6 July 1852, no. 66, OIOC P/249/6, BL.

the two Medical Officers appointed to its committee were to submit monthly reports to the Government Medical Board.[97] This arrangement nevertheless vindicated Scott's and the civilians' view that even regular government subscription to a hospital did not of itself turn that hospital into a state institution, subject to state supervision. It was an issue that would return later in the century when the Countess of Dufferin's Fund established women's hospitals independently of the state yet still subject to inspection by male government inspectors.

The second issue at stake centred around the importance of Scott's medical work. The value of Scott's work in parturition and midwife training was disputed by no one, though, as the Medical Board pointed out, "had only twenty patients been relieved it would have done good without exonerating the parties who might show on their records a false statement of twenty five".[98] Scott's civilian defenders on the Governor's Council, however, repeatedly drew attention to the special value attached to Scott's work in the field of uterine disorders. Eliott pointed out that in Lying-in cases alone the relief afforded by Scott's hospital was "at least equal to that of the Hospital maintained by Government", but he added that the latter, in contrast with Scott's hospital, "has afforded scarcely any other aid to women".[99] George Smith, a prominent Medical Officer and later Principal of the Medical College, visited the Black Town Hospital early one morning in May 1851 and found some forty-odd Indian women in-patients, of whom only a dozen or so were Lying-in cases; the rest were mostly uterine complaints. In the upstairs rooms he found "a few patients of the better class", all with uterine complaints and all happy with the care and conditions in the hospital. Smith commented to Scott:

> From my own very limited experience I am satisfied that uterine diseases are by no means infrequent in India, though I certainly was not prepared to find them so common as you have shown them to be.

[97] Minute by Thomas, 25 June 1852, no. 68, BL.

[98] Secretary, Medical Board, to Chief Secretary, GFSG, 24 April 1851, *Madras Public Consultations*, 17 June 1851, no. 44, OIOC P/248/69, BL.

[99] Minute by Eliott, 16 May 1851, BL.

> These are diseases which do not obtrude themselves upon notice for many obvious reasons, and consequently it is the more necessary that special institutions devoted to the treatment of such complaints be established. The demand for them exists and I hope that the day is not far distant when the necessity for their existence will be more abundantly recognised by the Government, by the profession, and by the public at large.[100]

The importance of Scott's work with uterine disease was only matched by his success at attracting caste women to come into his hospital. Acting Surgeon I. Crawford of the 51st Regiment commented on Scott's success in overcoming "the reluctance evinced by those who suffer from such diseases to seek relief at public Institutions of a more general character", and Edward Balfour, who knew the hospital well, having once stood in for Scott during a period of compassionate leave, thought that Scott's success in attracting high-caste women "alone sufficient to mark the good opinion entertained of the Institution, by respectable people of a class and station in society, well capable of learning its character and judging of its advantages. . . . That such people should consent to reside in an hospital seems to me one of the most extraordinary circumstances connected with your success."[101] Such was the hospital's fame that, according to the hospital's 1851 report, women were travelling to it from anything up to 300 miles.[102]

The importance of the medical work going on at the Black Town Hospital was clearly known to government. Eliott had criticised Key for ignoring the fact that at the Black Town Hospital "a novel and interesting experiment was being carried on" which government wanted to monitor closely; later he reminded his fellow Council members that "it was a chief object of this Institution to provide

[100] Smith to Scott, 13 May 1851, *Madras Public Consultations*, 17 June 1851, no. 44, OIOC P/248/69, BL.

[101] Crawford to Scott, 20 May 1851, *Madras Public Consultations*, 17 June 1851, no. 44, OIOC P/248/69, BL; Balfour to Scott, 19 May 1851, *Madras Public Consultations*, 17 June 1851, no. 44, OIOC P/248/69, BL.

[102] Report on Black Town Lying-in Hospital, *Madras Public Consultations*, 16 January 1852, no. 20, OIOC P/248/76, BL.

for the treatment of women labouring under sexual diseases".[103] This throws an intriguing sidelight onto Madras's policy towards female medicine in these middle years of the century. That European doctors were horrified by the delivery methods of the dai was well known in Anglo-Indian medical circles; moreover, since dais sometimes attended European women in labour and were widely used by Europeans as wet nurses it was not difficult even for a cost-conscious Governor like Pottinger, with no interest in the issue, to see how measures to undermine the dai's influence could benefit the state and the European population.[104] However, uterine disease among the Indian population was different. It was an Indian problem which did not affect Europeans either directly or indirectly; why, then, was Scott's work in this field of such importance to the Madras Government?

The answer seems to be that the Madras Government, or at least its increasingly important civilian strand, was more concerned with Indian female medicine than historical commentators have realised. Hospitals and the statistical reports they produced were undoubtedly instruments of control, by which the male colonial establishment was able to exert and maintain its dominance over the female population, but there was more to this official interest than crude manoeuvring for power. Madras's medical policy was based on the idea that Indian society could be transformed, and a close relationship forged between rulers and ruled, through exposure to Western science mediated through Western medicine. Acceptance of western medicine would lead Indians to turn away from the traditional healing of the *hakim* or the ritual role of the dai, and would eventually undermine caste itself.[105] Female medicine became a substitute for

[103] Minute by Eliott, 24 July 1851, *Madras Public Consultations*, 17 June 1851, no. 44, OIOC P/248/69, BL; Minute by Eliott, 22 March 1852, *Madras Public Consultations*, 4 May 1852, no. 20, OIOC P/249/4, BL.

[104] E. M. Collingham, *Imperial Bodies: The Physical Experience of the Raj, c.1800–1947* (Cambridge: Polity Press, 2001), 94–97.

[105] See, for example, Maneesha Lal, "'The Ignorance of Women is the House of Illness': Gender, Nationalism, and Health Reform in Colonial North India", in *Medicine and Colonial Identity*, ed. Mary Sutphen and Bridie Andrews (London and New York: Routledge, 2003); also Deepak Kumar,

rescuing women from sati or infanticide or other perceived forms of female oppression, especially in southern India, where neither sati nor infanticide had ever been widespread.

Central to this process of transformation were hospitals. Hospitals brought patients into direct contact with Western science and in their training role they transformed Indians into Western-thinking figures who would carry the message of Western medicine into the community. The Lying-in Hospital also acted as a forum within which Europeans could seek to understand and explain the workings of the Oriental female body. Given the symbolic importance of limiting access to women's bodies within both Hinduism and Islam, Western obstetrics were of great potential importance in bringing Western scientific philosophy into the heart of the Indian home. It was therefore essential that the Indian community should learn to have confidence in Western hospitals, but this would only come if a lead were given by high-caste women at the upper end of Indian society. The underlying thinking was well illustrated in a minute by J. F. Thomas, commenting on the practice of paying *batta* at the government hospital and on Scott's practice of presenting women with gratuities when they left:

> If European science is to make its way and be duly appreciated by all classes of the Native Community these gratuities must be abolished—a Patient who may receive the most signal benefit, cannot bear any testimony of value to the Institution as to the superior value of European treatment—her testimony rendered worthless in the eyes of the people, as she was paid for going there. The injury to the general progress of such Institutions is not to be estimated.[106]

Perhaps inevitably, the dispute over Scott's hospital ended unhappily. After Key was relieved of his responsibility for supervising the hospital he seems to have taken out his frustration on Dr

---

"Unequal Contenders, Uneven Ground: Medical Encounters in British India, 1820–1920", in *Western Medicine as Contested Knowledge*, ed. Andrew Cunningham and Bridie Andrews (Manchester and New York: Manchester University Press, 1997).

106 Minute by Thomas, 5 April 1852, *Madras Public Consultations*, 4 May 1852, no. 20, OIOC P/249/4, BL.

James Shaw, Superintendent of the Government Lying-in Hospital, who was pressing the Medical Board for accommodation for his apothecary despite having earlier had his request turned down. Key thought it impertinent of Shaw to question the Board's judgement by repeating the request; "Mr Shaw", he noted grimly, "deviated distinctly from the Board's injunctions, and it is my intention to put him right".[107] Scott found himself in further trouble with government when he explained that he had at first given women free money gifts when they left his hospital, in line with what he mistakenly thought to be the practice at the Government Lying-in Hospital, a practice Shaw emphatically denied ever having operated.[108] However, even with its government grant secure, Scott's hospital was forced to close in 1852 for want of funds.[109] The government was concerned enough about this to look into the possibilities of opening its own dispensary in Black Town, but nothing came of the idea, and in the end it was left to a local Indian charity, the Monegar Choultry, to open a Lying-in Hospital in Black Town in 1881. Apart from surfacing to ask for copies of his testimonials in 1859 Scott himself disappeared from the Madras medical scene and his hospital quickly faded from memory.[110]

Conclusions

The issue of maternity provision reflected the growing importance to state medical provision of accurate statistical returns. It was these that had alerted the Court of Directors both to the high rate of female suicide in Rajahmundry and South Arcot and to the discrep-

107 Key to Secretary, Medical Board, 21 October 1852, *Madras Public Consultations*,1 August 1854, no. 65, OIOC P/249/30, BL.

108 Third Annual Report to the Managing Committee of the Black Town Lying-in Hospital, 20 December 1851, *Madras Public Consultations*, 16 January 1852, no. 20, OIOC P/248/76, BL; Annual Return for Dr Scott's hospital for 1852 with commentary by Key, *Madras Public Consultations*, 4 May 1852, no. 18, OIOC P/249/4, BL; Shaw to Key, 17 February 1852, *Madras Public Consultations*, 4 May 1852, no. 18, OIOC P/249/4, BL; Shaw to Key, 17 February 1852, BL.

109 *Madras Public Consultations*, 26 October 1852, no. 26, OIOC P/249/7, BL.

110 *Madras Public Consultations*, 26 August 1859, no. 1, OIOC P/249/70, BL.

ancy between the intakes at the government and the Black Town Lying-in Hospitals. Eliott and Thomas claimed that the faults in Scott's record keeping had been exaggerated but it was clear that Scott had been caught out by the new statistic-driven efficiency drive in Indian administration. Statistical returns were a means by which the British authorities sought to define and control the Indian population, but they were also a means of controlling the subordinate servants of the state itself. Both hospitals ran into trouble with their statistical returns, but it was Scott who suffered more: he lacked both the resources and the mathematical skill to maintain the rate of statistical returns demanded by government. His note to Key accompanying his report for 1851 was disarmingly frank but was unlikely to impress a government which was increasingly measuring the efficiency of its agencies in purely statistical terms:

> The correct method of calculating the average daily number of sick was not understood by me, before the month of august, I am therefore unable to furnish with recovery [*sic.* "accuracy"?] any statement of the daily number of sick for the year.[111]

The Government of Madras clearly valued the midwifery work undertaken by its subordinates. The plight of Indian women in childbirth was accepted as the main reason for founding the government hospital, though the issue went wider than a humane concern to save life. The potential of maternity provision to spread Western medical science into the heart of the Indian community was quickly recognised, the more so when it was combined with a programme for training Indian women in Western midwifery; Scott was praised for setting this in motion and shortly after his hospital closed the government hospital finally got round to setting its own midwife training programme into operation. The proselytising potential of midwifery would soon be picked up by missionary societies, and the capacity of women's medicine to cement the ties between Britain and India would be an important theme within Dufferin Fund

[111] Black Town Hospital Report for 1851, *Madras Public Consultations*, 4 May 1852, no. 18, OIOC P/249/4, BL.

rhetoric towards the end of the century; in both cases Madras could claim to have anticipated them.

Madras was also quick to see the potential maternity work carried for bolstering its political prestige within India. The surgeons setting up the government hospital had cannily made use of the example of the Calcutta Lying-in Hospital to press their claim for government support: Madras should not deny itself what Calcutta had indulged in. The government hospital compared its first returns favourably against those of the Calcutta Hospital, and even at the height of the controversy surrounding Scott's hospital Eliott minuted that "the number of Confinements at both these institutions greatly exceeds the number of cases in the Lying-in Hospital connected with the Medical College in Calcutta".[112] The Government of Madras, or at least the civilian element within it, was setting in motion a process by which both Madras and Bombay would carve out separate identities for themselves as more liberal-minded, socially aware governments, compared with the rigidly hierarchical and remote Government of Bengal. In time the Madras Lying-in Hospital would become one of the presidency's best-known and most widely respected institutions, with an empire-wide reputation.

To benefit from the prestige of its Lying-in Hospitals, however, government had to sort out its own relationship with them. The government takeover of the original Lying-in Hospital seemed natural enough to the Government Medical Officers who established it; indeed, it is tempting to suspect that it was their desired outcome all along. However, this was not government's preferred course of action; nor could it take over any subsequent Lying-in Hospital that might be set up. Government in British India had a tendency to take over responsibility for the supervision of institutions while avoiding, where possible, the corresponding responsibility to pay for them, as the mission and Dufferin hospitals would later find out. Scott's hospital presented an intriguing, but to the military mind unacceptable, exception to the normal pattern in that it was a hospital government was helping to pay for but which was resistant to its supervision. The fact that the hospital closed so soon after its victory

[112] Minute by Eliott, 22 March 1852, BL.

over Key rather blunted any precedent it might otherwise have set, but the issue did show that the less rigidly hierarchical elements in government were prepared to give Scott's hospital a certain amount of leeway and benefit of the doubt in order to allow his important work to proceed unhindered. It was a flexibility of approach that would characterise the Madras Government's relations with its own Lying-in Hospital in the years that followed, and is a testament again to the importance the Madras Government was already giving in the 1840s to maternity provision.

4

The Mad in Their Midst: Accommodating Insanity and the Natal Government Asylum, 1880–1920

Julie Parle

The Ambiguity of Asylum

In December 1916, James Mkize, a *kholwa* (Christian) peasant farmer and preacher submitted a deposition to the Resident Magistrate of Umzimkulu, southern Natal, South Africa, detailing at some length the reasons why he believed that his brother, Bennie, was insane and should be legally detained in an asylum. James Mkize told the Magistrate: "My brother Bennie Mkize is of unsound mind. He first developed insanity while a youth."[1] He went on to list examples of Bennie's insanity, for instance, Bennie was given to interrupting the congregational services conducted by his brother. He was publicly committing 'intimate acts'. More worrying, he had also resorted to self-harm, deliberately chopping his right thumb off with an axe. James also recounted occasions of random, unprovoked violence. Once, Bennie had attacked his sister-in-law, Lena Mkize, "by hitting her on the face and shoulders with his fists and caused her to bleed through the nose and mouth." Only when James intervened did Bennie release Lena. James was then "smashed about the face." The children were becoming afraid of him; and his howling lasted through the night. In closing, James Mkize noted that Bennie's madness was becoming more frequent, more violent, and more burden-

[1] Attorney General to Registrar of Supreme Court, Minute RSCN (M), Mental Disorders Act, no. 38, 1916 (M) 8/16, Bennie Mkize of Rasmani's Location, Umzimkulu, 21 December 1916, Registrar Supreme Court (henceforth RSC) 1/27/1, Pietermaritzburg Archives Repository (henceforth PAR).

some to his family. He was also unambiguous in his demands that the state and its psychiatric institutions take responsibility for the restraint of this disturbed and dangerous family member

> we are now tired of him [Bennie] and ask the Government to look after him. I and my brothers are unable to support him whilst in hospital and cannot afford to look after our own families and himself. If Bennie will be allowed to be at large it will cause much trouble to one of the families of the above mentioned kraals. If he would be taken into custody at once it would be much better. . . . He used to be tied up for about a year before. We consider that his insanity and derangement increases as he gets older. Formerly he used to allow us to tie him up, now it is a great matter to get at him and have him tied up. The Government should surely relieve us of the responsibility we are in.[2]

The hospital to which James Mkize referred was the Natal Government Asylum (NGA) on the Town Hill at Pietermaritzburg, the capital of Natal. Between its construction in 1880 and 1927—when a second psychiatric facility, at the disused military barracks at Fort Napier, became available in the city, the NGA was the chief site of detainment in the region for those—white, African and Indian, men and women—who were certified as legally insane. Today, more than two hundred patients are still accommodated at what is now called Town Hill Hospital.

In 1868, Natal had been the first colony in what would later become South Africa to make explicit legal provision for the detention of lunatics. The NGA was also the region's first purpose built lunatic asylum. Although established at a time when the colonial state was most concerned with insanity and idiocy amongst white settlers, the NGA soon came to have a majority of patients who were black.[3]

[2] RSCN (M) 8/16, Bennie Mkize, 21 December 1916, RSC 1/27/1, PAR.

[3] Nineteenth- and early twentieth-century records from Natal use the then current terminology of "Europeans", "Natives", "Indians" and "Coloured" (called "Hottentot" in the early Natal Blue Book tables to refer to people of Khoisan origin, usually from the Cape Colony) and these terms have been replicated here. That they are now unacceptable is acknowledged, and their use is not intended to be offensive. This is also the case with such terms as "epileptic", "paralytic", "idiot", and so on. Here, I use "black" to refer to African, Indian and Coloured people. The Union Government and Cape

Institutional discrimination existed from the earliest days—in the form of accommodation in different, and inferior, wards (later separate buildings); inadequate food rations; restricted access to facilities and entertainments; as well as the greater exploitation of black asylum inmates as labour on the asylum estate. Nonetheless, the relatively early establishment of the NGA occurred at a time of liberal universalism, both in law and in psychiatry, and the NGA was never intended to be a whites-only institution (as was Valkenberg in the Cape) and the same professional and medical staff attended to black and white patients, on the same grounds, until racial segregation was temporarily achieved in the 1970s.[4]

By 1910, the NGA had the second highest asylum patient numbers in the new Union of South Africa. It was regarded as one of the country's pre-eminent mental hospitals and its Physician Superintendent—the charismatic and colonially well-connected James Hyslop—was widely recognised as one of the most respected 'mental specialists' in South Africa, and Pietermaritzburg remained a favoured posting for aspiring psychiatrists. In less than a decade, however, the Pietermaritzburg Mental Hospital (as the NGA was now being called, although the term asylum lingered for some time) had become a focal point for the anxieties of the city's white and Col-

records cited below sometimes use the term "Coloured" to include Africans. In Natal on the other hand by the 1920s "Coloured" referred to those who came from Natal and surrounding regions such as the Transkei and Eastern Cape and who were the descendants of intermarriages between persons of diverse origins including indigenous Africans, indentured or immigrant Indians, and "Europeans" (white, or both English settlers or Afrikaans-speaking peoples.)

[4] For histories of Valkenberg, see Sally Swartz, "The Black Insane in the Cape, 1891–1920", *Journal of Southern African Studies* 21, no. 3, 1995, 399–415; Sally Swartz, "Changing Diagnoses in Valkenberg Asylum, Cape Colony, 1891–1920: A Longitudinal View", *History of Psychiatry* 6, 1995, 431–51; Sally Swartz, "Colonialism and the Production of Psychiatric Knowledge in the Cape, 1891–1920" (PhD thesis, University of Cape Town, 1996); Shula Marks, "'Every Facility That Modern Science and Enlightened Humanity Have Devised': Race and Progress in a Colonial Hospital, Valkenberg Mental Asylum, Cape Colony, 1894–1910", in *Insanity, Institutions and Society, 1800–1914: A Social History of Madness in Comparative Perspective*, ed. J. Melling and B. Forsythe (London: Routledge, 1999), 268–91.

oured citizens, many of whom wished to have the hospital and its patients hidden from public view.

The accommodation of insanity thus has, in terms of the history of Western psychiatry in southern Africa, a relatively long history in Natal and one of my aims in this chapter is to sketch out a narrative of the history of the first, foundational decades of the NGA. Within this there are, however, indications of other ways in which such a history can be allied to the histories of Western medicine and hospitals beyond the West. There are at least three overlapping narratives and meanings to the term "accommodating insanity" reflected in what follows. The first concern is to chart what was often an ambivalent relationship between the state, the NGA and its patients and staff, and the city and the citizens of Pietermaritzburg in the decades between the late 1860s and 1920.

If asylums have long been regarded as ambiguous institutions, simultaneously sites of civic pride and of potential peril, in the context of South Africa in the early twentieth century, it is not surprising that it was the presence of a significant number of African insane, as well as black hospital staff, who were identified as posing a threat to the white rate-paying residents of Town Hill. As Africans, they were regarded as having only temporary rights to be in the city, and as black mental patients living in the midst of settler suburbs, they were seen to represent an even greater threat. Historians have also argued that asylums were profoundly foreign institutions for both the indigenous peoples of southern Africa and immigrant indentured workers from India, whose numbers equalled or exceeded those of settlers on the early 1900s. Much of the literature on the care of insane Africans emphasises the rupture with pre-colonial indigenous practices that incarceration in such an institution represented. Robert Edgar and Hilary Sapire, for example, write of "a major contrast between African healing cultures, with their emphasis on collective, social responses to afflictions and those of Western psychiatry [with] the absence in the former, of traditions of separating the deranged and disruptive from their communities." They quote the Reverend Henri Phillipe Junod's observations on Tsonga society, in which he claimed that segregation of lunatics from society was "unknown" and that "only in the most extreme instances, when dangerous madness seized a person, was physical restrain and forcible restraint adopted."[5]

Most recently, this stance has been underscored by Harriet Deacon, who writing of the Robben Island Lunatic Asylum from the mid-nineteenth century to 1910 comments: "How and why 'lunatics' entered mental institutions is related closely to the social function of the institution and the class, race or gender specific meanings attached to insanity." She goes on to detail the social profile of that Asylum which was, usually, mostly male; "disproportionately single"; and aged largely between twenty and sixty. The Robben Island Lunatic Asylum patient population was also, except for a short period in the 1860s and 1870s, predominantly African. Deacon attributes this in part to "the legal emphasis on dangerousness as a criterion (more often applied to men) for admission to scarce asylum beds and the way in which asylums were used by the state to empty gaols of disruptive criminals (who were predominantly men)".[6]

She goes on to explain that while

> white patients were overrepresented in asylum admissions compared to the general population [this] was explained at the time by racist theories that represented the white brain as more evolved and civilised, and therefore more susceptible to, and requiring more protection from, insanity than the black brain. . . . White insanity was feared within the colonial order because it denoted degeneration and threatened hereditary insanity. Black insanity was feared mainly in its contact with white communities—potentially disrupting employment relations or breaking the taboo in sexual contact with white women.[7]

Deacon and others thus emphasise the role of the colonial state and its medico-psychiatric practitioners in identifying and incarcerating the black insane in colonial South Africa, highlighting the

[5] Robert R. Edgar and Hilary Sapire, *African Apocalypse: The Story of Nontetha Nkwenkwe; A Twentieth-Century South African Prophet* (Johannesburg: Witwatersrand University Press, 2000), 45–46.

[6] H. Deacon, "Insanity, Institutions and Society: The Case of the Robben Island Lunatic Asylum, 1846–1910" in *The Confinement of the Insane: International Perspectives, 1800–1965*, ed. R. Porter and D. Wright (Cambridge: Cambridge University Press, 2003), 51.

[7] Deacon, "Insanity, Institutions and Society ", 52.

path to the asylum via the criminal justice system, transgressions of propriety in urban areas, and distance from "community networks of assistance":

> The black insane sequestered in relatively independent or isolated communities were thus not a major concern of the colonial state. African and Khoisan communities continued to use indigenous healing methods and to resist western medical treatment systems for mental illness well into the twentieth century.[8]

There is significant resonance with this picture in Natal, too. Nonetheless, and in a second concern of this chapter, I wish to argue that the NGA is of significance in the history of the management of madness both *of* and *by* blacks as well as whites in this region. The NGA should not be regarded simply as a "Western" institution, one that was imported and imposed on a passive African population for the purposes of state-sponsored social control. Rather, and as the deposition by James Mkize clearly indicates, by the early twentieth century, Western psychiatry and its institutions had become an option—one amongst many, to be sure—that could be utilised by African families and communities in their own quest for a means of controlling, if not curing, the mad in their own midst. After all, and as Megan Vaughan has commented: "Far from being destroyed by the joint assault of colonialism and biomedicine [African healing systems] tended rather to absorb and internalise, to 'indigenise', those elements of biomedical practice which seemed most effective and most impressive."[9] While her insight has been applied to practices employed by *izangoma* (diviners) or *izinyanga* (herbalists), such as injections, and diagnoses, such as hysteria, it has seldom been extended to include the role of Africans in initiating the process of committal of the deranged to a Western asylum.

There is yet another strand which I wish to point to, but it unfortunately cannot be developed here in any great depth. This involves a further play on the word "accommodating" in the title of the chapter: that is the outlining of the ways in which certain states

[8] Ibid.

[9] Megan Vaughan, *Curing Their Ills: Colonial Power and African Illness* (Stanford: California University Press, 1991), 24.

of mind came, in the decades before 1920, to be gradually accepted as being more appropriately within the realm of psychiatrists and their institutions than matters for law courts. In Natal and Zululand, such acceptance occurred at different rates and different times for whites and for Africans and for Indians. While the most striking example of this was perhaps colonial attitudes towards those settlers who were alcoholics or who attempted suicide, the story, in as much as we know it today, of James and Bennie Mkize serves as just one powerful example of how both medicine and hospitals beyond the West were the subjects of shifting understandings of their place, power, and promise.

From "that miserable place" to a "Model Asylum for the Insane": Accommodating Insanity in Colonial Natal

At no time in the history of southern Africa, or anywhere else, have the majority of those who suffer from mental illness been accommodated in formal institutions such as hospitals, clinics or asylums. [10] From the 1860s onwards, however, the colonial state in Natal began to assume responsibility for the definition of and provision of facilities for those it designated "lunatics". This followed imperial promptings by the Colonial Office in London, which was becoming increasingly concerned with the reform of hospitals and lunatic asylums throughout the empire. [11] In 1864, Secretary of State for the Colonies, Edward Cardwell, sent a Circular Despatch to the Governors of the Colonies referring to a request he had sent out the previous year requiring answers to one series of interrogations respecting public hospitals, and to another respecting Lunatic Asylums. In his despatch he commented:

[10] For the limits to the influence of colonial psychiatry, and the variety of other strategies for managing madness and for seeking "mental health" in Natal and Zululand in this period and beyond, see Julie Parle, *States of Mind: Searching for Mental Health in Natal and Zululand, 1868–1918* (Pietermaritzburg: University of KwaZulu-Natal Press, 2007).

[11] Edmund H. Burrows, *A History of Medicine in South Africa up to the End of the Nineteenth Century* (Cape Town: A. A. Balkema, 1958), 216.

> I regret to find that, generally speaking, the state of these Institutions in the Colonies, though not perhaps worse than in England at a former period, is yet widely and deplorably different from what would be now considered in this country to be consistent with the humane objects they are designed to promote; whilst in some cases, though not I trust, in very many, the state of Colonial Hospitals and Lunatic Asylums would seem to be such as can hardly be deemed to be consistent with humanity itself.[12]

The despatch went on to outline how the majority of hospitals and asylums in Britain had their origins in the "bounty and philanthropy of private persons" but that in the colonies the responsibility for establishing and maintaining such institutions would have to be "founded and supported from public funds" being "dependent for their well-being on the Executive and Legislative Authorities."[13] Cardwell closed by asking for further information on the progress that had been made in the provision of public hospitals and lunatic asylums, statements on what was still required, and by saying that he was "confident that in the interests of humanity the exposition of the subject thus afforded will command, not only your own serious attention, but also, if necessary, that of the Legislature."[14]

In response to this request, Lieutenant Governor Scott had been able to supply information on the recently completed Grey's Hospital in Pietermaritzburg, but had nothing to say about institutions for lunatics in the Colony, for there were none. Lunatics were detained either at the city's gaol, or—for those of melancholic rather than murderous disposition—at Grey's Hospital. Four years after Cardwell's despatch, in 1868, the government of the Colony of Natal, by now headed by Lieutenant Governor Robert W. Keate, passed southern Africa's first legislation that formalised the detention of persons "dangerously insane" or "of unsound mind".[15]

[12] Circular Despatch from Secretary of State for the Colonies, 6 April 1864, Government House (henceforth GH) 359, PAR.

[13] Circular Despatch from Secretary of State, 6 April 1864, GH359, PAR.

[14] Ibid.

[15] Natal Custody of Lunatics Law 1 of 1868, "To make provision for the safe custody of persons dangerously insane, and for the care and custody of persons of unsound mind". In the Cape, the legal basis for the detention of

Before his arrival in Natal, Keate had been the Governor of Trinidad. From there he too had replied to the Despatch of 1863, and in May 1864, on the day before his departure to take up his new appointment in Natal, he had written to Cardwell about the Trinidad Lunatic Asylum in which he had "evidently taken much interest."[16] Keate's report had represented the asylum there as the exemplar of mid-nineteenth century enlightened psychiatric thinking and practice, using no mechanical restraints, but instead resorting occasionally to the seclusion of patients in rooms—padded or otherwise—as the only "discipline resorted to." Patients were kept occupied and amused in "household services, washing, needlework, working at trades, gardening, reading and writing, various games, music and dancing."[17]

In Natal, even for the white insane, these luxuries were probably unknown until the opening of the NGA in 1880. Throughout the 1860s and 1870s lunatics, dangerous or otherwise, continued to be housed as they had before, at Grey's or in the gaol, or at home, or in a series of makeshift asylums where the accommodation was basic, cramped and custodial. The inadequacy of such measures for managing the mad was becoming increasingly evident, however, and it is not coincidental that the early lunacy law in Natal was passed at a time when economic depression had made poverty among white settlers publicly visible for the first time. During "the dismal sixties", more particularly between 1865 and 1871, Natal experienced a sharp economic setback accompanied by many bankruptcies, widespread unemployment and destitution, especially acute in the urban areas.[18] For the first time, the existence of settler poverty and the colony's lack of welfare provisions became glaringly obvious. Grey's Hospital became, so the Town Council frequently complained, effectively a poor house, taking in the elderly, the indigent, the disso-

lunatics was questionable until the passage of the Cape Lunacy Act 20 of 1879, which was a very close copy of the Natal 1868 Act.

16 Edward Cardwell, Secretary of State for the Colonies, to Governor Keate, 1 July 1864, *Despatch* 45, GH 359, 105, PAR.

17 Ibid.

18 Julie Parle, "The Impact of the Depression upon Pietermaritzburg During the 1860s" (M. A. thesis, University of Natal, Pietermaritzburg, 1988).

lute, and the demented. In 1866 the Town Council drew attention to the number of people, who were not necessarily "proper subjects for admission" to Grey's: These included ". . . the insane —in some instances mild cases—where proper care and kind treatment might produce speedy recovery; yet it is to be regretted that no satisfactory provision has been made to meet their cases".[19]

According to a historian of medicine in South Africa in the nineteenth century, Edmund Burrows, in the following year, 1867, Keate was moved to appeal to the Cape to admit Natal's lunatics to the Robben Island Asylum.[20] When this was refused, "the Natal Government decided to erect a temporary lunatic asylum at the Pietermaritzburg gaol which was already in use when Law no. 1 of 1868 made provision for the custody of lunatics within the Colony."[21] The conditions for the care and even custody of the mentally ill were woefully inadequate: it was here, for instance, that on the night of 29 October 1876 the quixotic Thomas Phipson, former Sheriff of Natal and outspoken critic of the colonial government, hanged himself from the window bars. The contagion of craziness and criminality that tainted Phipson's death, according to his biographer, "caused a sensation", but the shame of his madness, the meanness of the temporary asylum, and the stigma of suicide, meant "his family dropped a curtain of silence over the whole affair."[22] For many, too close association with madness was a terrifying prospect.

It was also under Keate's curatorship that Natal's first temporary lunatic asylum that was not attached to the gaol, or part of Grey's Hospital, was opened. This property, at 525 Longmarket Street, was purchased by the government at a cost of £1,112, and con-

[19] Mayor's Minute, 4 August 1866, Pietermaritzburg Corporation (henceforth PC) Town Council Minutes 1/1/3, PAR.

[20] Burrows, *History of Medicine in South Africa*, 218. Unfortunately, Burrows gives no sources for this claim beyond, "Personal Communication, Dr M. Minde". Max Minde was a psychiatrist who between the 1950s and 1970s wrote a series of articles for the *South African Medical Journal* on the early history of psychiatric services in South Africa.

[21] Burrows, *History of Medicine in South Africa*, 218.

[22] R. N. Currey, ed., *Letters and Other Writings of a Natal Sheriff, 1815–1876* (Cape Town: Oxford University Press, 1968), 22–23.

sisted of "about eight-and-a-half acres of ground and a house."[23] Somewhat ironically, this had once been the home of a prominent Natal Judge.[24] By the mid-1870s, this temporary asylum housed between thirty and forty inmates, but it seems doubtful that it was a significant improvement on the gaol: the Colonial Secretary, for instance, was said to have referred to it as "that miserable place", where mechanical restraint by wrist straps and iron handcuffs was still practised.[25]

As in the Cape, in Natal during this time the majority of persons detained or restrained as lunatics were men; and of these there were roughly equal numbers of Europeans and Africans, and very few Indians. African males formed the greater number of psychiatric patients in Natal from the late 1890s, but until then white men were the single largest category of legally-detained lunatics. Indeed, rather than being designed to nullify the growing numbers of African insane that were endangering the emerging capitalist colonial social order it was the presence of the mad in the midst of colonial society which was most troubling. This echoed the situation in nineteenth-century India, where as Waltraud Ernst has described, the European insane were regarded as potential transgressors of class and racial borders, and early asylum construction was largely in response to the need to prevent the undermining of the colonial image of fitness to rule.[26] Unlike India, however, as a settler colony, in Natal mad whites were not repatriated, and there was apparently a growing need for their acceptable accommodation. Instead, indentured Indians in Natal who

[23] Max Minde, "Early Psychiatry in Natal", *South African Medical Journal* 30, no. 12, 1956, 287.

[24] Report of the Commissioner of Mentally Disordered and Defective Persons, Union of South Africa U. G. 31-'20 (Cape Town: Government Printer, 1920), 25.

[25] Alan F. Hattersley, *A Camera on Old Natal* (Pietermaritzburg: Shooter and Shuter, 1960), 59.

[26] Waltraud Ernst, "The European Insane in British India, 1800–1858: A Case-study in Psychiatry and Colonial Rule", in *Imperial Medicine and Indigenous Societies*, ed. David Arnold (Manchester: Manchester University Press, 1988), 27–44. Ernst has subsequently elaborated this argument in several other articles and in her book, *Mad Tales from the Raj: The European Insane in British India, 1880–1858* (London: Routledge, 1991).

were found to be unsuitable for work by reason of insanity were returned to India to face an uncertain future there. This meant that the number of Indian inmates in the formal institutions of insanity in colonial Natal was kept artificially low.

The Natal Custody of Lunatics Act of 1868 was important in establishing a framework for the institutionalisation of insanity in colonial Natal and elsewhere in this region, for despite recognition of several important shortcomings in the Act (including by the emergent psychiatric profession in Natal) and with only a small modification in 1891, it remained in force until 1916, when it was superceded by the Union of South Africa's Mental Disorders Act. During the half-century that followed its enactment, the state and medicine would strengthen the alliance between them that had been first formally established in 1868, and the Natal government would honour the promptings of the imperial government to provide a lunatic asylum that, in avowed intent at least, was "consistent with the humane objects" that such institutions were, by the mid-nineteenth century, "designed to promote."[27]

It took recovery from economic depression and an eventual return of prosperity, almost a decade after the passage of the "Lunacy Act", before the Colonial Secretary was, in 1877, finally able to authorise the expenditure of £20,000 for the construction of a new lunatic asylum on the Town Hill, then on the outskirts of Pietermaritzburg. He had been nagging the colony's Civil Engineer for at least a year to put forward building plans and estimates. When these were finally delivered, there were three alternatives: "For No. 1—£20,000, For Nos. 2 and 3, £15,000 each. Each of these would accommodate about 100 patients."[28] Lieutenant Governor Bulwer opted for No. 1, which he deemed to be "the latest and most approved design."[29] In 1878 actual construction began: it was this

[27] Circular Despatch from Secretary of State for the Colonies, 6 April 1864, GH 359, PAR.

[28] Civil Engineer for the Colony to Colonial Secretary, 18 July 1876, Colonial Secretary's Office (henceforth CSO) 539, 1876/96, New Lunatic Asylum, PAR.

[29] G. Fouché, "Mental Health in Colonial Pietermaritzburg", in *Pietermaritzburg: A New History of an African City*, ed. J. P. C. Laband and R. Haswell

building which, though considerably expanded and reconstructed over the following decades, formed the nucleus of the Natal Government Asylum. District surgeons for the City, Charles Gordon and Charles Ward were optimistic that with the appointment of a permanent resident medical officer and a "new system of superintendence" there could be no reason why it "should not become, in every respect, a Model Asylum for the Insane".[30] This "New Asylum" was formally opened in February 1880: it housed just under sixty patients.

The location of the NGA on the Town Hill had not been the first choice of the Pietermaritzburg Town Council, but was the result of a compromise it had been forced to make in order to accommodate the objections of some of the city's citizens. For, despite the commitment of the imperial and the colonial governments to the provision of lunatic asylums, the people of the city of Pietermaritzburg soon expressed mixed feelings about the permanent presence of madmen in the borough. An early proposal, made in 1865, had been for the public asylum "in extent not more than ten acres" to be situated near the base of the garrison at Fort Napier, on land where the railway station (which has subsequently become famous for its association with Gandhi) stands today.[31] Nothing came of the matter until 1873, when, this time, the government asked for 100 acres. This proposal met, however, with resistance from a significant number of white burgesses, and 115 petitioners persuaded the Town Council to withdraw its offer to donate any land within the city. The Council bowed to the pressure, and decided to offer the state 50 acres of land "provided that it be not within 1 mile of the City, and does not abut on any of the main roads."[32] Later that year, a site of fifty acres on the Town Hill, then a mile and more to the west of the town, was mooted and eagerly accepted by the Council.

(Pietermaritzburg: University of Natal Press and Shooter and Shuter, 1988), 186.

30 Natal Blue Book (henceforth NBB) 1879, Lunatic Asylum Return.

31 Minutes, Town Council Meeting, 8 March 1865, Pietermaritzburg Corporation (PC) 3/PMB 1/1/3, 1031, PAR.

32 Minutes, Town Council Meeting, 14 March 1873, PC 3/PMB 1/1/4, 802, PAR.

A temporary asylum was established here, marking the beginning of a permanent accommodation of the legally-defined mentally ill on the hill overlooking the city.

The NGA did not have an especially auspicious beginning. The site allocated on the Town Hill was, at the time, largely barren and there was a single well, which provided sufficient water for cooking and drinking purposes only. Water for laundry and bathing had to be carried in buckets from a stream about 350 yards away. Sewage was received into wooden buckets, which were emptied daily in a trench sunk for the purpose in the grounds. Light was supplied by oil lamps.[33] The NGA's first Physician Superintendent, James Hyslop, a newly-minted twenty-six year old, fresh from graduating from Edinburgh University and a three-year stint "specialising in mental diseases at Berlin, Vienna, and Munich"[34] was later recorded as being so "much disappointed with the primitive arrangements that he seriously considered the advisability of resigning and returning to Scotland." The design of the asylum buildings did not impress him either.[35]

Nor did he find the colonial government willing to lay out further funds: without official support, he obtained "a few barrows and a few spades and set to work laying out the grounds and tree planting. In 1883 over 2,000 trees were planted and a start made with road making."[36] Over the next several decades Hyslop oversaw the expansion of the buildings, which became more imposing, combining nineteenth-century thinking about asylum construction with the especially aesthetically pleasing Victorian salmon-pink brick architecture for which Pietermaritzburg became well known.

Originally intended to accommodate a hundred patients, the NGA was always filled to capacity, often beyond. In 1887, there

[33] Report of the Commissioner of Mentally Disordered and Defective Persons, U. G. 31-'20, Report of the Commissioner of Mentally Disordered and Defective Persons, 25.

[34] "Obituary: James Hyslop", *South African Journal of Science* 14, 1917–1918, 312–14.

[35] U.G. 31-'20, Report of the Commissioner of Mentally Disordered and Defective Persons, 25.

[36] Ibid.

were 112 patients. Ten years later, there were 263 patients; and in 1909, 589.[37] Hyslop and his successors constantly commented upon the "overcrowding" that was a "more or less prevalent condition." Some temporary wards were constructed out of wood and iron, at times patients slept in the corridors, and several houses on properties adjoining the asylum estate were purchased, both for private patients and for staff. It was, however, a point of pride for Hyslop, that no one was turned away, provided they were accompanied by the correct documentation.

As the asylum facilities were expanded, they increasingly reflected the social stratifications of late-colonial Natal. From the beginning, white and black patients were accommodated in different wards or "quarters"; later, in separate buildings. In 1891, the imposing and attractive Main Building—which still today acts as the most prominent public face of the hospital—was completed. The front part of the building was "occupied by Europeans".[38] At the beginning of the next decade, the original kitchen was replaced; a "general bathroom" and laundry were built, and a drawing room, recreation rooms and two new dining rooms—one being for private patients—were added.

Men and women were accommodated in separate wards and wings, but there was no strict segregation of the sexes as appears to have been the case at some other asylums. Indeed, men and women were encouraged to mix, sharing the dining rooms, recreation facilities, and at the weekly dances.[39] To what extent, if any, black patients were permitted to use the private or recreation facilities, we do not know, but it seems unlikely. African and Indian patients did

[37] I have discussed the social profile of the NGA patients in detail in Chapter 2 of *States of Mind: Searching for Mental Health in Natal and Zululand, 1868–1918*, and an analysis of the asylum patient statistics was published in Julie Parle, "The Fools on the Hill: The Natal Government Asylum and the Institutionalisation of Insanity in Colonial Natal", *Journal of Natal and Zulu History* 19, 1999–2001, 1–39.

[38] U.G. 31-'20, Report of the Commissioner of Mentally Disordered and Defective Persons, 26.

[39] SC. 14- '13, Report of the Select Committee on Treatment of Lunatics, May 1913 (Cape Town: Cape Times Limited, Government Printers, 1913), 54. Evidence of Dr J. Hyslop, 16 April 1913.

not sleep in beds, but on mattresses on the floor.[40] Dietary provisions were less varied, and less nutritious, than those received by white patients, more of whom in any case were able to supplement their hospital food with items bought or brought by visiting friends or relatives.

In 1904, Hyslop commented on the building then underway—"the Male side being completely occupied at the end of 1905 and the Female side in 1906"[41]—to provide "new quarters for the Native and Indian patients". He explained that although the construction of separate amenities appeared to be costly in terms of the duplication of facilities, in fact, through economies achieved by the deployment of black patients on the estate grounds (which now produced vegetables, milk and eggs, and kept cattle and pigs, as well as having a quarry) this arrangement would ultimately be a beneficial one. For white patients, the assumption was that minimising contact with black patients was in and of itself conducive to their better state of mind.[42]

At the same time, the number of private patients was increasing. At the end of 1904, Hyslop reported that there were seventy "European private patients, nineteen of whom were paid for at rates varying from £104 to £200 per annum." He added that this was a "very high proportion", especially of the white women patients at the NGA, of whom just over 50 per cent were privately paid for, while this was the case for only 19 per cent of the men.[43]

When building of the NGA first began in the late 1870s, the site of 50 acres on the Town Hill was somewhat remote from the city, though its elevated position on a bare hill made it visible for some miles around. Until the extension of the railway up the Town Hill in the early twentieth century, many of the staffs travelled to and from town on horseback and, later, by rickshaw. Hyslop's merging of his passion for horticulture and the regimes of moral management, es-

[40] Select Committee on Treatment of Lunatics, 1913. Evidence of Dr J. Hyslop, 16 April 1913.

[41] U.G. 31-'20, Report of the Commissioner of Mentally Disordered and Defective Persons, 26.

[42] Report of the Medical Superintendent, NBB 1904, NGA.

[43] Ibid.

pecially purposeful work by patients meant that, by the 1890s, the grounds were well planted with trees and shrubs. All patients were encouraged to become involved in the gardens and fieldwork or in the laundry on the asylum farm or at the quarry. Hyslop once remarked that "You might as well deprive the inmates of the institution [asylum] of medicine as deprive them of work, and the most suitable work for most is on the land. I regard useful employment for inmates of an asylum as quite as important as medicine."[44]

By the early twentieth century, the asylum grounds had come to represent a country estate, both reassuring and desirable for a city that sought to establish its colonial credentials. The opening of the Main Building in 1891 added substantially to the image of the NGA as a monument to the civilising influence of British culture and bourgeois values. Moreover, as we have noted, the racial geography of the estate soon reflected that of the city and the country in which it was rooted.

In the decades that bracketed the turn of the twentieth century, the NGA was often referred to in approving terms. No doubt Hyslop's character, his deep involvement in the colonial military, the town's civic affairs and social life, helped to alleviate any elite suspicions of the institution he so dominated. From 1887, for instance, comes the following comment:

> The Lunatic Asylum at Pietermaritzburg, to which insane persons are sent from all parts of the Colony, is a fine, brick building situated on a hill about one mile north-west of the city, in well-kept grounds, 50 acres in extent, commanding a beautiful view of the city and its suburbs. Female patients are housed in a separate block. . . . We carefully inspected all the arrangements of the institution, and we now record, with great satisfaction, that under the care of Dr. Hyslop, who assumed charge in 1882, the comfort and welfare of the inflicted inmates are sought to be secured by all means which ability and experience can suggest.[45]

[44] Select Committee on Treatment of Lunatics, 1913, 42. Evidence of Dr J. Hyslop, 16 April 1913.

[45] Report of the Commission appointed to inquire into and report upon the Indian Immigration Laws and Regulations of the Colony, and on the general condition of the Indian population of Natal, Chapter XXVIII, 59,

In 1906, the glossy publication, *Twentieth Century Impressions of Natal*, devoted some space to both the NGA and to Hyslop, and expressed similarly approving sentiments. The tributes paid to Hyslop after his death in 1917 also made frequent mention of the manner in which the asylum grounds added to the aesthetic and architectural appeal and prestige of the city. So long as the asylum remained on the outskirts of the city, madness was segregated and domesticated. When the city encircled the asylum, however, the mad in the midst were once more to be feared.

"The Night Long Song of a Hundred Mad Natives": The Mad in the Midst of Pietermaritzburg, 1910–1920

By 1910, Natal had the "highest ratio of white [mental] patients to general population" in the Union of South Africa.[46] Hyslop attributed this to the smooth, if not to say lax, operation of the 1868 Custody of Lunatics Act, and not to any greater incidence of insanity in Natal and Zululand. While the growing numbers of private patients would seem to indicate that the asylum was gaining in respectability as a place to which mentally ill whites could be sent, this did not necessarily mean the stigma and shame of having an insane relative had disappeared. Indeed, testifying before a Parliamentary Select Committee on the Treatment of Lunacy in 1913, Hyslop emphasised that "people"—meaning whites—"are very averse to sending their relatives to an asylum . . . it is regarded as a sort of disgrace to have relations in an asylum."[47] Perhaps more surprisingly, however, he went on to say "but I fancy the natives are not at all averse to sending theirs and that they take full advantage of the opportunity of getting rid of the troublesome relatives in this way. I have noticed

Government Notice no. 430, 1887, Natal Government Gazette, no. 2262, 20 September 1887.

[46] Memorandum from Dr J. T. Dunston and Mr P. Eagle to Acting Secretary for the Interior, 22 December 1912, 8, Public Health: Extension of Lunatic and Leper Asylums, Prime Minister's Office (henceforth PMO) 1/1/322 184/2/1913, National Archieves Repository, Pretoria (henceforth NAR).

[47] Select Committee, 1913, 52–53. Evidence of Dr J. Hyslop, 16 April 1913.

more especially of late cases are being sent to the asylum which at one time would not have been sent."[48]

This is an intriguing statement. A dearth of extant patient records—especially those of African and Indian patients—unfortunately makes it difficult to gauge with accuracy the extent of family involvement in initiating asylum committals. Nonetheless, snippets of documentary evidence indicate that some African families were beginning to regard the asylum as the appropriate place where those of unsound or disturbed states of mind could and should be sent. The family of Bennie Mkize were not alone: in 1913, to take just one example, Johannes Mhlongo, a plantation worker from the Natal Midlands, was "consigned to the Asylum by the Magistrate of the Lions River Division at the express request of his relatives who were living in considerable fear of him."[49] The threat of violence was uppermost in this appeal, but who was most at danger is not specified.

If African families and communities were beginning to turn to Western psychiatric institutions for their own protection, from the early twentieth century, dangerousness—to oneself and not necessarily to others—became a common reason for the committal of white patients to the NGA: of the 251 European admissions recorded between 1904 and 1908, more than forty persons were identified as being "suicidal". Many of these were admitted as private patients.[50] Along with alcoholism, which was coming to be spoken of as a "disease" rather than a mere moral failing, attitudes towards suicide, for upper-class whites at least, were by this time beginning to undergo a shift towards a more sympathetic understanding.[51] For several more decades, however, Africans or Indians who attempted or threatened self-destruction were more likely to be gaoled or fined

[48] Select Committee, 1913, 52–53. Evidence of Dr J. Hyslop, 16 April 1913.

[49] John A. Lidgett to Medical Superintendent, NGA, Maritzburg, Accession Papers of John Lidgett, Letter Book, October 1911 to February 1914, p. 908 (uncatalogued), 9 January 1913, PAR.

[50] Patient Case-book XI, NGA (European). This is a conservative estimate as I have not included those who were said to be "probably suicidal".

[51] L. R. Anderson, "Society, Economy and Criminal Activity in Colonial Natal, 1860–1893" (PhD thesis, University of Natal, Durban, 1993), 282.

than regarded as mentally frail. Nonetheless, in the early decades of the twentieth century, for some people, in some states of mind, the NGA now came to represent a less shameful alternative to incarceration. Particularly in cases where the deranged could afford private quarters or personal nurses, the stigma of suicidal behaviour began to lessen, or at least began to be regarded as more appropriately the domain of the doctor than of the magistrate.

More patients meant an even greater strain on the existing facilities of the NGA and a need for more extensive buildings and grounds. In 1909, another 36 acres of ground had been acquired for the asylum, and in 1910 building began on new housing for both paying patients and the white male staff. This coincided with a new phase of thinking about both psychiatric practice and asylum construction. In tandem with international trends, in South Africa, doctors, psychiatrists and law-makers shifted away from fears about an apparently general increase of madness, to a concern with "mental hygiene" as a vital strand in the effort to preserve racial purity. In South Africa, these fears contributed, both directly and indirectly, to the elaboration and implementation of segregationist legislation.[52] Moreover, class distinctions amongst white South Africans acquired great salience, as poorer class whites—even more so if they were mental patients—were viewed with increasing suspicion along with the perceived threat they supposedly posed to the vitality and mental vigour of "the white race".

With some justification it might be said that, by 1920, South African psychiatry although still bearing the imprint of its nineteenth-century origins had taken on a different orientation, one that was more carefully directed in the interests of a state that was concerned to systematise the segregation of its citizens and its subjects. In this, the boundaries of race, gender and class continued to be potentially

52 The general South African picture—of the eugenics and mental hygiene movements, concerns about degeneration, "poor whiteism", the "feeble-minded" and racial purity—is well covered in Saul Dubow's *Scientific Racism in Modern South Africa* (Cambridge: Cambridge University Press, 1995). See also P. Rich, "Race, Science, and the Legitimization of White Supremacy in South Africa, 1902–1940", *The International Journal of African Historical Studies* 23, no. 4, 1990, 665–86.

threatened by those who exhibited insanity or idiocy, a concept and a category that was now more broadly understood to include the "feeble-minded". These concerns would come to be reflected in the spatial organisation of the asylum. The new thinking favoured several small "villas" on a larger hospital estate, with different "classes"—both in terms of social and psychiatric classifications—of patients accommodated according to their different requirements and to the state's willingness to provide facilities. This was an arrangement that Hyslop endorsed, believing that a move away from the "block system"[53] would increase the therapeutic value of the asylum, especially for the growing numbers of private patients.

In the years following the Union the South African asylum system was placed on a national footing and reorganised according to a scheme first articulated by a newer generation of psychiatrists. The most influential of these was Dr J. T. Dunston, the Union's Commissioner for Mentally Disordered and Defective Persons, whose office fell under the Department of the Interior.[54] Addressing the 1913 Select Committee, Dunston explained that the new "science" and "economy" of psychiatric classification required hospitals on a substantial scale. While an older generation of asylum superintendents—such as Hyslop at Pietermaritzburg and W. J. Dodds at the Cape—feared the creation of huge "monster asylums", Dunston recommended economies of scale both within individual asylum estates and across the new Union. This necessitated the enlargement of some asylums, and also the more efficient allocation of different categories of patients around the country. Accommodation of criminal lunatics would be centralised at a new facility at Bloemfontein in the Orange Free State; Fort Beaufort in the eastern Cape was for troublesome, but not criminal, black patients; Valkenberg and Grahamstown were to be for white patients only; and until it could be closed down (which was finally achieved in 1921) the Rob-

[53] Select Committee, 1913, 13. Evidence of Dr W. J. Dodds, 14 April 1913. This term was also used by the Chairman of the Select Committee to describe the "huge asylums" in America and elsewhere that had around 2,000 patients.

[54] From the 1920s, the Commissioner for Mental Hygiene.

ben Island Asylum housed black patients; only chronic, long-term patients were sent to Port Alfred.[55]

Underpinning Dunston's design was the revolutionary reordering of psychiatric classification under the system advocated by Emil Kraepelin. Key to the success of recovery from insanity was its early detection, classification, and the allocation of the patient to the correct facility. It was important that "Class 1" patients, the neurasthenics and those vulnerable from stress, worry or other enervating conditions, should never have to come into contact with "Class 2" patients, who were "troublesome" but, who after a time spent at a "special psychopathic hospital" or treated as out-patients, stood a reasonable chance of recovery. They, in turn, needed to be kept separated from patients categorised as "Class 3", who were described as being prone to mental disturbance because of "hereditary and constitutional weakness". The fourth and final "class"—the imbeciles, degenerates, the demented, those who suffered from secondary dementia following epilepsy, and from general paralysis of the insane—were, Dunston believed, "from the beginning incurable". Their prognosis, he said, was hopeless and all that could be hoped for was custodial care to prevent them from being dangerous to themselves and to others.[56] Ideally, for each of these categories of patient, different wards, even hospitals, were required.

Clearly, this suggested overhaul of South African psychiatry could clearly not be achieved overnight. An asylum arrangement that combined different elements of the overall scheme was therefore mooted. Based on what was termed the "villa" or "village" system, it had already begun to be implemented at a number of older asylums. At Pietermaritzburg, private patients (who were invariably white) were housed separately from non-fee paying white patients as well as African and Indian inmates. The distinction between patients was on the basis of race and class, not necessarily on clinical categories. Nonetheless, it was recognised that dangerous, manic and disruptive white

[55] Select Committee, 1913, 134. Evidence of Mr E. H. L. Gorges, 25 April 1913.

[56] Select Committee, 1913, 78. Evidence of Dr J. T. Dunston, 18 April 1913. See also Public Health, Extension of Lunatic and Leper Asylums 78, PMO 1/1/322 184/2/1913, NAR.

patients needed to be kept apart from those whites who were quiet and more melancholic. This led to a proliferation and multiplication of wards and buildings.

Dunston, and the Commissioners of Mental Hygiene who followed him, were primarily concerned with the prevention of the propagation of the white "mentally unfit", and had relatively little interest in those already detained as mental patients in the country's asylums. This meant that there was even less concern with the provision of treatment for black asylum inmates.[57] Instead, they were to provide a pool of unpaid labour for the upgrading of mental hospital grounds and buildings. Under this new, less liberal, regime, discriminatory practices that had been initiated under colonial governments became an even more entrenched component of asylum administration and practice.

By 1914, when Hyslop retired, the Pietermaritzburg Mental Hospital was no longer on the outer boundaries of the city. Its patient numbers had increased vastly more than the hundred originally envisaged. Keeping pace with the expanding asylum population with the attendant need for staff, room for recreation, as well as, increasingly, for land upon which to grow food for the patients, Hyslop had gradually expanded the grounds. By purchasing lands adjoining the original grant, by 1913, the asylum estate covered 140 acres. Following the Union an even more concerted effort was made to acquire a number of properties abutting the asylum lands. During the years of World War I this became more important even still as the country's mental hospitals were urged to become as self-sufficient as possible.

In 1915, in accordance with the recommendations put forward in the Select Committee Report, part of one of the older buildings at the Pietermaritzburg Mental Hospital was converted into an admission ward for the reception of "acute cases", and it was put under the charge of female nurses. This, Hyslop's successor, Dr Robert Sinclair Black would later comment, "was the first real attempt in Natal at Hospital treatment for the Mentally Disordered,

[57] See Swartz, "Colonialism and the Production of Psychiatric Knowledge", 31–32.

and though it was makeshift [*sic*] it was a very great advance and improvement on previous conditions."[58]

Work on further accommodation for black patients began in 1917, but was considerably delayed because of materials shortages experienced during the War. New quarters for black men were opened in 1918, though not before the "overcrowding" there had accounted for a high death toll following the Spanish Flu epidemic of that year.[59] In late 1918, work commenced on "New Female Native Quarters". This was finished in 1919. For these constructions, all the labour was performed by patients. While some white inmates did join the work gangs, it was mostly African and Indian patients who were engaged in the heavy work of tilling, digging, and building. Moreover, the accommodation given to black patients was of an inferior standard to that for whites. This had been firmly established in 1913 when the vast discrepancy between the officially calculated rates providing for the facilities of white and black mental patients was clearly stated: Secretary for the Interior, Edmond Gorges, had told the Select Committee, "[w]e have made provision on the basis of £250 a bed for Europeans and £75 a bed for natives."[60] Pressure for segregated facilities within the hospital complex came not only from administrators, state officials and psychiatrists, however, but also from the families of patients, including on occasion, some who would later be officially classified as being "not European". In 1920, for instance, Coloured voters in Pietermaritzburg petitioned the state for a greater measure of racial segregation within the mental hospital, asking that their relatives who were patients should not be housed with African inmates, and stating that they, the families, were "prepared to pay substantially towards the maintenance costs of these Coloured patients."[61]

[58] U. G. 31-'20, Report of the Commissioner of Mentally Disordered and Defective Persons, 25.

[59] Ibid., 27.

[60] Select Committee, 1913, 140. Evidence of Mr E. H. L. Gorges, 25 April 1913.

[61] Asylums: Coloured People at the Mental Hospital, Pmb, Accommodation, Mr Benjamin, 376 Greyling Street, Pietermaritzburg to Private Secretary, 4 May 1920, Department of the Treasury 4009 F21/53, NAR. The petitioner

All this meant for a sizeable community of people—patients, medical and nursing staff, attendants, gardeners and workmen—who were permanently resident at the Pietermaritzburg Mental Hospital. In 1910, there were 619 patients; in 1914, 643; and then, in the next four years, there came a large jump to 797, of whom only 355 were classified as "Europeans". In 1918, there were also more than 140 staff, many of whom were black. The ambivalence towards the asylum shown in the 1870s by the white citizens of Pietermaritzburg was now turning to antipathy, if not hostility. For not only had the asylum expanded far further than had originally been anticipated, it was also increasingly anomalous as an institution housing large numbers of blacks in the midst of what were now predominantly white suburbs.

Opposition to the asylum coincided with its expansion during the years of World War I. This was also a time when the city of Pietermaritzburg was characterised by growing numbers of African workers, Indian traders and artisans, and an expanding, though still relatively small, community of "Coloureds". Suburban settlements were also accelerating, and competition for the most economically favourable land was closely tied to racial politics.[62] These suburbs included the Town Hill, and the plans to extend the asylum ignited a flash of protest in which concerns about class, race and gender were given an extra edge by the prospect of the presence of the insane in the midst of a white residential area.

The first signs of organised protest came in November 1916, when some twenty-four petitioners, "and others", submitted a memorial to the Pietermaritzburg City Council in which they objected to an impending grant of a section of the town lands, at the back of

---

was told that accommodation for "Coloureds" would, in the future, be provided at Valkenberg.

62 Trevor Wills, "The Segregated City", in *Pietermaritzburg: A New History of an African City*, ed. J. P. C. Laband and R. Haswell (Pietermaritzburg: University of Natal Press and Shooter and Shuter, 1988), 39. Also T. Wills, "Segregation, Separation and Desegregation: Pietermaritzburg since 1910", in *Receded Tides of Empire: Aspects of the Economic and Social History of Natal and Zululand Since 1910*, ed. B. Guest and J. Sellers (Pietermaritzburg: University of Natal Press, 1994), 283–309.

the Mental Hospital. The Council, as it had done forty years before, bowed to the pressure of its rate-paying constituents, and passed a resolution refusing to enter into further negotiations on the matter with the government. Over the next few years, opposition to the extension to the hospital grounds became if anything more virulent and the demands for safeguards more specific. Furthermore, whereas the earlier objections had been to the asylum and its inmates in general, now the attempts to highlight the grievances of the residents became couched in overtly racialised terms that stressed the "dangerousness" that "mad Natives" posed to "innocent" and "peaceful" whites, especially women and children.

Further petitions in 1917 and 1918 spoke of "the strength of the opposition to the grant of land in the midst of a popular residential area to the Mental Hospital" and of their fears that the suburb would soon become "a total wreck".[63] They pointed out that the number of patients at the Mental Hospital had originally been "comparatively small" but that

> [w]ith the present growth with patients brought from other Provinces—the Cape and the Free State—the residents' disabilities and disadvantages had become very marked . . . the number of natives is on the increase and that it would be readily admitted that no one desired a Native Location in the neighbourhood. The residents were being saddled with a growing Native location in which the Natives are mad and while the night-long song of a 100 mad Natives is not too agreeable, the nuisance becomes far more than ten times as bad when the number is increased to 1,000. The same applies to the risk of escape.[64]

Combining white fears of black men making unprovoked sexual attacks on white women and popular stereotypes of mental patients as being dangerous, the head of a 1918 delegation, a Mr Bigby, told the Town Council that his deputation "had thought out certain conditions a) to secure protection and a sense of security for ladies and

63 Land for Natal Mental Hospital, Minutes of the Meeting of Finance and General Purposes Committee, 26 September 1918, at 2:30 p.m. 877/18. Grant of Land to Mental Hospital, 2767 4/78, Department of Health [Afrikaans Gesondheid] (henceforth GES), NAR.

64 Minutes of the Meeting of Finance and General Purposes Committee, 26 September 1918, GES, NAR.

children living or having occasion to use the road in the vicinity and b) to call a halt to the 'peaceful penetration' and so preserve the suburb as a residential area."[65] These conditions included a screen of trees and that "the Government shall erect and maintain in good repair a double fence along the whole of the boundaries", the outer fence to be constructed of wire and the inner, a "'Pale' unclimable [*sic*] steel fence." The two were to be "no less than 100 feet apart", and the belt of ornamental trees should be planted between them. Nor was there to be any new entrance to the Mental Hospital on the new grant of land, which was in any case only to be used for grazing purposes. Furthermore, no patients—unless "under strict observation" while engaged in agricultural labour—were to be allowed on the land. These patients would, by and large, have been African and Indian. Finally, the government was not to seek to acquire any further land for the hospital on the Howick Road or in the remaining lands that approached the city.[66] In November 1918, the Department of the Interior agreed to the conditions requested by the Deputation.[67]

The limits to any significant future expansion of the Mental Hospital in the midst of the city were thus established by 1918. In the next decade, a solution to the perennial overcrowding of patients that had characterised the asylum on the Town Hill almost since its inception in 1880 was sought by converting the former military barracks at Fort Napier into a mental hospital. The first group of patients were moved to this most unsatisfactory facility in 1928.[68]

Epilogue and Conclusions

The history of the accommodation of insanity in Pietermaritzburg is simultaneously one of expansion and of contraction. While between the mid-1870s and 1920, the material facilities for the institutional

65 Minutes of the Meeting of Finance and General Purposes Committee, 26 September 1918, GES, NAR.

66 Ibid.

67 Land for Natal Mental Hospital. Acting Secretary for the Interior to Secretary for Lands, 16 November 1918, 2767 4/78 GES, NAR.

68 See G. Fouché, "Mental Health in Colonial Pietermaritzburg", 188.

care of the mentally ill were enlarged, under the Union, and later, the Republic, of South Africa, psychiatric patients in Natal arguably received less concern than they had under the colonial state. Located at some distance from the political and economic hub of Rand, Natal's "mental services" and its psychiatrists no longer occupied the position of prestige enjoyed by and under James Hyslop. Even as some forms of derangement were becoming, albeit gradually, accepted as treatable, significant stigma remained attached to mental illness. Under great strain during the War years and after, facing escalating patient numbers, increasing bureaucratic burdens, and frugal finances, Hyslop's successors complained to state officials of overwork, official neglect, and extreme fatigue.

Since the late nineteenth century, the majority of patients accommodated at the Pietermaritzburg Mental Hospital were black—African, Indian and Coloured—and the overriding interest of the emerging national South African psychiatric profession and scientific practice lay in a concern for whites. Nonetheless, numbers at the Pietermaritzburg Mental Hospital continued to rise: by 1918, nearly eight hundred patients were accommodated, in a variety of different buildings, wards, and wings, on the Town Hill. Of these, there were 294 "Natives", 31 "Coloured" and 117 "Asiatics": "European" patients had long been in the minority.[69] In the absence of committal papers or patient records for the period before the implementation of the Mental Disorders Act of 1916, it is impossible to establish accurately the grounds on which patients, especially black patients, were admitted. The number of Indian patients at Pietermaritzburg had begun to escalate from the early 1900s. The reasons for this acceleration lie in both the dire economic circumstances experienced by Natal Indians at this time and, possibly, a gradual shift of attitude amongst Indians themselves towards Western psychiatry and medicine. Certainly, the constantly rising numbers of African inmates, as well as testimonies such as that by James Mkize, suggest that to see the asylum on the Town Hill simply as an alien institution that was imposed on subject peoples does not do justice

[69] U. G. '31 –20, Report of the Commissioner of Mentally Disordered and Defective Persons for the Union of South Africa, 32.

to questions of medical pluralism, African agency, or to the complex social history of Western medicine in contexts far from its genesis.

The continued accommodation of several hundred black patients, as well as black staff who worked at the asylum, had, by the years of World War I, aroused the resentment and animosity of a number of white Pietermaritzburg residents, who fused fear of the insane inmates, racial stereotypes, and avaricious interests in the, by now extensive and economically desirable, lands that the Mental Hospital occupied at the heart of the city. While the asylum had always been regarded with ambivalence, by 1918, the mad in the city's midst were regarded as a nuisance at best, and a danger, at worst.

Even after further expansion of the Pietermaritzburg Mental Hospital was halted, the city's ambivalent attitude towards the accommodation of the mad did not disappear. Indeed, in the 1960s, by which time most of the patients at Town Hill Hospital were white, the Pietermaritzburg City Council again bowed to pressure from local rate payers to approach the government to "release" the 305 acres that the hospital then occupied. Arguments put forward ostensibly prioritised the needs of the patients for more "modern" facilities, as well as the desire to run the city's two psychiatric hospitals on a more "efficient" basis.[70] In a submission made in Parliament on 20 September 1966, Mr Bill Sutton, the M. P. whose constituency included Town Hill, gave voice to the concerns of the white citizens of Pietermaritzburg that can be seen as continuing to reflect the same motivations that had prompted the petitioners of the 1870s and of 1918. Sutton asked whether it was the government's intention to move some of the African mental patients from the city since "both Town Hill and Fort Napier were now in the centre of Pietermaritzburg."[71] Racial segregation of psychiatric patients was not sufficient however, and he pointed out that Town Hill occupied prime city land, which could be developed for residential purposes. There is an irony in the insane of Natal and Zululand occupying land that came to be highly desired by the citizens of the city. There is perhaps another irony in that it was the *apartheid* Minister

[70] "Council Gets MP Support Over Hospital", *Natal Witness*, 18 June 1966.

[71] "Minister Rejects Town Hill Plea", *Natal Witness*, 21 September 1966.

of Health, Albert Hertzog, who rejected the request to close down Town Hill Hospital, saying that "The plea for the hospital to be moved resulted from 'glittering eyes on that ground.'"[72]

Today, Town Hill and Fort Napier continue to be regarded with some ambivalence by the citizens of Pietermaritzburg, and a series of recent tragedies and scandals involving patients has revived public concerns about the potential for abuse that exists in psychiatric hospitals.[73] Considerably reduced in extent from more than 300 acres of grounds that it occupied in the 1960s, Town Hill Hospital is now bounded by the "new" Grey's Hospital, an upmarket retirement complex, an exclusive hotel and restaurant—on the site of Hyslop's former residence—and a busy road that borders on a burgeoning commercial and light-industrial area. The two hundred or so patients who are still accommodated at Town Hill are thus both more in the midst of the city than ever before, and as removed from it as they were in the past.

72 "Minister Rejects Town Plea."

73 See, for example, "A Conspiracy of Silence: A Little Boy was Murdered at Fort Napier and No Official is Taking the Rap", *Natal Witness*, 13 February 1999; and "When Patients Come Last", *Natal Witness*, 13 April 2002.

5

Medicine Between Religious Worlds: The Mission Hospitals of South-East Tanzania During the Twentieth Century

Walter Bruchhausen

The difficulty or even impossibility of separating medicine from religion in African societies has always puzzled European observers, from participants of pre-colonial sea voyages until today's medical anthropologists.[1] However, the attempt to delimit a European category of 'medicine' was and probably had to be repeated by all endeavours to introduce European medicine to East Africa. In the case of mission medicine, where medicine and religion were more closely connected with each other than in secular colonial medicine, the relationship between the two caused considerable confusion and discussion on the European as well as on the African side. The hospital was for the mission, much more than for the colonial state with its emphasis on disease control, the main focus of medical work. For the majority of the rural African population the hospital, initially in the form of the mission hospital only, was the main place to encounter European medicine. This can be seen from the native terms for the new type of medicine from Europe. *Dawa ya hospitali* (hospital medicine), is—besides *dawa ya kizungu* (European medicine), and *dawa ya kisasa* (modern medicine)—one of the common Swahili names for what anthropologists call biomedicine i.e., the science-based type of health care dominating in industrialised

[1] Susan Reynolds Whyte, "Anthropological Approaches to African Misfortune: From Religion to Medicine", in *Culture, Experience, and Pluralism: Essays on African Ideas of Illness and Healing*, ed. Jacobson-Widding and David Westerlund (Uppsala: Acta Universitatis Upsaliensis, 1989), 289–301.

nations. The specific problems and chances of the mission hospital are thus very instructive in questions on the "Hospital Beyond the West".

My own research on past and present medical pluralism in south-east Tanzania [2] did not focus upon the hospital. It was devoted to all kinds of medical services from all sides—colonial and national governments, Christian missions and churches, Muslim and traditional African experts—in a particular region over the past hundred years. However, in the course of study the mission hospital was identified to be a major point of reference for traditional healers and for government health policy, too. In order to explain the specific relationship between other agents in health care and the mission hospital it is necessary to briefly describe the local population.

South-eastern Tanzania is peculiar for its recent combination of matrilineal peoples and a Muslim majority. The main ethnic groups are Mwera, Makua, Makonde and Yao. [3] The region of the Lukuledi valley and the adjacent Rondo and Makonde plateaux are densely populated compared to the surrounding areas, but did not develop any high condensation of political and economic power or larger settlements. Before colonial rule the local 'big men' had followers of different ethnic origin which prevented the formation of dynasties and made the German conquest in this region after 1889 rather a campaign against these 'big men' labelled as slave traders and rebels than against kingdoms or peoples as in other parts of the new protectorate German East Africa. [4] Therefore between the World Wars the British attempts to introduce "Indirect rule" in their new League of Nations' mandate Tanganyika Territory, i.e., modern administration based on local 'traditional' authorities, failed in this area com-

[2] This research was mainly done from 2000 to 2003 in a project generously funded by the German Volkswagen Stiftung, Az II/76050.

[3] For their general history and ethnography John A. R. Wembah-Rashid, *The Ethno-History of the Matrilineal Peoples of South-east Tanzania,* Acta Ethnologica et Linguistica 32, Series Africana 9 (Wien: Stiglmayr, 1975).

[4] Felicitas Becker, "Traders, 'Big Men' and Prophets: Political Continuity and Crisis in the Maji Maji Rebellion in South-east Tanzania", *Journal of African History* 45, 2004, 3–8.

pletely.[5] Only since the socialist policy of enforced villageisation in the 1970s the traditional scattered settling in small hamlets or single houses surrounded by the own plantations has been changed to villages of several thousand inhabitants. As the population had been already ethnically mixed before, these villages are always inhabited by members of more than just one ethnic group. The traditionally more independent position of women in these groups has been changed by conversion to Islam, with the Yao already since the late nineteenth century,[6] with the other groups mainly between the two World Wars. Thus confrontations in healing did not only develop along the boundaries of European vs African medical practices, but also between Christian, Islamic and various local religious affiliations and between patriarchal and matrilineal attribution of social roles.

The Missions Between Medicine and Religion

Two Christian missions in one region

For both the relevant missionary societies the mission stations in south-east Tanzania had not been the first attempt to start work in the interior of East Africa. The "Oxford and Cambridge Mission to Central Africa", later renamed "Universities' Mission to Central Africa" (UMCA), was initiated by David Livingstone's book and speeches in 1857, chose the region of Lake Nyasa, today the borderland between Malawi and Tanzania, as its original destination and tried to reach it via Portuguese East Africa up the river Shire.[7]

5 William Malcolm Hailey, *East Africa: Uganda, Kenya, Tanganyika*, Part I, *Native Administration in the British African Territories* (London: H.M. Stationary Office, 1950), 303.

6 Edward A. Alpers, "Towards a History of the Expansion of Islam in East Africa: The Matrilineal Peoples of the Southern Interior", in *The Historical Study of African Religion with Special Reference to East and Central Africa*, ed. Terence O. Ranger and Isaria Kimambo (London: Heinemann, 1972), 172–201.

7 Michael Gelfand, *Livingstone the Doctor, His Life and Travel: A Study in Medical History* (Oxford: Basil Blackwell, 1957), 124–219; for the general development of this mission society, Anne Elizabeth Mary Anderson-Morshead, *The History of the Universities' Mission to Central Africa, 1859–1909*, vol. 1 (London:

After hostilities and several deaths due to disease they withdrew to the British influenced island of Zanzibar with its ancient Muslim city. More than a decade later, with freed slaves from the interior on a different way to Lake Nyasa parallel to the Rovuma river, the Anglican missionaries founded a Christian village at Masasi, today south-eastern Tanzania, in 1876. Minor mission stations in Newala, Lulindi and other places followed later.

Twenty to thirty years later the German Benedictine Fathers, invited by a Roman Catholic member of the colonialist *Deutsch-Ostafrikanische Gesellschaft* (the German Chartered Company for East Africa), followed the Anglicans' pattern of first failed attempt in the interior, recovery in the city and second successful attempt to settle in the interior of today's south-east Tanzania.[8] The Benedictines started their first mission station near the coastal town Dar es Salaam in the Pugu Hills where soon the mission members were either killed, captured or expelled by the Arab-led uprising against the Germans in 1888. A new group of missionaries started again in the town of Dar es Salaam which soon became the capital of the new German protectorate. A few years later, during their second attempt to found Christian communities in the interior, they decided to stay in the well populated area near the Anglican settlement of Masasi. They had their main centre first in Lukuledi, due to lack of water later in Nyangao and finally, after the Maji Maji war, in Ndanda.

Both mission societies started their stations by arrangements with the local 'big men', as control of the south-eastern hinterland by the colonial power was only established after 1897.[9] In retribution, the 'big men's' families received favourable services in education and health care. Most of the first UMCA's African clergy belonged

---

Universities' Mission to Central Africa [henceforth UMCA],1909); George Herbert Wilson, *The History of the Universities' Mission to Central Africa* (London: UMCA, 1936).

[8] Frumentius Renner, "Die Benediktinermission in Ostafrika", in *Der fünfarmige Leuchter. Beiträge zum Werden und Wirken der Benediktinerkongregation von St Ottilien*, ed. Frumentius Renner (St Ottilien: EOS, 1992), 4: 126–34; Bernita Walter, *Sustained by God's Faithfullness: The Missionary Benedictine Sisters of Tutzing* (St Ottilien: EOS, 1992), 2: 13–118.

[9] Becker, "Traders, 'Big Men' and Prophets", 8.

to these families, and the local ruler, Sultan Hatia was visited by Benedictine sisters several times for several days at a time during his periods of illness.[10] Thus two missionary societies of different denominations and nationalities, but both with celibate missionaries and a similar catholic theology and liturgy, worked at a distance of just 20 miles of each other, among the same ethnic groups, under the administration of first the one's and then—after World War I—the other's nation. As the colonial central government was hardly present and the so-called "native administration" here was notoriously weak in influence and finances, the missions were the only obvious European representatives for many decades. This setting produced continuous rivalry between the two missions—and presents an ideal opportunity for the historian to make a comparative study. As other historians already did sound work on the UMCA's medical work my research was rather devoted to the Benedictines in order to allow such comparison. The comparison has to end in the 1960s as the two mission societies or churches went different ways in the process of nationalisation. The new national Anglican church handed its hospitals in Masasi, Newala and Lulindi over to the independent state, whereas the German and Swiss Benedictines, following the example of church hospitals in the public sector at home in Germany, kept the responsibility for Ndanda hospital and transferred the two other hospitals in Nyangao and Mnero to the Catholic bishop of Lindi.

Death toll and scepticism towards modern medicine

As Mike Jennings has shown for the UMCA[11] and could be confirmed with similar, even higher figures for the Benedictines,[12]

[10] Diary entries 2 January 1908 and 26/ 27 October 1910, Kongregationsarchiv St Ottilien (KAStO), Z.1.2.34 Chronik der Schwestern von (Lukuledi, Nyangao und) Ndanda, 1895–1917.

[11] Mike Jennings, "'This Mysterious and Intangible Enemy': Health and Disease Amongst the Early UMCA Missionaries, 1860–1918", *Social History of Medicine* 15, 2002, 65–87.

[12] Rochus Schroth, "Personalliste (Patres und Brüder) in der Ostafrikamission bis zum Ersten Weltkrieg", in *Der fünfarmige Leuchter. Beiträge zum Werden*

death and infirmity by disease was the major threat to the missionaries. Depending on effective health protection and care for themselves, however, not all of them did embrace modern medicine. Missionaries had several grounds for scepticism towards academic medicine and a certain preference of naturopathy. The secular and materialist tendencies of late nineteenth-century's academic medicine deeply disturbed the Christian clergy responsible for missionary activities.[13] Generally, German experts of missiology were more critical towards "Western materialism" than the British and Americans, as Marcia Wright noted.[14] It was something in the very nature of this kind of medicine that deterred medical laymen especially in Germany with its heavy romantic heritage in the ideas of health and healing. Many contemporary Germans not only in the colonies feared the severe side-effects of pharmaceuticals like *Antipyrine*. Preventable deaths were attributed to their use without or against medical advice.[15] The administration of such drugs as *Phenacetine* and Antipyrine was explicitly discouraged in the Latin Constitutions of the Missionary Benedictine Fathers, whereas the herbal by Father Sebastian Kneipp, the most famous contemporary naturopath and Bavarian Roman Catholic priest, was strongly recommended.[16] This precaution mainly concerned the unqualified use of pharmaceuticals by lay people. For some lethal diseases like dysentery, however, detailed written prescriptions circulated on the

---

und Wirken der Benediktinerkongregation von St Ottilien, ed. Frumentius Renner (St Ottilien: EOS, 1992), 2: 151–54; Walter, *Sustained by God's Faithfullness*, 337–44.

13 Wolfgang U. Eckart, *Medizin und Kolonialimperialismus. Deutschland, 1884–1945* (Paderborn: Schöningh, 1997), 92–93; Christoffer H. Grundmann, *Gesandt zu heilen! Aufkommen und Entwicklung der ärztlichen Mission im neunzehnten Jahrhundert* (Gütersloh: Verlagshaus Gerd Mohn, 1992), 124–25.

14 Marcia Wright, *German Missions in Tanganyika, 1891–1941: Lutherans and Moravians in the Southern Highlands* (Oxford: Clarendon Press, 1971), 3.

15 *Gouvernement* Dar es Saalam to Colonial Department Berlin, 28 February 1894, Bundesarchiv Berlin-Lichterfelde R 1001/854, 76.

16 *Constitutiones Congregationis Ottiliensis O. S .B. pro missionibus exteris cum appendice* (St Ottilien, 1897), 193–94.

use of strong drugs like morphine and ipecacuanha.[17] The preference for Father Kneipp's naturopathy also developed from regional and personal ties: Kneipp's residence Wörishofen was close to the Missionary Benedictines' home abbey St Ottilien and their superior general since 1896, Abbot Ildefons Schober, had served as a secretary to Kneipp when the first book *Meine Wasserkur* ("My Hydropathy"), published in 1887, had been written.[18] Until today, Missionary Benedictine Fathers of St Ottilien heavily rely on herbal medicine, promote it on TV and publish books on it.[19] Even in Tanzania today this preference is well known to the public, as some members of the order propagate the 'Uvemba pastilles', preparations containing a herbal antimalarial (from *Artemisia annua*) in a low dose, while the country's medical experts, also the only physician among the Benedictine Fathers, want to apply this substance *Artemisinine* only in a dosage sufficient to avoid resistance development.

Other reasons for sceptical distance to academic medicine were the increasing conflicts in Europe between professional medicine and other healing activities which often led to accusations against Father Kneipp and other clergymen practising naturopathy. Even the first superior of the Missionary Benedictine Sisters, Sr Katharina Scheins, had problems with the Bavarian police for "illicit practice of medicine".[20] The quarrels also concerned the training of missionaries in basic health care. Medical students refused to sit in the same courses with students of a protestant missionary institution in the university town of Tübingen.[21] The short medical training

[17] "Einiges über Dysenterie", hectograph copy, 24 June 1912, KAStO, folder Dar es Salaam 4, Regierung [Government].

[18] Frumentius Renner, "Vom Missionshaus Reichenbach zur Benediktiner-Kongregation von St Ottilien", in *Der fünfarmige Leuchter. Beiträge zum Werden und Wirken der Benediktinerkongregation von St Ottilien*, ed. Frumentius Renner (St Ottilien: EOS, 1992), 1: 253.

[19] Johannes Gottfried Mayer/Bernhard Uehleke/Kilian Saum, *Handbuch der Klosterheilkunde* (München: Zabert Sandmann, 2003).

[20] Renner, "Vom Missionshaus", 66.

[21] "Demonstration der Medizinstudierenden gegen die Zulassung von Missionszöglingen zu medizinischen Vorlesungen", *Münchner Medizinische Wochenschrift*, 1910, 335.

of missionaries gave rise to the accusation of quackery.[22] Yet the contemporary concern about quacks did not particularly impress the German mission societies. A German protestant mission even employed a mission doctor for East Africa who was without proper academic education and had been accused of quackery at home in Germany.[23] Where missionaries had been trained in basic medical skills by doctors, as in the Cologne Academy for Practical Medicine, the therapeutic methods taught usually comprised less dangerous therapies, among them one that was practised by the Africans, too: cupping.[24]

With the UMCA the attitude towards academic medicine was different as this mission society was an offspring of four British universities.[25] The mission's first expedition had been accompanied by four doctors, one of them, Dickinson, being a formal member of the mission society[26] and the others, Livingstone, Kirk and Meller, as well as the later lay superintendent Horace Waller, contributing to scientific medicine by their observations and publications about the "fevers".[27] The leading authority on tropical medicine, Patrick Manson, joined the UMCA's Medical Board in 1898.[28]

Despite such ideological differences between these two Roman Catholic and Anglican mission societies, the daily self-treatment of the missionaries seems to have been similarly arbitrary in both denominations. In the UMCA the physician and bishop John Edward

[22] Eckart, *Medizin und Kolonialimperialismus*, 108, ff 61.

[23] Ibid., 372–73.

[24] For example, Catholic missionaries according to Cölner [Cologne] Akademie für praktische Medizin, "Ankündigung eines medizinischen Kurses für Missionare" (Announcement of a medical course for missionaries), no. 3370, 5 September 1906, KAStO, folder Lindi 4.

[25] Besides Cambridge and Oxford later also Durham and Dublin.

[26] Wilson, *History of the Universities' Mission*, 14.

[27] Meller's articles in the *British Medical Journal* 1862 and *The Lancet* 1964 are reprinted as Appendices D and E in: Gelfand, *Livingstone the Doctor*, 304–21; Horace Waller, *Remarks on the Bilious Remittant Fever of East Africa: Its Treatment, and Precautions to Be Used in Dangerous Localities* (London: UMCA, 1873).

[28] Patrick Manson, Letter, 27 January 1898, Rhodes House Oxford (henceforth RHO), UMCA A3 Medical History and Reports, 1882–1934, 11.

Hine complained in 1904 about his missionaries' attribution of fancy health rules to an alleged "Dr Manson's advice", their irrational use of "dangerous poisons like Antipyrine", Quinine and Phenacetine and their hostility towards professional advice by doctors and nurses.[29] Similarly as in Germany, the Association of Medical Officers of Missionary Societies demanded in a resolution of 1908, obligatory certificates in first aid for all missionaries, preferably also hygiene and sanitation and, for female staff, also a certificate in nursing, to be acquired with the Ambulance Associations of St John or St Andrew.[30]

Health care for the local population

For followers of David Livingstone as well as for monks and nuns in the tradition of medieval monastic medicine, health care was not only intended for the members of the mission, but also as a service to the poor. Whenever the Anglican or Roman Catholic sisters arrived one of their first activities was the care for the sick. They did many home visits when invited to do so but soon they also offered out- and in-patient services in special rooms close to their convents. While after World War I these rooms for treatment started to be built from more endurable materials than the usual wattle-and-daub huts, the patients' and staff's (sometimes even the Europeans'[31]) accommodation remained in buildings constructed in the local tradition often until after World War II. The Benedictines with their impressive ancient tradition of solid construction and their emphasis on skilled manual work by the brethren started solid construction of buildings besides the central churches much earlier than the more academic Anglicans. Whether we call these institutions for health care, "hospital" or not, depends on the specific meaning of

[29] Bishop John Edward Hine, "To the Members of the UMCA in the Diocese of Zanzibar" (Zanzibar: UMCA Printing Office, 1904), 2–5, RHO, UMCA A3 [also in RHO UMCA A1 (XIII), 138].

[30] Secretary of the Association of Medical Officers of Missionary Societies, Letter and resolution, 20 May 1908, RHO, UMCA A3, 48–50.

[31] Leader Stirling, *Come Over and Help Us—A Doctor in Africa* (Dar es Salaam: AMREF, 1995), 69.

this word which has its own history in East Africa. Around 1900 a mission station for treatment was often called *Spital* in German, or in the ancient English meaning "hospital", as it fulfilled the function of the medieval hospital or hospice: the care of the outcast and homeless. People were not only given medicines and dressings, but also food and clothing. When the service was rather confined to out-patient medicine, the German term *Poliklinik* and the English dispensary or French *dispensaire* came into use, the Latin word for the reports to Rome being *pharmacopolium*. A few decades later, after local health staff had been trained, the difference became a rather racial one: a health care unit run by a European nurse was called a "hospital", whilst one with an African in charge was named a "dispensary".[32] Only after World War II the medical profession offered the decisive distinction: with doctor it was a "hospital", without him or her only a "dispensary" or later also "rural health centre", even when the unit had more than twenty beds. Today, services in major surgery or the responsibility for a health district are the decisive criteria for upgrading a health centre to a hospital. A qualified surgeon's private establishment, even with in-patient beds, would remain a dispensary.

The missionaries' and sisters' first patients were usually among the Christian converts but health care soon became much more popular than religious services and religious instruction. Further expansion of health care services, however, was limited by the lack of qualified staff for several reasons. Qualified doctors were too expensive for most missions, especially for the Catholic missions as they usually came from poorer regions in their European home countries. A doctor as a lay person could not be subjected, as a regular member might have been, to the strict rules and very modest lifestyle of the religious order. On the other hand the Anglican mission was a society of equals devoted to sharing the same very modest means for their living. Also on the Catholic side, nuns were restricted by Canon law. They were usually qualified nurses, but were not allowed to be trained and to work as midwives. As for the missionaries

32 Timotheus Wilhelmus Joseph Schulpen, "Integration of Church and Government Medical Services in Tanzania: Effects at District Level" (Diss., University of Nijmegen, 1975), 49.

local customs around birth constituted an area where "pagan" practices proved to be especially strong and many deaths could be prevented, they longed for access to this field. Finally the Benedictine bishop got permission from the sisters' superiors in Germany to have some of them trained in midwifery.[33] Yet the Archbishop of Cologne did not want them to be seen in religious habit during the obstetric activity. Therefore they were trained in the occupied French territory of Metz. However, their midwifery service was not much sought after by African women for about two decades.

Thus the main practical limit to more health care by missionaries was not Canon Law, but the population's reluctance which was again partly due to the lack of very obvious success. For before World War I, the missions in the South-east could not offer the more impressive procedures of modern medicine, for example, major surgery including Caesarean section, as well as injections of arsenicals which were already offered by German government doctors at that time. The mission's treatment consisted mainly of the cleaning and dressing of wounds, from ulcers, accidents and animals. In the remote South-east it was only in the late 1920s that the mission doctor's injections and major surgery were added to the treatment already being provided by the nurses in the form of tablets and dressings. During this time time the cheap injection therapy became available for one of the main health problems, the disfiguring and often crippling infectious disease yaws, making the need for a mission doctor more imperative. After a female doctor of the UMCA's headquarter in Zanzibar had introduced this new technique in the Anglican and Catholic hospitals of the South-east, both remote missions got doctors of their own, Dr Frances Taylor for Masasi in 1926 and Sr Dr Thekla Stinnesbeck for Ndanda one year later. The latter first had to pass an additional exam in Britain as German qualifications were not acknowledged in British Tanganyika. The two doctors worked in their missions until the early 1960s and thus deeply influenced the medical development of the region. Despite their religious commitment, they and their later medical

[33] Walter, *Sustained by God's Faithfulness*, 279–84.

colleagues were strong proponents of medical science in the debates to be considered next.

Health care in the missionary strategy

The world-wide discussions of the Medical Mission Movement about medicine as a strategy in missionary work took place in East Africa, too. In 1911 the Benedictine Bishop of the area, Thomas Spreiter, emphasised

> that we do not have our hospitals and dispensaries just to administer emergency baptism, but as well not only in order to heal. The missionaries are mainly care-givers and physicians of the soul. The care for the body is not the main aim, but only a very important means for the great apostolic aim of saving souls. It is similar to the school. [34]

In the early years the strategic use of health care for conversion had sometimes led to a kind of blackmailing unacceptable to later times. A famous example is the Anglican Mrs Williams in Zanzibar who in 1880 refused the treatment of a child as long as the mother did not cut off its charms. [35] Such instances disappeared from later missionary records, but even the academic mission doctors' motivation remained biased towards the fate of the soul. Characteristic is the story of Sr Dr Thekla's first major surgery:

> A young man with a rotten leg lies in the camp. I advise the amputation to which he agrees. As he is in a miserable state, I instruct him a little and give him the emergency baptism. A severe disapproval by the Father Prior follows, as all catechumens have to attend the instruction for three years first. We put the patient on the table. What happens? Inhaling the

[34] Bishop Thomas Spreiter, "Allgemeiner Visitationsbefund", 25 March 1911, KAStO, folder Daressalam 1, *Bischof Rundschreiben* [Bishop Circulars], 14.

[35] Terence O. Ranger, "Godly Medicine: The Ambiguities of Medical Mission in South-eastern Tanzania, 1900–1945", *Social Science & Medicine* 15B, 1981, 262. Abbreviated version in Steve Feierman and John M. Janzen , eds., *The Social Basis of Health and Healing in Africa* (Berkeley: University of California Press, 1992), 256–82.

first drop of ether he expires his soul. When I met the Father Prior later, we were both very happy, but who the most?[36]

In Sr Thekla's case the obligation to save souls certainly did not interfere with her medical duties as she became famous for her dedication to patients and especially mothers-to-be, irrespective of their religion. The local Indian community even included her picture in the shrine of venerable beings in their local temple.[37] The little story, however, clearly states an important part of motivation to devote one's whole life to such remote mission hospitals—the "supernatural ends".

When Africans used ritual practices that Europeans regarded as religious for healing and physical protection, religious Europeans could also consider the application of their own spiritual means for such purposes in Africans. This is especially the case where, before the arrival of religious sisters as nurses and of mission doctors, the priest's care for the sick often had included the administration of drugs as well as of sacraments. In this question, however, denominational differences became obvious. More than twenty years ago, Terence Ranger argued in his seminal study on mission medicine in southern Tanzania that with regard to their protestant, low or broad church supporters at home, the Anglicans of the high church UMCA had to refrain from such use of spiritual matters.[38] As they might face the charge of introducing a magical version of Christianity into Africa, they avoided any suspicion of a magical understanding of ecclesiastical rites. Of course, they could not prevent their parishes and their African clergy from doing so, as the African concepts held their power within the local population. Even in 1969 some of the members of the higher Anglican clergy, who hoped to become the first African Bishop of Masasi, used sacrifices and magic to promote their success.[39]

36 Thekla Stinnesbeck, *33 Jahre Missionsärztliche Tätigkeit im Ndandagebiet in Tanganyika* (c. 1960), 3.

37 *Jubilei ya Miaka 100. 1896–1996 Parokia ya Nyangao* (Jubilee of 100 years Parish of Nyangao [Ndanda-Peramiho: Benedictine Publications, 1996]), 26.

38 Ranger, "Godly Medicine", 273–75.

39 Wembah-Rashid, *Ethno-History of the Matrilineal Peoples*, 156.

The Roman Catholic Benedictines were less constrained by accusations from their home country than the UMCA, at least until World War II, as most of their Bavarian supporters accepted religious means for healing and protection. In particular the Benedictine sisters and brothers, who formed the majority and, unlike the fathers, had no theological education themselves, strongly believed in the physical effects of sacraments. The chronicle of Ndanda notes in 1910: "Sr Hieronyma has severe fever with vomiting gall. She received the sacrament of the extreme unction whereupon she accordingly recovered soon." [40] The sisters found similar expectations among the local population, as the African priest and church historian Sebastian Napachihi noted about the first mission station, Lukuledi:

> Sometimes the missionaries decided to baptise people especially children without even consulting the parents of those children nor even explaining to them what they were doing to the sick. People simply took the whole rite of such baptism to be a manner of curing the sick. A case is told in which Sr Afra Gillot administered such secret baptism to a child whom she had believed was going to die. The child recovered on the following day. The child's mother came and asked the sister to apply the same medicine as the previous day for the child got much better but the sister could not repeat it. [41]

The theologians among the Benedictines openly discussed the question of using religious means for healing. Again in 1910, the East Africa missionary Father Ambros Mayer, the Benedictines' expert in ethnography as well as religious instruction, declared on the problem of female infertility:

> I don't see why we should not completely accommodate the religious desires of the Negro, be it that he regards the sterility as Godly Providence or demonic influence—and we cannot maintain that this is not the case—and why we should not—like our pious ancestors—apply

[40] Chronikeintrag 3.-11.6.1910, KAStO Z.1.2.34.

[41] Sebastian Wolfgang Napachihi, *The Relationship Between the German Missionaries of the Congregation of St Benedict from St Ottilien and the German Colonial Authorities in Tanzania, 1887–1907* (Ndanda, Peramiho: Benedictine Publications, 1998), 91.

> religious means. Even if they—which we do not wish to suppose—had no other value than the psychological of calming the nervous system and enhancing self-confidence . . . they had fulfilled their purpose.[42]

One year later, in 1911 Bishop Spreiter officially took up these arguments, even more generally in view of all medical problems:

> As we give care to the sick for supernatural reasons and are firstly directed towards supernatural ends, we should apply those supernatural means that our sender, the Holy Church, gives us for the achievement of our natural and supernatural ends. These are the prayers and blessings of the Roman Ritual Book. With this we do not introduce anything new, but on the contrary something old and we accommodate the Negro's desire to use besides the natural remedy also a supernatural one.[43]

Bishop Spreiter recommended blessed water for the sick in honour of St Albert, in honour of St Hubert for rabies, or more generally the assistance of St Ignatius and St Mary as blessings of the sick, of the linen, the medicines, the oil and of meals, and finally medals of saints.

Although such blessings by Christian rituals were accepted as additional means to fight evils like witchcraft, malicious spirits and disease, they could not replace the traditional customs altogether. In order to secure the mission's success, i.e., to enable the converted Christians to lead a Christian life without breaking with tradition completely, some adaptation was inevitable. Again the Anglicans set the example, and the Benedictines followed soon after. The first bishop of the new Anglican diocese of Masasi, Vincent Lucas, wrote a *Kitabu cha Ibada Mbalimbali* (Book of Various Liturgies), in which he stated that priest and holy water should protect in dangerous situations such as childbirth and the fight against 'all harmful forces'.[44] Although only by inference, this phrase would probably have been understood by Africans and Europeans alike as also referring to the

[42] Ambros Mayer, Nambiligya Blättle April 1910, Abteiarchiv Ndanda, Nambiligya Blättle, 1910, 44.

[43] Bishop Thomas Spreiter, "Allgemeiner Visitationsbefund".

[44] Andrew J. Clayton, "Christianity and Islam in South-East Tanzania: A Study of Religious Appropriation Among Makonde" (Diss., John Rylands University of Manchester, 1993), 167.

dangers of witchcraft. Much more renowned became his attempt to introduce a Christian version of the socially very important puberty rites of passage, the *unyago*.[45] The Benedictine Abbot-Bishop Joachim Ammann soon imitated this adaptation. This conservation of the boys' circumcision in the bush—female circumcision had never been practised in these matrilineal societies—while only substituting certain rituals with Christian prayers and prohibiting some dances, caused considerable conflict with the initially Anglican, later Catholic mission doctor Leader Stirling—although this later African nationalist politician was himself quite Africanised in other matters.[46] Stirling criticised the preventable deaths by unhygienic conditions and unskilful operations. The female doctor Taylor had never been accepted for performing circumcision. Until today, only a minority of adolescents are circumcised in the hospital but the biomedical training in hygiene and surgical skills for the experts performing circumcision in the camps *(wagariba)* has been advanced.

Despite their adaptation of such rites, both bishops confirmed that 'traditional' medicine in general—apart from the exclusive use of herbal medicine—was not acceptable for Christians.[47] African Christians were to be temporally excluded from the sacraments because of participating in ceremonies of divination and healing. Yet even devout Christians continued many old practices besides their otherwise ardent and sincere adherence to the Christian church whereas among the missionaries opposite options for replacing the 'traditional' could be observed. Even after World War II some Benedictine priests continued the successful use of

45 Lyndon Harries, "Bishop Lucas and the Masasi Experiment", *International Review of Missions* 34, 1945, 389–96; A. M. Hokororo, "The Influence of the Church on Tribal Customs at Lukuledi", *Tanganyika Notes and Records* 54, 1960, 1–13; Terence O. Ranger, "Missionary Adaptation of African Religious Institutions: The Masasi Case", in *The Historical Study of African Religion*, ed. Terence O. Ranger and Isaria Kimambo (London: Heinemann, 1972), 221–51.

46 Stirling, *Come Over and Help Us*, 98.

47 William Vincent Lucas, "The Christian Approach to Non-Christian Customs", in *Christianity and Native Rites* (London: Central Africa House Press, 1950), 19.

Christian rites for physical protection and exorcism,[48] while the new Abbot-Bishop Viktor Haelg of Ndanda who had studied medicine for some years himself and wrote Swahili text books on infectious diseases for teachers, resented any appearance of magical healing. The first African Benedictine Abbot in southern Tanzania, Gregory Mwageni, demonstrates African pragmatism when he recommends the substitution of 'superstition by scientific and revealed truths and means such as scientific medicines, sacraments, sacramental rituals and Christian prayer'.[49] The increasing split between medicine and religion on the European side might have contributed to a more relaxed attitude towards African attempts of preserving and restoring health, too. Thus changing ideas in international health and in missionary theology weakened the earlier fear of unscientific practices and paganism at many places. Even mission hospitals today include referral to traditional healers by the hospital's psychiatrist, spiritual healing and charismatic groups by the hospital chaplain, training courses for traditional healers on hygiene and necessities for referral. Despite the fact that the mission hospitals had followed the racist and economy-orientated German and British policy of separate wards for European, Asian and African patients (which was sometimes resented by the religious doctor[50] and broken by the hospital admission of sick African clergy and nuns to the European wards), the main discrimination of Africans seems to have taken place along lines which were not racial, but were regarded as religious or cultural by Europeans. This insight into the changing European attitude towards African healing[51] leads to the question: how did the African population view European medicine?

48 Lambert Doerr, ed., *Peramiho, 1898–1998: In the Service of the Missionary Church* (Ndanda-Peramiho: Benedictine Publications, 1998), 1: 259–60.

49 Gregory Mwageni, "Ein Benediktinerkloster in einer afrikanischen Gesellschaft", in *Zukunft aus empfangenem Erbe. 100 Jahre benediktinische Missionsarbeit*, ed., Siegfried Hertlein and Remigius Rudmann (St Ottilien: EOS, 1983), 79.

50 Stinnesbeck, *33 Jahre Missionsärztliche Tätigkeit*, 2.

51 For the early attitudes in German East Africa, Walter Bruchhausen and Volker Roelcke, "Categorising 'African medicine': The German Discourse on East African Healing Practices, 1885–1918", in *Plural Medicine, Tradition and*

"Traditional" Medicine and the Mission Hospital

The people's perception of the hospital

As demonstrated above, local customs surrounding sexual life, birth and early infancy had been the main reasons for the earlier missionaries to call for nurses and doctors.[52] As Europeans could not do all the necessary work themselves, education and training of African staff became a prominent means in fighting allegedly 'pagan' and 'unhealthy' practices. However, training did not always contribute to a 'rational' understanding of medicine but contributed to new myths. The use of dead bodies in the education of African staff created fears of ritual murder as known from some areas of African medicine while the white staff of the mission did not understand this relationship.

'Vampire stories' that relate European institutions and their African staff to the criminal use of human bodies are well known in East Africa and often use the Swahili term *mumiani*.[53] Taken from the medieval Latin word *mumia*, mummy, for medicinal substances prepared from Egyptian mummies, (mummies') pitch or clotted human blood, this concept projects African medicine's use of dead bodies into supposed European sources of power. An incidence of such suspicions of mumiani is reported from Ndanda, in two different versions. At Christmas in 1933 the African Christians from the villages did not attend the midnight mass as they feared a supposed band of killers headed by a white person were active during the night. The priest's story focuses the superstition without mentioning

---

Modernity, 1800–2000, Routledge Studies in the Social History of Medicine 13, ed. Waltraud Ernst (London: Routledge, 2002), 76–94.

52 For the importance of child care in the development of health care services Walter Bruchhausen, "Practising Hygiene and Fighting the Natives' Diseases: Public and Child Health in German East Africa and Tanganyika Territory, 1900–1960", *Dynamis. Acta Hisp. Med. Sci. Hist. Illus.* 23, 2003, 85–113.

53 Luise White, *Speaking with Vampires: Rumor and History in Colonial Africa* (Berkeley: University of California Press, 2000), 3–11.

any real event as possible origin,[54] while the doctor Sr Thekla tells her conservation of a human brain for teaching purposes and local fears and uncertainties arising from this without referring to the common stories and even practice of ritual murder.[55] Both accounts—that of the priest as well as that of the doctor—reveal that the common European attitude towards problematic foreign beliefs was still inclined towards confrontation, disregard and contempt rather than the settling of conflicts by understanding and dialogue.

Changes in local healing

So-called 'acephalous' or 'stateless' societies, living in groups of families without strongly centralised authority, do not tend to develop very professionalised health care such as those famous experts who did abdominal surgery in the kingdoms of the East African Great Lakes' Region during the nineteenth century.[56] When the 'stateless' societies of south-eastern Tanzania were increasingly Islamised and thus 'Swahilised', communal ancestor veneration, an important means for preserving and restoring health, was substituted by 'possession cults' in the area of healing ceremonies.[57] The

[54] Alkuin Bundschuh, *Ost-Afrika. Land und Leute. Aufzeichnungen aus der Sicht eines langjährigen Missionars* (St Ottilien: EOS, 1976), 264–66.

[55] Thekla Stinnesbeck, *33 Jahre Missionsärztliche Tätigkeit*, 7.

[56] Jack Neville Phillips Davies, "The Development of 'Scientific' Medicine in the African Kingdom of Bunyoro-Kirara", *Medical History* 3, 1959, 47–57.

[57] In the vast literature on spirit possession or *ngoma* in southern and eastern Africa there is no study on one of the four ethnic groups relevant here. Studies for neighbouring people include, Jessica Erdtsieck, *Pepo as an Inner Healing Force: Practices of a Female Spiritual Healer in Tanzania* (Amsterdam: Royal Tropical Institute, 1997); Jessica Erdtsieck, "In the Spirit of Uganga: Inspired Healing and Healership in Tanzania" (Diss., Amsterdam, 2003); Linda Giles, "Possession Cults on the Swahili Coast: A Re-examination of Theories of Marginality", *Africa* 57, 1987, 234–57; Linda Giles, "Spirit Possession on the Swahili Coast: Peripheral Cults or Primary Texts"? (Diss., University of Austin, 1989); Linda Giles, "Spirit Possession and the Symbolic Construction of Swahili Society", in *Spirit Possession: Modernity and Power in Africa,* ed. Heike Behrend and Ute Luig (Madison: University of Wisconsin Press, 1999), 142–64.

comparison between ethnographic accounts from the 1930s[58] and my field research reveals fundamental changes in healing over the past half a century. The original local monstrous spirits causing specific diseases or epidemics and the ancestral spirits, who might trouble members of their clan in their search for sacrifices, for averting risks to health and welfare or for the call to healing, were replaced by foreign spirits.[59] These new spirits were believed to issue from eminent Muslim experts, members of other ethnic groups or even animals. While some of these spirits just disturbed those they possessed and should have been appeased by music, dance, drinks and other gifts, it was believed that others wanted to assist the sick by passing their own healing powers and knowledge through the healer as a spirit medium. By this contact with several spirits who are each supposed to have different expertise in healing, today the usual healer in the South-east, the *mganga (wa jadi)*, combines all the classical tasks in healing that were formerly separated functions and done by different experts using divination and oracles, recommending herbal remedies, communicating with spirits and fighting witchcraft.

My field research including interviews with about eighty traditional healers demonstrated major differences in the healers' attitudes towards the hospital. The greatest difference was marked by gender. The vast majority of the interviewed healers (about 75 per cent) were female spirit mediums.[60] The specific motivations and

58 Meinulf Küsters, "Die Wamuera" (unpublished script, 1931), to be edited by Maria Kecskési, Staatliches Museum für Völkerkunde München; Joachim Ammann, "Sitten und Gebräuche bei den Wamwera" (unpublished script, 1955), to be edited by Maria Kecskési, Staatliches Museum für Völkerkunde München.

59 Beatrix Heintze, *Besessenheits-Phänomene im mittleren Bantu-Gebiet* (Wiesbaden: Franz Steiner, 1970), 255.

60 The figure seems to be rather representative for the healers of this region as samples of healers taken in four different ways rendered about the same result. These four ways were the registration lists for a licence to healing with the District Cultural Officer, the mission hospital's list for training courses in hygiene and eye care for 'traditional healers', the recommendation by field research assistants and acquaintances and the enquiry in villages for their waganga which is a gender neutral term.

roles of female and male healers have to be considered in order to understand their relation to hospital medicine.

Female healers: Referral and assistance to the hospital

Regarding the preponderance of female healers, several reasons can be discussed here. Within Islamic societies it is common for women to dominate activities related to spirits. Being in fact excluded from the official Friday prayer in the mosque, women have often developed their own religious meetings related to extra-Islamic tradition and custom, to graveyards and spirits. This could lead to a special female expertise in spirits. Yet Islamic influence could exclude women from the healing business. This was observed for the ethnic group of the *Wazaramo* in the Tanzanian capital Dar es Salaam where hardly any women practised as mganga, whereas in the rural surroundings where the traditional religion flourished side by side with Islam the same ethnic group had many women holding this office of healing.[61]

Another possible explanation might lie in social history. As the ethnic groups of south-eastern Tanzania belong to the so called 'belt of matrilineal people' in south-eastern Africa, the women—or rather the matrilineal relatives as opposed to those on the husband's lineage—had a strong economic position. The title *Der Mann als Bettler* ("The Husband as Beggar") of an article by the Swiss anthropologist Rupert Moser[62] might be exaggerated but these 'acephalous' societies were certainly less patriarchal than the coastal Islamic groups influencing them. Thus women could feel themselves as the losers of Islamisation and might have found ways to counteract this. By their own staged introduction into healing women extend initiation—so

[61] Lloyd W. Swantz, *The Medicine Man Among the Zaramo of Dar es Salaam* (Uppsala: Scandinavian Institute for African Studies and Dar es Salaam University Press, 1990); Marja Liisa Swantz, *Ritual and Symbol in Transitional Zaramo Society with Special Reference to Women*, Studia Missionalia Uppsaliensia 16 (Lund: Glerup, 1970).

[62] Rupert R. Moser, "Der Mann als Bettler. Geschlechterbeziehungen bei den mutterrechtlichen Mwera von Südtanzania", in *Sie und Er. Frauenmacht und Männerherrschaft im Kulturvergleich,* ed. Gisela Völger (Köln: Rautenstrauch-Joest-Museum für Völkerkunde, 1997), 381–86.

important in matrilineal groups for pregnancy, delivery and puberty—into the realm of disease and affliction. All the female healers had started healing by being sick from spirit possession themselves while none of the male healers admitted to this unmanly weakness. By completing the initiation of spirit possession, women are given a chance to return to society and to render a service which gives them a raised status. They sometimes even adopt the names of deceased or fictive famous male healers whose spirits advise them in healing. As a result of their initial disease women are thus able to gain a status otherwise unobtainable to them in a patriarchal society.

It might be due to this religious and social background that female healers have less problems with the hospital, for they remain different from men in healing. None of the female healers, even the obviously prosperous ones, had erected buildings similar to dispensaries or hospitals. For them, *uganga,* the art or practice of healing, is not simply a business as one of them expressed in her complaints about the necessity to have a permit from the government: "Why do they trouble us? We did not choose this."[63] Their healing was enforced on them by the healing spirits who looked for a medium. Thus healing by spirits is a calling, even against one's will, and a service to the community and the sick.

The supposition that such healing with the spirits is not a business is confirmed by other data. For example, the money given for calling the spirit is just a symbolic sum, today sometimes of no value at all, such as the old two-penny coin. If more is demanded the spirit threatens to leave the medium forever. When people are asked which way of healing costs most, the consultation of Islamic scholars, an exclusively male profession, is regarded as the most expensive kind of medicine. The spirit medium is not expensive, although it has to be admitted that paying for a *ngoma* (drums, dance or music), one of the forms of healing with regard to spirits, with the requisite male drummers for several nights, demands a high sum.

Not doing healing mainly for money gives the female healers a more relaxed position towards the hospital. They can and must be more interested in their patient's health than in their own wealth.

[63] Interview with S. D. B. alias D. in Mkangu, 3 November 2001.

They have less fear to lose patients to the hospital, as the difference as well as the complementary function of healing by spirits and hospital medicine is obvious to all. Many female healers—or more precisely, their spirits—recommend the hospital, especially for surgery and for the treatment of fever. The hospital is easily included into the repertory of means to be revealed by divination. A special, often mentioned task of the healer which makes her more of a family doctor as opposed to the specialist is the removal of spells from investigations. When the hospital has not found a cause for complaints by a diagnostic procedure, the healer treats the patients and sends them back to hospital, and it is expected that this time the X-rays or the lab results detect the problem.

Male healers: Competition and ideas of co-operation with the hospital

All the twenty interviewed male healers were different from the women in their healing practices, but not in their basic attitude towards biomedicine. None of them rejected the hospital. On the contrary, all of them were keen to praise the advantages of hospital medicine and readily used it for their own health problems. On closer examination, however, they were obvious imitators of and competitors with hospital medicine. Four of them had erected or rented buildings for their patients similar to health centres and hospitals, building them from brick and cement, some even with single bedrooms for those better off.[64] The quality of accommodation was an important factor for attracting patients, as focus group discussions with patients and their relatives indicated.[65] Some of the healers wore white coats and sat behind a desk during consultation. Several sold prepared medicines, including pharmaceuticals such as painkillers or antimalarials, and stored herbal drugs in glass bottles for injection. In contrast, none of the female healers had similar buildings, and all of them when using herbal therapy selected roots

[64] Interviews and visits with N. in Masasi-Mkuti, 1 November 2001; M. S. M. in Mkwera-Pwawani, 3 November 2001; B. N. in Mahuta, 16 November 2001; M. in Chinatola-Lengo of Kitangali, 4 December 2001.

[65] Focus Group Discussions in Mkwera and Ndanda, 26 January 2002.

and herbs from their shelves or in the bush under the influence of the 'spirit'. Male healers especially liked to use the word X-ray for describing their mode of divination. The male healers' wish to be equal to the hospital is expressed by their ideas of co-operation. Some refer their patients to the next mission hospital, in order to get investigations and surgery done there. Yet they expect these patients to return to them and stay for other kinds of treatment in their buildings which are supposed to offer a more spiritual environment and perhaps cheaper accommodation.

The healers not only sought cooperation with the hospital in the care of patients, but several herbalists expressed their interest in having their herbal remedies examined by hospital doctors. *Kupimo*, Swahili for measuring, is regarded as the decisive advantage of hospital medicine and lacking in traditional healing. The word can be interpreted as meaning both quantitative and/ or qualitative analysis. Accordingly some of the healers rather want a better way of finding the right dosage, while others want to have the efficacy of their remedies proven by a laboratory.

A special type of male healer, identified in four among the twenty interviewed men, is the Muslim Koran scholar and teacher, the *mwalimu*.[66] He is highly respected and active as a healing expert, too. Having gained knowledge on the Koran and the Islamic tradition during several years in a *medresa* (Swahili Koran school) at the coast, usually in Kilwa, he is not so much sought after as an expert for healing in the Graeco-Arabic humoural tradition, i.e., *Yunani-Tibb*[u] ('Ionic medicine'),[67] but for writing amulets in Arabic, calculating horoscopes and exorcising demons. Writing amulets is derived from a more mystical or religious type of Arabic medicine, the *Tibb-ul-Nabbi* (prophet's medicine).[68] Differing from the common female

66 Interviews with I. A. N. in Njenga, 5 November 2001; A. T. in Chiungutwa, 8 November 2001; S. M. M. S. in Chikundi, 5 November 2001; and A. S. M. alias M. in Chilangala, 6 November 2001.

67 For an introduction to Unani medicine Altaf Ahmad Azmi, *Basic Concepts of Unani Medicine: A Critical Study* (Hamdard Nagar, New Delhi: Jamia Hamdard, 1995).

68 For an introduction to prophet medicine J. Christoph Bürgel, "Secular and Religious Features of Medieval Arabic Medicine", in *Asian Medical Systems: A*

spirit medium, for the orthodox Muslim any friendly dealing with spirits is *shirk*, i.e., strictly prohibited pagan practice. Therefore the only right answer for the mwalimu is exorcism. Half of those Koran scholars we visited did not only use spiritual and magical methods, but also herbal therapy. One of them, an influential Sheikh, sold medicinal drugs and spices imported from India in a well furnished shop at a larger trade centre,[69] while his more locally oriented colleague on the Makonde plateau used the knowledge of forty trees inherited from his father.[70]

The Koran scholars were very much interested in hospital medicine and public health. They demonstrated a high degree of biomedical information on common diseases, their prevention and cure. This knowledge does not only stem from personal interest and general education, but also from their common function as local intellectuals, political leaders and members of various committees. So these men had different reasons for their favourable attitude to the hospital from those of the female healers. It was not a benevolent spirit who recommended the hospital for the patient's benefit, but the scientific, non-spiritual and politically approved character of this medicine which recommended itself to the rationally minded responsible men, as they saw themselves.

Conclusion: The African Incorporation of the Mission Hospital

After the encounter between Christian hospitals and African practices around sickness and healing had often been marked by misunderstanding, suspicion and confrontation from both sides the relationship became much more relaxed after political independence. On the European side developments in theology and missiology as well as in the medical discussion enhanced an open contact and even co-operation with 'traditional healers'. On the African side

---

Comparative Study, ed. Charles Leslie (Delhi: Motilal Banarsidass Publishers, 1998 [Reprint of Berkeley: University of California Press, 1976]), 44–62.

69 Interview with S. M. M. S. in Chikundi, 5 November 2001.

70 Interview with A. S. M. alias M. in Chilangala, 6th November 2001. Forty is a symbolic figure in healing, for example, the Neem tree is also called mwarobaini (the forty), for healing this number of diseases.

the ready acceptance of the apparent superiority of some biomedical methods—leading to imitation as well as to recommendation—prevented continuing confrontation. The healers cosmopolitanised their practice with regard to Islam and to European modernity and found their market niches in more 'local', 'spiritual' or 'natural' ways of healing. The mission hospital, with its vast majority of African staff today, is no longer a foreign body but an integral and indispensable part of the local healing universe. Even religion does not constitute an obvious obstacle for the Muslim patient to consult the Christian hospital and for the hospital staff to reach the population. Having achieved this within just a few decades is impressive proof of the African ability to adapt and incorporate the new and the foreign.

6

The Mission Hospital, 1880–1960

David Hardiman

The Medical Mission Journal, *Conquest by Healing*, noted in an editorial of 1947 that mission hospitals provided a focal point for health care in many parts of the world. There were, it estimated, about three hundred mission hospitals in China, making up about half of the total biomedical hospitals there. At the same time in India there were 256 mission hospitals and 250 branch dispensaries, providing about a third of all hospital beds throughout the subcontinent. These hospitals were not, it was argued, there merely to fill a gap left by colonial and other governments. They provided not only "the best that modern medical science can provide," but were also imbued with a unique Christian spirit. "It is this atmosphere of ungrudging service, this willingness to extend to the very poorest the hand of welcome, this keen personal interest in the individual body and soul of each patient, which stamps the mission hospital as different from the ordinary medical centre, and which so profoundly affects those who come into contact with it." The editor went on:

> It is not only the work actually done in the hospital wards—the careful diagnosis of obscure disease, the impressive list of major operations, the X-ray and pathological investigations, and the nursing back to life of hundreds of sufferers. More than this is its daily message of unselfish service to the community among which it is placed. First-aid work for the local townspeople; visitation of outlying dispensaries and rural areas; the organisation of preventive measures in times of epidemic and distress; the training of citizens in a sense of social responsibility for their sick—all this forms part of the hospital's regular routine. [1]

[1] Editorial, "Medical Missions in the World of Today", *Conquest by Healing* 24, no. 4, December 1947, 76.

The heyday of the Protestant mission hospital was from about 1880 to 1960. The paper focuses on these European and American Protestant missions. The Catholic Church was a latecomer to such work, only becoming strongly involved in the period after 1920.[2] Before the 1880s, Protestant missionary societies had lacked interest in putting their resources into such institutions. Thereafter, hospitals became the keystone of what they defined as their "healing ministry." During the first three decades of the twentieth century, mission hospitals were built all over the globe. Some began to specialise in particular diseases or complaints, a few became the centres for Christian medical schools. This strategy came into crisis with the depression of the 1930s, which stifled such expansionist strategies. Thereafter, mission hospitals were on the decline. With the end of formal colonialism in the second half of the twentieth century, the hospital-based strategy for Christian healing became increasingly unviable.

Medical Missions became a major element within Protestant missionary work only in the last quarter of the nineteenth century. Although a number of medically qualified men had served as missionaries—the most notable being David Livingstone—they were very few in numbers and not given any significant support in the field by their missionary societies. It was rare that funds were made available to establish hospitals. Attitudes towards medical missions began to change as biomedicine gained a new status and sense of moral direction in the second half of the nineteenth century. Policies of public hygiene and the implementation of preventive health measures were bringing observable benefits, and breakthroughs were being made in surgery and immunisation.[3] As the Comaroffs have noted, medicine began to replace the church as the guardian

[2] Catholic priests and nuns were forbidden to study medicine formally. This prohibition was relaxed in the case of nuns only in 1936. Dana Robert, *American Women in Mission: A Social History of Their Thought and Practice* (Macon, Georgia: Mercer University Press, 1996), 372.

[3] Editorial, "God's Hand in Medical Missions", *Medical Missions at Home and Abroad*, February 1914, 68–69. This article depicts these medical advances as providential; God's purpose being that biomedicine would become "a

of public and private health.[4] Missionary organisations responded to this development by trying to keep a foot in both camps—the spiritual and the medical.

Increasingly, medicine came to be viewed as a powerful aid to conversion. It was argued that in the "heathen" mind, religion and healing went hand-in-hand. As John Lowe stated in 1886: "In India, China, Africa, Madagascar and in almost every heathen land, crude systems of medicine are intimately associated with the religions of the people, and the treatment of disease, such as it is, is monopolised by the priests, or by others under their control."[5] In the words of another missionary, writing in 1901: ". . . among all rude races, magic and medicine are wedded, the priest and the doctor are one."[6] Twelve years later R. Fletcher Moorshead argued that western medical treatment undermined the superstitions on which "false religious systems" depended:

> It follows, therefore, that no more fatal blow can be dealt at this awful evil, cursing alike body and soul, than by proving by living demonstration the fallacy, fatuity, and powerlessness of the superstitious methods of treatment employed by the medicine man. Destroy the faith of the non-Christian man in his "doctor" and you have very frequently taken the surest and simplest course towards the destruction of his faith in the superstition of his religion.[7]

---

mighty instrument to open up the way and keep open the way for the Gospel of Christ."

[4] Jean Comaroff and John Comaroff, *Of Revelation and Revolution: The Dialectics of Modernity on a South African Frontier* (Chicago: Chicago University Press, 1997), 2: 325.

[5] J. Lowe, *Medical Missions: Their Place and Power* (Edinburgh: Oliphant, Anderson and Ferrier, 1886),148; quoted in Rosemary Fitzgerald, "'Clinical Christianity': The Emergence of Medical Work as a Missionary Strategy in Colonial India, 1800–1914", in *Health, Medicine and Empire: Perspectives on Colonial India*, ed. Biswamoy Pati and Mark Harrison (New Delhi: Orient Longman, 2001), 115.

[6] J. Wells, "The Sixth Gospel", *Medical Missions in India*, 27 October 1901, 73; quoted in Fitzgerald, "Clinical Christianity", 115.

[7] R. Fletcher Moorshead, *The Appeal of Medical Missions* (Edinburgh: Oliphant, Anderson and Ferrier, 1913), 76.

Miss M. Andrews wrote five years later that: “Every attendance at the dispensary is a defiance of evil spirits.”[8] Heathenism, in other words, had to be attacked on the medical front as well as through belief-systems, and Christianity had to provide “an all-encompassing cosmology that addressed the needs of body, mind and soul.”[9]

For these ends, the Medical Missionary Association was established in London in 1878.[10] It provided grants for potential medical missionaries to study medicine, and it opened a hostel for their residence in the city while they studied.[11] The New York Medical Missionary Society (later the International Medical Missionary Society) was founded in 1881. It provided funding to students undergoing training, and the first of them graduated in 1884. The American Medical Missionary society was established in Chicago in 1885, and, in Germany, the Medical Missionary Society of Stuttgart was founded in 1898 as an auxiliary of the Basel Missionary Society.[12]

Earlier in the nineteenth century, most mission healing had been carried out by missionaries who had no medical qualifications. By the later years of the century there was a growing criticism of such “amateurism.” Some missionaries were worried that poor standards of treatment were compromising their work in general. Colonial doctors often felt that the incompetence of the mission healers might

[8] Miss M. Andrews, “Speech to the Anniversary”, *Central Africa* 36, 1918, 149, quoted in Terence O. Ranger, “Godly Medicine: The Ambiguities of Medical Mission in Southeast Tanzania, 1900–1945”, *Social Science & Medicine* 15B, 1981, 262.

[9] Fitzgerald, “Clinical Christianity”, 115.

[10] This was not the first medical missionary organisation; the Medical Missionary Society in China was founded in 1838 and Edinburgh Medical Missionary Society in 1841. These bodies failed, however, to develop into major forces within the missionary movement in the 1840–75 period. Michael C. Lazich, “Seeking Souls Through the Eyes of the Blind: The Birth of the Medical Missionary Society in Nineteenth-Century China”, in *Healing Bodies, Saving Souls: Medical Missions in Asia and Africa*, ed. David Hardiman (Amsterdam: Rodopi Press 2006), 59–86; and John Wilkinson, *The Coogate Doctors: The History of the Edinburgh Medical Missionary Society, 1841 to 1991* (Edinburgh: The Edinburgh Medical Missionary Society, 1991).

[11] Wilkinson, *Coogate Doctors*, 22–23.

[12] Ibid., 23.

discredit biomedicine itself, particularly if they attempted surgery. The indigenous elites within the colonies were also becoming more discerning towards biomedicine, and could give vent to their frequent hostility towards Christian missionaries by accusing them of being charlatans. [13] In the words of a mission doctor: "The people of India are quick to detect a sham. They can soon determine whether or not persons are qualified for the position they are trying to fill." [14] This all created a demand for medically qualified missionaries. Although many medically unqualified missionaries continued to provide rudimentary medical care as a part of their work, such people were no longer considered to be "medical missionaries." This title was now reserved in missionary parlance for those who had full medical training and qualifications. In this way, medically qualified missionaries distanced themselves from untrained missionary practitioners. [15]

The number of medical missionaries grew rapidly. In 1858 there had been only seven such missionaries in India and China, this rose to 28 in 1882, 140 in 1895, and 280 in 1905. By the 1890s there were 680 medically qualified Protestant missionaries working worldwide, of whom 338 were American, 288 British, 27 Canadian, 7 Australian, and 20 from continental Europe. By 1916 the Protestant medical mission force worldwide had grown to 1,052 doctors and 537 nurses. Of these, 420 (40 per cent) of the doctors were serving in China and 281 (27 per cent) in India; while 127 (24 per cent) of missionary nurses were in China and 108 (20 per cent) in India. [16]

Until the 1870s, few missions had purpose-built medical facilities. Missionaries saw patients in their own houses or in rented buildings that had not been built with this purpose in mind and which were often poorly suited to the task. They also treated patients on tour.

13 Fitzgerald, "Clinical Christianity", 125.

14 A. Manwaring, ed., *Report of the Third Decennial Missionary Conference Held at Bombay, 1892–93* (Bombay: Education Society, 1893), 1: 328, quoted in Fitzgerald, "Clinical Christianity", 125.

15 A. Neve, "The Calling of a Medical Missionary", *Mercy and Truth*, December 1911, 398–400; 'C. F. H.', "Principles and Practices of Medical Missions", *Mercy and Truth*, February 1912, 48–49.

16 Fitzgerald, "Clinical Christianity", footnote 10, 77, and 67.

Some set up field hospitals where they performed surgery, such as amputations and cataract operations. The patients had to recover in a hospital tent, and when the doctor moved on, they had to be carried to the next camp.[17] With the growth of formal medical missions run by qualified doctors, there was a growing demand from such doctors that the mission societies pay for the building and running of permanent purpose-built hospitals at a central location in a mission. In part this development occurred because biomedical treatment was becoming increasingly complex and sophisticated. It was argued that with high-quality facilities, mission doctors could perform wonders of healing that would bring credit to their missions. In the past, a high proportion of patients who underwent surgery had died from post-operative infections. With the advent of antiseptics, long-term success rates had soared. Once this became the norm in the mission field, the occasional failure would not tell against the mission.[18] As the Rev Dr John Lowe stated in 1886: "... it is in the hospital that the most satisfactory and successful medical and surgical work will be accomplished—work which will produce the deepest impression, and direct public attention most favorably to the higher objects of the mission."[19]

The hospital was seen to be of particular spiritual value for missions, as patients were confined and underwent a possibly life-changing experience. In his history of the hospital, Guenter Risse has noted how going to a hospital is often regarded as being like a journey to a foreign, exotic and perhaps hostile and frightening land in which there are strange rites, miraculous interventions and frequent deaths. He argues that: "Like many other lifestyle journeys,

[17] J. M. Macphail, "Medical Missionary Village Work in India", *Medical Missions at Home and Abroad*, October 1895, 40.

[18] Editorial, "The Hand of God in the Direction and Development of Modern Medical Mission", *Medical Missions at Home and Abroad*, October 1919, 270–71.

[19] Lowe, *Medical Mission,* 48, quoted in Rosemary Fitzgerald, "A 'Peculiar and Exceptional Measure': The Call for Women Medical Missionaries for India in the Later Nineteenth Century", in *Missionary Encounters: Sources and Issues*, ed. Robert A. Bickers and Rosemary Seton (Richmond: Curzon Press, 1996), 192.

hospital stays can induce profound personal mutations, including changes in lifestyle and spiritual growth . . . the once key issues of sinful causality, need for penance, and some form of redemption still echo powerfully through the wards of the modern hospital."[20] Even in ostensibly secular institutions, nineteenth-century doctors believed that the experience could be turned to good Christian advantage. As the trustees of the Massachusetts General Hospital stated in 1842: "It must be obvious to every reflecting mind that seasons of bodily infirmity and sickness present peculiarly favourable opportunities for making useful impressions upon the character and for affording Christian comfort and consolation."[21]

Risse has also noted how hospitals originated as monastic institutions in which there was a strict hierarchy enforcing a strong discipline and conformity to institutional rituals on all inmates, and that this model was extended to later secular institutions.[22] Mission hospitals had a clear agenda in imposing their own forms of discipline and ritual on their patients. The hospital wards were designed to demonstrate Christian order and cleanliness, with their beds in neat rows with clean white sheets. It was hoped that the patient would learn to be punctual, self-disciplined and sober—virtues that were seen as preconditions for what was seen as "Christian" rationality and civilisation.[23] Religious ritual was a part of the everyday life of the institution, with frequent bedside prayers and services in the wards on Sundays. Often, Holy Communion were deliberately placed next to Christians so that they could witness the non-believers. Scenes from the Bible decorated the walls.

The downside to the hospital-oriented strategy was that running such an institution placed great burdens on mission doctors. The place had to be equipped and staffed with doctors, nurses and trained local assistants. The mission societies generally lacked funds either to employ adequate numbers of medical missionaries

[20] Guenter B. Risse, *Mending Bodies, Saving Souls: A History of Hospitals* (New York: Oxford University Press, 1999), 10.

[21] Risse, *Mending Bodies, Saving Souls*, 347.

[22] Ibid., 6.

[23] Ranger, "Godly Medicine", 262.

for the work available or to provide state-of-the-art hospital facilities. Often, there was only one fully qualified doctor at a hospital. A survey in 1929 of the 175 mission hospitals in India with over ten beds found that they were staffed by only 228 medical missionaries, which meant that 122, or 70 per cent must have had only one doctor.[24] When he or she went on leave, the place had to close down, so that there was no continuity in the work. Even when there was more than one doctor available, they had to turn their hand to many areas that would have been considered specialised in their home countries. General practice was frequently combined with surgery, eye, ear, dental and laboratory work. In addition, they had to administer the hospital and raise funds. Money was a perennial problem. The 1929 survey of mission hospitals in India estimated that a fifty-bed hospital required an annual budget of at least Rs 20,000 to function properly, while the actual average was Rs 14,000, nearly a third less than the requirement. Few of these hospitals were as a result adequately equipped. Only 7 per cent had X-ray equipment. Many lacked the laboratory facilities needed to make accurate diagnoses. Record-keeping facilities were frequently poor, so that no research was possible. Medical libraries for the staff were a rarity. There were not enough bathrooms or water closets, and often no piped water or septic tanks. Although steam laundries were considered best in point of hygiene, the rule was for local women to be employed to carry out the washing by pounding it on rocks.[25]

These problems continued into the 1940s. At Ranaghat, a mission hospital run by the Church Missionary Society (CMS) in India, there were officially 108 beds, but rarely less than 180 in-patients. Between five hundred and a thousand out-patients also came each day. The hospital served an area with a population of five and a half million. The superintendent in the late 1940s, Dr Frank Lake, remarked that they never turned away a single patient and

24 R. H. H. Goheen, "Indian Medical Missions: The Lessons of the Survey", *Conquest by Healing*, March 1929, 12.

25 Goheen, "Indian Medical Missions", 12–13.

were often working from seven in the morning to seven at night seeing them.[26]

Burdened by having to run a hospital on a shoestring, and driving themselves too hard, many medical missionaries broke down under the strain. Between 1913 and 1919, for example, five doctors of the Baptist Missionary Society in China—mostly young men—died at their posts as a result of overwork and illness.[27] In other cases—unable to develop their institutions in the manner they felt necessary for efficient and effective medical work—they gave up the struggle. John Stanley, in a study of a medical mission in Weixian in China, has shown how one such doctor in China abandoned the mission to which he had devoted many years of his professional life due to his frustration with the dismal conditions in which he was forced to work and after his attempts to raise funds for improvements to the hospital failed due to lack of support from his mission organisation.[28]

Due to these pressures, the standard of medical treatment provided in mission hospitals was frequently inferior to better-funded government institutions. The mission doctors, because of their arduous schedule, had little time to keep up-to-date with the medical literature or refresh their skills in other ways, so that their methods were often decades out of date. For example, Dr Margaret Johnson went to India in 1941 as a highly skilled surgeon to take charge of a CMS mission hospital, but never developed her techniques, and was surprised to find on a visit to the Wellcome Museum in London in 1963 that many of the instruments she had continued to use were now museum pieces.[29]

[26] Frank Lake, "The Realignment of Medical Missions in the Face of Changing Conditions on the Basis of Spiritual Priorities", *Conquest by Healing*, December 1950, 79.

[27] A. F. Walls, "The Heavy Artillery of the Missionary Army: The Domestic Importance of the Nineteenth-Century Medical Missionary", in *The Church and Healing*, ed. W. J. Sheils (Oxford: Basil Blackwell, 1982), 291–92.

[28] John Stanley, "Professionalising the Rural Medical Mission in Weixian, 1890–1925", in *Healing Bodies, Saving Souls*, ed. David Hardiman (Amsterdam: Rodopi Press, 2006), 122–27.

[29] Rachel Mash, "Margaret Fitzhugh Johnson, Doctor and Missionary, 1941–1963: Her Work and Family Life in the Context of Pre-independence and Post-Imperial India" (BA. thesis, University of Brighton, 2001), 31.

It was realised that many of these problems could be overcome if missions developed their own training facilities. Standards would be raised and converts could be trained and then employed to assist and relieve the white medical missionaries. In this, however, there were problems, given the frequent arrogance and racism of the white mission doctors towards their subordinates. The first medical mission to employ a medically trained convert was in Hong Kong, where the London Missionary Society (LMS) appointed Wong Fun to work in their hospital in 1857. He resigned after a year in protest against the way in which his supposed "colleagues" treated him. He set up a private practice in Canton that was extremely successful.[30]

Doctors such as Wong Fun were trained in the West. By the later years of the nineteenth century it was becoming clear that facilities were needed to train converts locally. In India, Dr Colin Valentine, a Scottish medical missionary, established the Agra Medical Missionary Training Institution in 1881. Christian converts were provided with grants to stay in Agra, and housed in a special Christian hostel while they trained at the Government Medical College in the city. Many indigenous Christian doctors were trained there, and without their work many of the medical missions in India would have been unable to function.[31] Others were trained at government medical colleges in their own regions. In Gujarat, for example, a local convert called Dalpat Makanbhai qualified as an assistant surgeon in the 1890s, becoming the first local Christian doctor. He was appointed initially as a medical evangelist. In the early years of the twentieth century he was promoted to house surgeon at the important mission hospital of the Irish Presbyterians at Anand.[32] By the 1920s, Indian Christians were being sponsored by missions to receive medical training, so that they could work as fully qualified doctors in mission institutions.

[30] Timothy Man-kong Wong, "Local Voluntarism: The Medical Mission of the London Missionaray Society in Hong Kong, 1842–1923", in *Healing Bodies, Saving Souls*, ed. David Hardiman (Amsterdam: Rodopi Press, 2006), 92–93.

[31] Wilkinson, *Coogate Doctors*, 30–31.

[32] Robin Boyd, *Church History of Gujarat* (Madras: The Christian Literature Society, 1981), 216–18.

Measures were also taken to provide training for young Indian Christians who could act as assistants in mission hospitals. The American Presbyterian Mission established a medical school at Miraj, and the LMS, two such schools in Travancore and at Jammalamadugu. Students trained in medicine and theology for four years, receiving a diploma at the end that enabled them to become "Medical Evangelists". They generally went on to work as subordinates of Western-trained medical missionaries in mission hospitals, or to run branch dispensaries in outlying mission stations.[33] Similar training institutions were opened for women at Ludhiana and Vellore. The Women's Christian Medical College, Ludhiana, was founded in 1894, and by 1932 had trained 227 medical assistants, 125 compounders, 166 nurses, 367 nurse midwives and 56 indigenous midwives. They had gone to work all over India.[34] The Scudder Missionary Medical School for Women was established at Vellore in 1918. These institutions admitted non-Christian as well as Christian students. They provided only licentiate-level training, that was inferior to the M. B. degree. The medical assistants who were so trained played a critical role in medical missions. Being able, as a rule, to communicate with greater facility with the patients in their own language, they could explain forms of treatment and unfamiliar hospital practices—for example, that the bedding and utensils that was provided for patients had to be returned when their stay was over. They often played an important role in popularising Western medicine more generally in their society.[35]

The mission hospitals provided training for local pastors and school teachers employed by the mission so that they could provide basic treatment in the villages in which they worked. They were provided with medicine chests and medicines to give or sell at low rates to villagers. Follow-up training was provided in further short courses at the hospital at regular intervals. This work was,

33 Moorshead, *The Appeal of Medical Missions*, 98–99.

34 Edith Brown, "Preventive and Welfare Medical Missionary Service", *Conquest by Healing*, June 1932, 47.

35 David Arnold, "Disease, Medicine and Empire", in *Imperial Medicine and Indigenous Societies*, ed. David Arnold (Manchester: Manchester University Press, 1988), 2.

for example, carried out in Dornakal in South India, where there were around 1,400 teachers and catechists employed by the mission throughout the diocese. Once such people were trained, the medical work that was focussed on the hospital could be extended over an extremely wide area.[36]

Mission hospitals established their own medical schools initially in China. The first initiative in this respect was taken by a leading Christian in Hong Kong called Ho Kai, who had qualified as a doctor in London. He played a critical role in establishing a new mission hospital for the LMS in 1886, followed in 1887 by a medical college that used the premises of the hospital. Many of its students were Christians or from Christian families, the most notable being Sun Yat-sen, the future nationalist leader. A lot of the money for the hospital and medical school was raised locally, being a noteworthy early example of a self-sustaining initiative by local Christians.[37] Further Christian medical schools were founded in the following years. The premier institution in this respect was the Peking Union Medical College (PUMC), founded as a mission institution in 1906, and supported by the Rockefeller Foundation's China Medical Board from 1915. This funding allowed it to gain a reputation as the best medical college throughout eastern Asia. It was co-educational.[38] By the time of the communist takeover there were in all six such institutions run by missions in China.[39]

India lagged behind China in this respect. By the 1920s, mission hospitals were finding it increasingly difficult to recruit doctors from the home countries, and also very hard to attract fully qualified Indian Christians to work in them. Although Indian Christians made up a disproportionate number of medical students in India, they preferred to work in government hospitals or in private practice

[36] Henry Whitehead, "Medical Work in the Villages of India", *Conquest by Healing*, June 1931, 53.

[37] Timothy Man-kong Wong, "Local Voluntarism", 93–96.

[38] Ruth Compton Brouwer, *Modern Women Modernizing Men: The Changing Missions of Three Professional Women in Asia and Africa, 1902–69* (Vancouver: UBC Press, 2002), 43.

[39] Harold Balme, "Medical Missions in the World Today", *Conquest by Healing*, March 1948, 9.

as the pay was much better. This was a time of strong nationalist sentiment, and working in mission hospitals also carried a stigma of being anti-nationalist.[40] By the late 1920s, demands were being made in India for a Christian medical college that would qualify students to be full-fledged doctors. Indian Christians were finding it increasingly hard to gain admission to the government medical colleges. The medical profession was growing in prestige, attracting a wider range of elite students. Also, as nationalists gained more power within provincial governments, they sought to allocate places in medical colleges according to the proportion of each religious group within the population as a whole, and the Christians—who were in a small minority—were losing out. It was moreover felt that the government colleges inculcated a materialist attitude and poor ethical standards, and that doctors trained in Christian institutions could give an ethical lead to the profession as a whole.[41]

These plans fell through in the 1930s. One reason was that no money could be spared for such an expensive initiative at a time of economic depression. Another was that some influential Indian Christians opposed the idea on the grounds that evangelism must take priority over impressive but expensive medical projects. The Anglican Bishop of Dornakal, V. S. Azariah, took the lead in this. He was committed to mass-movement evangelism amongst the poor in India, and was not convinced that higher education would help much in this task. As it was, he believed that the professionalisation of the middle classes was leading to a general decline in spiritual values. He himself had no degree. Another reason for his lack of enthusiasm was possibly that his son, a doctor, had been refused an appointment in a CMS medical mission in North India in the early 1930s on the grounds that it hired only Europeans for higher-grade positions.[42] As a result, Christian missions failed to take the lead in university-level medical education in India, as they had done in China. Even at Indian independence in 1947, none of the Christian

[40] Brouwer, *Modern Women Modernising Men*, 34.

[41] Ibid., 34–35; W. Paton, "A Problem in India Medical Missions," *Conquest by Healing*, June 1931, 45.

[42] Brouwer, *Modern Women Modernising Men*, 46.

medical colleges had upgraded themselves to full university status. The first to do so was Vellore, in 1950.

In Africa, the missions found it hard during the early years to recruit local people to work as medical assistants, as the work was regarded as lowly and demeaning. The majority at that time were former patients who had become converts and who had stayed around the mission compound after they were healed.[43] Later, most came to be recruited from those who had studied at the mission schools. They were almost always male, and were known as *dawa* (medicine) or dispensary "boys." The mission doctors in Africa generally held a low opinion of the abilities of their assistants, commonly regarding them as hard to train, lazy in their work and often guilty of misdemeanours. They felt that such work was not "natural" to natives. Those who were considered to have made a success of the job were a cause for rejoicing.[44]

The paucity of African medical personnel was even more apparent at more senior levels. There were almost no African doctors working for the medical missions before the 1960s. Terence Ranger has argued in the context of Tanzania that educated African Christians tended to shun the medical profession until after World War II as they resented the intolerant way in which the mission doctors tried to impose their cultural values in the sphere of healing. Instead, they preferred to become teachers or priests.[45] This situation was to cause some embarrassment to the missions as independence loomed in the different colonies, leading to some hasty measures to train Africans to work at this level alongside the missionaries.

Nursing was developing as a profession at the same time. In the early years many unqualified women had turned their hand to this task, but by the early years of the twentieth century the occupation was becoming more professionalised. Nurses were expected

[43] Megan Vaughan, *Curing Their Ills: Colonial Power and African Illness* (Cambridge: Polity Press, 1991), 61.

[44] Vaughan, *Curing Their Ills*, 64–66. Also Linda Beer Kumwenda: "African Medical Personnel of the Universities' Mission to Central Africa in Northern Rhodesia", in *Healing Bodies, Saving Souls*, ed. David Hardiman (Amsterdam: Rodopi Press, 2006), 193–226.

[45] Ranger, "Godly Medicine", 270–72.

to have undergone a three-year course of training in a recognised school, and to have obtained extra qualifications in areas such as midwifery, dispensing and tropical diseases. Nurses were in strong demand, more so even than women doctors. They were needed to staff hospitals for women and children, and to educate local women to become nurses.[46] By getting in first in developing nursing in the colonies, missionaries saw an opportunity to exert a Christian influence over women's medical and nursing education. This would, it was hoped, imbue their future professional practice with an ethos of selfless service and devotion to duty rather than with a spirit of commercialism.[47] The training element in medical mission work became seen as being a prime purpose of such work in general and training programmes for nurses were established. In India, the missions were in the vanguard of such work; by World War II, some 90 per cent of Indian nurses were Christians, and 80 per cent of all Indian nurses had been trained in mission hospitals. This "proved to be one of the most enduring legacies of the female medical missions of the colonial era,"[48] and it laid the basis for the profession of nursing in India since then.

In Africa, most of the nurses in government and mission hospitals were male until almost the end of the colonial period. In some areas, missions rather than the colonial governments took the lead in trying to attract women into nursing. In northern Rhodesia, for example, a new Anglican Bishop who was appointed in 1941 championed this measure for the first time.[49] Mission girl's schools provided the best recruiting ground for trainee nurses. One major problem was finding qualified nurses who could train the recruits. Even then, the new nurses often ended up only half trained and holding an inferior certificate. In northern Rhodesia, the first course designed to turn

[46] Rosemary Fitzgerald, "Rescue and Redemption: The Rise of Female Medical Missions in Colonial India During the Late Nineteenth and Early Twentieth Centuries,' in *Nursing History and the Politics of Welfare*, ed. Anne Marie Rafferty, Jane Robinson and Ruth Elkan (London: Routledge, 1997), 74–75.

[47] E. K. Paget, *The Claim of Suffering: A Plea for Medical Missions*, London 1913, 87–90, quoted in Fitzgerald, "Rescue and Redemption", 75–76.

[48] Fitzgerald, "Rescue and Redemption", 76–77.

[49] Kumwenda, "African Medical Personnel", 211

out fully qualified female nurses only started in 1964.[50] However, even an inferior certificate provided immense openings for young women who held it, as they were in demand from not only missions, but also from other medical institutions, both in Africa and in Europe.

Being evangelising institutions, missions were always active in taking their message to the surrounding population, and this ethos informed their medical work also. Missionaries saw it as their task to inculcate biomedical knowledge with a zeal similar to that of their evangelising colleagues.[51] The mission hospital provided the focus for such work. As the editor of the medical missionary monthly, *Conquest by Healing*, remarked in 1932: "The hospital is not a costly piece of Western medicine maintained at an unnecessary expense in certain needy places on the Mission Field. It is the vital pivot upon which the activities of any well-considered scheme of medical mission must depend."[52] From this base, medical missionaries toured the villages providing treatment and giving lectures on modes of infection, preventive measures and means of treatment. They handed out or sold literature on health issues. They organised functions at their hospital for the same purpose. In 1928, for example, a health week was organised at the mission hospital in Dornakal in South India. About 350 attended from surrounding villages to be lectured on ". . . such subjects as hookworm, tuberculosis, leprosy, plague, child-feeding, small-pox and vaccination. The grand finale was a health musical drama composed by a school teacher and performed by the school girls."[53]

There were, nonetheless, dangers in bringing too much pressure to bear to change local sentiments. As the Belgian Congo medical missionary Clement Chesterman remarked in a medical mission journal in 1932, hospitals could get a "reputation of being the centres of organised interference with venerated native customs or

[50] Ibid., 216.

[51] Clement C. Chesterman, "Preventive Medicine and the Mission Hospital", *Conquest by Healing*, March 1932, 13.

[52] Editorial, "The Truth is, Both are Essential", *Conquest by Healing*, September 1932, 70.

[53] Whitehead, "Medical Work in the Villages of India", 52.

as running a sort of inquisition into personal and social hygienic heresies."[54] He himself was actively engaged in a campaign to reduce the incidence of sleeping sickness in the Congo. In a detailed study of the medical mission in which Chesterman worked, Nancy Rose Hunt has shown how he was quite prepared to use coercion when persuasion failed, beating Africans with a vicious hippopotamus-hide whip when he discovered cases of sleeping sickness that were being concealed from him. He later bragged about this before an audience of specialists in tropical medicine in London. Hunt provides evidence of similar cases by other medical missionaries, observing that: "Each of these missionary doctors strayed far from Great Physician idioms in these scientific circles, where they spoke proudly—code switching into a register of imperial masculine bravado impossible in missionary magazines—that they acted as agents of colonial discipline, using flogging to punish those who dared to defy them."[55] Such people were inevitably perceived as agents of the colonial state, and thus a threat to whatever power the local elites still retained. In some areas—most notably in Africa—they often became like an alternative local state, with mission stations that were centres for education, medical treatment, relief provision during periods of dearth, agricultural activity (which might include the provision of cooperative credit for farmers), and local craft production.[56] In such a situation, there could be conflicts over medical treatment that had a strong political dimension.

Such battles were often depicted in mission literature as ones between the mission doctor and the "witchdoctor" or "wizard." When called to treat a patient in their hut, the missionary was frequently shown as being drawn into an encounter with such practitioners of the "dark" arts. The struggle became one between the Light of Christian Reason and the Forces of Evil. In some cases the missionary triumphed, in others he or she was forced to withdraw, for the time being at least. Unlike the "rational" patient of Europe, the

[54] Chesterman, "Preventive Medicine and the Mission Hospital", 14.

[55] Nancy Rose Hunt, *A Colonial Lexicon: Of Birth Ritual, Medicalization and Mobility in the Congo* (Durham: Duke University Press, 1999), 95.

[56] I am grateful to David Arnold for this point.

native was depicted as being frequently too "primitive," stubborn and ignorant to heed the doctor's wisdom. This was shown to be deeply frustrating, requiring a staunch Christian forbearance on the part of the missionary.[57]

Medical mission work could provoke a backlash directed by local spirit mediums who felt threatened by such ideas. When a mission hospital was completed by the Society for the Propagation of the Gospel at Pondoland in South Africa in 1923, local "wizards"—as the missionaries described them—spread a rumour that evil spirits had pursued the patients and were now haunting the wards. The patients fled, and people avoided the hospital. Confidence was restored only after a visiting bishop carried out services of exorcism in each ward.[58] Though effective, the measure hardly represented a victory for biomedical values. In general, mission medicine appears to have had only limited success in mounting a challenge to the local wielders of supernatural power. Although they tried to insist that those who took advantage of their medical facilities, whether Christian or non-Christian, should disavow the so-called "witch doctors," they often found themselves waging a losing battle in this respect. There were after all many maladies that they were powerless to cure, so that people inevitably looked elsewhere for treatment. As a result, their form of treatment came to be viewed as one alternative among many, with people tending to approach the mission doctors only in cases of certain diseases, such as yaws, which biomedicine was fairly effective against. There was thus a change in consciousness in relationship to certain diseases, that came to be seen as treatable by drugs. Beliefs about supernatural agency in the case of many other diseases and ills were not however undermined. Certainly, this provided no revolution in the popular understanding of disease causation, or provided any great challenge to the patriarchal power of elders.[59]

[57] Vaughan, *Curing Their Ills*, 162–66.

[58] H. R. Henrich, "Training African Nurses", *Conquest by Healing*, December 1942, 52–53.

[59] Ranger, "Godly Medicine", 262.

With growing medical specialisation in the early twentieth century, an increasing number of medical missionaries developed skills in treating particular diseases and maladies. For example, the Baptist medical missionary, Paul Brand, pioneered hospital-based treatment for leprosy patients in the late 1940s and 1950s. Missionaries already ran leprosy colonies, but these were hardly hospitals, and the medical care provided for inmates was often rudimentary.[60] Brand was trained as a hand-surgeon in London and worked at the Vellore Christian Medical College hospital from 1946, where he pioneered new techniques of reconstructive surgery on those who had been deformed by the disease. This was the first time that leprosy patients had been admitted to a general hospital, and this in itself helped to remove some of the stigma attached to the disease. Brand gained a worldwide reputation for this work.[61] Tuberculosis was another disease for which specialist care was at that time considered necessary. Medical missionaries established special sanatoria for sufferers, the best known of which was located at Arogyavaram in Madras. Most of the staff were fully qualified Indian doctors who were encouraged to publish research papers on their work. In the late 1940s, missionaries provided about half of all beds in such sanatoria in India.[62] Missions also ran eye hospitals that specialised in cataract-removal. This was considered a particularly effective area for medical mission work, as the surgeons appeared to be walking in the footsteps of Christ giving "sight to the blind." The mission eye-hospital at Shekapur, near Quetta, was one such place, where by 1948 almost thirty thousand successful cataract operations had been performed.[63]

As the medical missionaries focussed more on prestigious specialist work, the day-to-day running of the hospitals became more and more the responsibility of indigenous medical workers. By the 1940s this was creating situations of increasing tension. Ruth

[60] S. Kakar, "Leprosy in British India, 1860–1940: Colonial Politics and Missionary Medicine", *Medical History* 40, 1996, 217–22.

[61] John Young, *Paul Brand and His Leprosy Work* (London: SCM Press, 1980); Michael Waters, "Paul Brand: Obituary", *The Guardian*, 27 August 2003.

[62] Balme, "Medical Missions in the World Today", 10.

[63] Ibid., 12.

Brouwer has noticed how, even after missionaries replaced earlier intolerance and racism with an attitude of greater circumspection and humility, they frequently retained a conceit about their superior professional training and resulting skills: "An exemplary 'life lived' could breed its own kind of arrogance; zeal in applying Christianity through social reforms and the application of Western techniques and technologies could, in practice, be even more culturally invasive than a narrowly focused zeal for conversions; and it always proved easier to 'talk the talk' of devolution than to put it into effect." [64] At the Ranaghat mission hospital in India, Dr Frank Lake of the CMS found himself in one such conflict with a hospital union supported by the Communist Party of India. About a quarter of the staff—whom Lake described as "mostly nominal Christians"—joined this union and went on strike. Pamphlets described Lake as "a secret agent of arrogant imperialism," and "an oppressor of the nurses with various forms of tyranny." The tension continued after Lake was replaced by Dr Hatt, culminating in the shooting of the latter by a young male nurse. There were similar protests in other mission institutions at the time of Indian independence. [65]

With the waning of European colonial power and influence in the period after World War II, there were often political pressures for the mission hospitals to be either closed down or taken over and run as government institutions. In China, the new communist rulers were hostile to mission work of any sort, and medical missionaries were soon forced to leave. Dr Chris Maddox, for instance, had worked in the mission hospital at Paoning in Sichuan Province since 1938, and had remained there right through the war with Japan, communicating with the outside world through Vietnam. He and his wife found the communists to be far more concerned with the welfare of the local people than the former nationalist regime, and they donned Maoist outfits and participated enthusiastically in the "barefoot doctor" scheme. The Korean War, however, saw all

[64] Brouwer, *Modern Women Modernizing Men*, 4.

[65] Frank Lake, "The Realignment of Medical Missions", 77.

Westerners in China being stigmatised and in 1952 the couple left to practice in Thailand.[66]

Many mission hospitals had to close in India too, though the process was spread over a longer period than in China. During the 1950s and 1960s, the Indian government became increasingly hostile towards foreign missionaries, whom they saw as agents of western neo-colonialism. More and more, it refused to issue visas to missionaries. Controls were placed on foreign funding, and mission-run institutions found it increasingly hard to obtain clearance for donations. The government also began to develop its own network of Primary Health Centres, which were often located near to mission hospitals and in direct competition with them. Mission hospitals had a choice of either closing down or deciding to become entirely indigenous organisations, staffed and financed by Indians.[67] The former choice was, for example, made by the CMS, which had run a mission hospital at Lusadiya in Gujarat since 1905. Local Hindu politicians connected with the ruling Congress party turned against the work because of the mission connections. When the hospital superintendent, Dr Margaret Johnson, left in 1963 the atmosphere deteriorated as the Indian medical staff quarrelled with the remaining white missionaries. The CMS decided that the place was no longer viable, and promptly closed it down, so that the staff as a whole had to find alternative employment.[68]

By the 1960s, it was clear that Christian missionary organisations had to review their strategy towards medical missions. The topic was debated in Tübingen in Germany at a special meeting on medical mission convened in 1964 by the World Council of Churches. Lesslie Newbigin, a former Bishop of the Church of South India, argued that in many respects the work begun by medical missions had been fulfilled as the state took responsibility for such work in Asia and Africa. "The whole business of secularisation and the

66 Ray Porter, "Chris Maddox: Obituary," *The Guardian*, 31 January 2004.

67 R. K. M. Sanders, "Metamorphosis of Medical Missions in India: The Emmanuel Hospital Association", *Saving Health*, June 1972, 33.

68 Interviews with Surji Timothibhai Suvera, Lusadiya, 15 December 2002, and with Rajnikant Christian, Nava Rewas, 17 December 2002. Rajnikant's father Daniel had worked as a doctor at Lusadiya hospital.

Welfare State is obviously something which could never have arisen out of the ancient pagan religions of Asia. It is a by-product of Christianity."[69] Now that missionaries had achieved this objective, he wondered whether the distinctive elements to Christian medical mission work were sufficient to justify a continuation of the work. It was perhaps best to encourage Christian doctors and nurses to act as good Christians within a secular medical system. Erling Kayser, a Norwegian who had served as a medical missionary in Indonesia, pointed out that medicine had lost some of its lustre in recent years, with scandals such as the thalidomide affair, "which was in a sense, an epidemic of a very handicapping disease, brought about by a modern drug, the result of the physician's work." There was a widespread feeling that something was seriously wrong with modern medicine. Much disease was hardly understood, and it was increasingly realised that many maladies were psychosomatic. This being the case: "Can the medical profession . . . continue to ignore or look askance at pre-scientific forms of healing?" Citing Freud, he argued that disease was likely to develop if strong emotions were repressed or were in conflict. "The point is that there is no dichotomy between soul and body." The real dichotomies were those of creation and destruction, the urge to life and the urge to death, God and the devil, and crucifixion and resurrection.[70] The implication here was that Christianity might be better served if it focussed on spiritual rather than biomedical healing.

In its heyday, medical mission work had been strongly hospital-centred and mission hospitals had a reputation as a beacon for health care in poor countries. By the 1960s and 1970s, this strategy was in crisis. Hospitals were becoming more and more expensive to maintain at a time when donations to missions were in sharp decline. The work was becoming hazardous in many parts of the world, due to political strife and civil wars. Armed gangs were a growing

[69] Lesslie Newbigin, "The Healing Ministry in the Mission of the Church", in *The Healing Church: The Tübingen Consultation, 1964*, ed. Frank Davey (Geneva: World Council of Churches, 1965), 10.

[70] Erling Kayser, "Medicine and Modern Philosophy: An Introduction", in *The Healing Church*, ed. Frank Davey (Geneva: World Council of Churches, 1965), 18, and 20–21.

danger in many parts of Africa, and medical missionaries located in isolated hospitals were in some cases ill treated, taken hostage, and even murdered.[71] It was also seen that the much ill health in mission regions was caused by poverty, malnutrition, poor sanitation, a lack of education and social depravation. Hospitals could hardly provide a solution to these multiple problems. Church resources were—it was argued—best used in preventive campaigns, rather than in providing high-level care to a fortunate few.[72] Although excellent Church-supported hospitals continue to this day to operate in many parts of the world, their importance for medical care in poor countries in general has for all these reasons become increasingly marginal.

[71] H. H. W. B., "Perils and Pressures", *Saving Health*, September 1973, 45.

[72] James C. McGilvray, *The Quest for Health and Wholeness* (Tübingen: German Institute for Medical Missions, 1981), 50–51.

7

Medicine and Witchcraft in South Africa: Initiatives at Victoria Hospital, Lovedale

Anne Digby

Thirty one years ago [in 1898] this hospital was started as a venture of faith. At that time there was no hospital [e]specially for natives south of the Zambezi and no natives were being trained as nurses. The pioneer days were difficult. At the outset native patients were afraid to enter the hospital and native women would not undertake nursing. The change in these three decades is tremendous. Four times the hospital has had to be enlarged; some twelve thousand in-patients have been treated in its wards; almost 100,000 out-patient attendances have been dealt with; twenty-six native probationers are in training today. . . . The trained native nurses who have gone out are doing good service in town locations and other centres in the four provinces of the Union and in South-West Africa.[1]

Victoria Hospital, Lovedale was situated near the eastern frontier of South Africa, which from the early eighteenth century had been a zone of interpenetration where contact between white and black increased, continual friction escalated periodically into war, and the government tried different strategies to stabilise the frontier.[2] Vig-

[1] Stewart papers, funding appeal, Cory MS 16,457 n.d. (1929), Rhodes University (henceforth RU).

[2] Monica Wilson, "Cooperation and Conflict: The Eastern Cape Frontier", in *The Oxford History of South Africa*, ed. M. Wilson and L. Thompson (Oxford: Oxford University Press, 1969), 1: 233, 238; L. Switzer, *Power and Resistance in an African Society* (Madison: Wisconsin University Press, 1993), 43; W. M. Macmillan, *Bantu, Boer, and Briton: The Making of the South African Native Problem* (Oxford: Clarendon Press, 1929), 20, 27, 41, 53–54; Anne Kelk Mager, *Gender and the Making of a South African Bantustan: A Social History of the Ciskei, 1945–1959* (Oxford and Cape Town: James Curry, 1999), 1–5;

orous missionary activity also occurred on and beyond the frontier, and it was near a frontier military station at Fort Hare that the Lovedale missionary institution was created in 1826 by the Glasgow Missionary Society (which soon after joined the Free Church of Scotland or FCS.) The Governor of the Cape Colony, Sir George Grey, had developed an assimilationist strategy within a segregationist spatial framework in which the local African population—the Xhosa—were to benefit from the colonial order through an innovatory development of education and medicine. Grey decided to set up a pioneering hospital in the main frontier of King Williams Town as a showcase for 'Western' medicine.

Dr John Fitzgerald was chosen to head this agency, and in 1858 a 120-bed Native Hospital (later re-christened the Grey Hospital), opened its doors.[3] The hospital was envisaged as an important instrument of Western civilisation with Fitzgerald enthusiastically adopting his role as agent of empire.[4] Fitzgerald intended his work to "destroy a great and diabolical delusion." "By keeping one object ever in view, viz., the cure of the sick, that witchcraft and witch doctors in a few years will cease to have much influence within the sphere of our practice."[5] Indeed, in what became a classic trope in such accounts, Fitzgerald pointed to an African traditional doctor who "consulted and received medical treatment."[6] Significantly, Fitzgerald stressed that he practised a secular medicine, recording that "I told the natives that we were here for the Body and not for the Soul".[7] Although opposed to the witch doctor, Victoria Hos-

Allan Lester, "The Margins of Order: Strategies of Segregation on the Eastern Cape Frontier, 1806–1850", *Journal of Southern African Studies* 23, no. 4, 1993, 638, 650–51.

[3] J. P. Fitzgerald MRCS (England), MD (Glasgow); D. Gordon, "Science, Superstition and Colonialism: Disease and Therapy at King Williams Town, Xhosaland, 1847–91" (unpublished paper).

[4] Letter to resident magistrate, 12 March 1858, letter books of J. P. Fitzgerald, Cory PR 3624, RU.

[5] Letter book entry, 23 May 1856, and May 1858, Cory, PR 3624, RU.

[6] Letter book entry, 30 September 1856, Cory PR 3624, RU.

[7] Letter book entries, 8 October 1857, 3 August 1856, and 8 June 1856, Cory PR 3624, RU.

pital, Lovedale that opened 50 kilometres away in 1898, envisaged the biomedical treatment of a patient providing the opportunity for Christian conversion.

Cultural Frontiers

The missionary ethos and philosophy of the founding educational institution of Lovedale permeated its later creation—Victoria Hospital—and the two coexisted symbiotically with overlapping membership of their governing bodies. Principal James Stewart's clear but paternalistic vision for Lovedale—later carried over into Victoria Hospital—fused a religious imperative with secular improvement. "We try to fit young men and women to become useful and industrious citizens and to become also missionaries of Christianity and civilisation to other natives of Africa."[8] In educating pupils from fourteen ethnicities in one school, Lovedale showed to the outside world the potential of building a common society in South Africa.[9] But Lovedale's role was ambiguous in that, while the institution broadly supported black aspirations, it subtly limited them by making its backing conditional on activity being congruent with the mission's overall objectives. Hierarchical but caring relationships institutionalised a view of African culture as deficient. A distinguished alumnus, Z. K. Matthews (later Professor of African Affairs at Fort Hare), recollected his brief schooling at Lovedale (1916–18) in

> the resentment we felt at the implied acceptance of the inferiority of Africans as students and as people. This was an integral part of the atmosphere of the school as a whole, which was one of a highly self-conscious benevolence. Its avowed purpose was to do things *for* Africans, and Africans . . . were not supposed to allow any extraneous feelings of our own to get in the way of the essential emotion of gratitude.[10]

[8] James Wells, *Stewart of Lovedale* (London: Hodder and Stoughton, 1909), 198.

[9] Z. K. Matthews, *Freedom for My People: The Autobiography of Z. K. Mathews; Southern Africa, 1901–1906*, ed. M. Wilson (Cape Town: David Philip, 1983), 35; F. Wilson and D. Perrot, eds., *Outlook on a Century: South Africa, 1870–1970* (Braamfontein: Lovedale Press, 1973), 11.

[10] Matthews, *Freedom for My People,* 42.

In Matthews' view Lovedale failed to show that it was "possible for black and white to live together and work *with* one another as equals in practice as well as in theory". [11] Lovedale missionaries and teachers were concerned to imprint the mission's distinctive ideas on the people of the surrounding area and when they encountered traditional African cultural attitudes or practices, they attempted to exclude them as undesirable. [12] Despite its humanitarian and liberal reputation Lovedale and its later institution, the Victoria Hospital, could thus play a culturally coercive role. [13]

This socially conservative view—of a limited African agency that needed continued European oversight—became increasingly outdated. It was made redundant by the success of Lovedale and Victoria Hospital themselves in helping to create a black elite, as well as by wider changes in society by the mid-twentieth century that had produced a self-confident and assertive black political agenda. So a liberal paternalism that elite pupils and student nurses would once have seen as protective or supportive, could appear to members of later cohorts as oppressive, although staff still continued to see their actions as altruistic. From the 1940s—when what staff perceived to be legitimate authority was interpreted by students or nurses as tipping over into undesirable social control—a crisis of incompatible expectations sparked unrest. [14]

[11] Mathews, *Freedom for My People*, 44–45.

[12] *Isidimi*, February 1871; J. Opland, "The Drumbeat of the Cross", in *Christianity in South Africa,* ed. R. Elphick and R. Davenport (Oxford: James Currey, 1997), 308.

[13] W. A. Saayman, *A Man with a Shadow: The Life and Times of Professor Z. K. Mathews; A Missiological Interpretation in Context* (Pretoria: Unisa Press, 1996), 27–28.

[14] P. Ntantala, *A Life's Mosaic: The Autobiography of Phyllis Ntantala* (Bellville: Mayibuye Centre, 1992), 122–23; Mager, *Gender and the Making of a South African Bantustan*, 197–205; Shula Marks, *Divided Sisterhood: Race, Class and Gender in the South African Nursing Profession* (Johannesburg: Witwatersrand University Press, 1994), 111; Helen Sweet and Anne Digby, "Race, Identity and the Nursing Profession in South Africa, 1850–1958", in *New Directions in the History of Nursing: International Perspectives,* ed. B. Mortimer and S. McGann (London: Routledge, 2005), 113–20.

In tracing this history of Lovedale in order to provide the context for more specifically medical events, this narrative has moved ahead of the chronology of medical development. Even before Victoria Hospital opened in 1898, the medical work of Dr James Stewart, Principal of Lovedale (1870–1905) displayed the effectiveness of 'Western' medicine to local people. James Stewart had been inspired by David Livingstone, who had said, "I have opened the door; I leave it to you to see that no-one closes it after me." Stewart was sufficiently motivated by Livingstone's visit to Scotland in 1857, to begin a course of medical training at Edinburgh to fit himself for work in Africa. He interrupted his studies for a couple of years for a journey to Central Africa and then South Africa where he visited Lovedale. Stewart confided to his journal that "I have the impression that I have a work to do in this quarter of the world." Doubtless his commitment would have been strengthened by Livingstone's personal letter to him stating that "The effects of missions are cumulative. You here begin a work which in influence and power will go on increasing to the end of time. . . . Africa must be Christianised from within outwards." Stewart believed that biomedicine was invaluable to the white man in Africa in this process of conversion, because it would open closed doors to him, and oppose what was perceived as the malignant influence of the witch doctor. He thus had every motivation to resume his medical studies in 1864 before qualifying two years later, and in the following year taking up an appointment at Lovedale. [15] During his first two decades there Dr Stewart developed a large medical practice although, as he became ever busier with the general administration of a growing institution, these activities diminished.

Stewart's personal charisma drew very able people to work at Lovedale, including Jane Waterston, who became the first Lady Superintendent of the girls' boarding school in 1867. Soon deciding that medicine rather than education should be her priority, Waterston returned to Britain to seek medical qualification. [16] When the combined medical and educational post that the Free Church

[15] Wells, *Stewart of Lovedale*, 21–36, 54, 86, 92–97.

[16] Licentiate of KQCPI, 1878; MD Bruxelles, 1888, LRCS, Edinburgh.

of Scotland (FCS) had designated for her (at Livingstonia on Lake Nyasa in Central Africa) did not work out, because the presence of an existing doctor meant that she found little medical work to do, she came back to Lovedale in 1880. But those in mission headquarters in Scotland did not absolve her from breaking her engagement in leaving her post, and so declined to sanction a medical mission at Lovedale. James Stewart then set up a dispensary for her to run at Lovedale but without Scottish mission funding.[17] Waterston was therefore forced to support herself from private medical practice, although most of her time and energy was devoted to the Lovedale Dispensary where she treated over six thousand cases during her first two years. "This large amount of human suffering would [otherwise] have gone unrelieved or fallen into the hands of native or witch doctors", commented Dr Stewart.[18]

Clinical Work

James Stewart had wished to found a medical mission, a hospital, possibly a medical school, but for almost two decades the FCS mission headquarters gave no encouragement to these aspirations.[19] A breakthrough came when funds collected for Queen Victoria's Jubilee were skilfully built up, thereby enabling one of the first mission hospitals in South Africa to open in 1898.[20] Under the dedicated superintendence of Neil Macvicar, who came in 1902 and stayed until his retirement in 1937, the hospital became a national institution.[21]

[17] Note by Dr Stewart on medical missions, 1883, accession 7548 D80, National Library of Scotland (henceforth NLS).

[18] In order to make an adequate medical living, Waterston was forced to move to Cape Town. R. H. W. Shepherd, *Lovedale South Africa: The Story of a Century, 1841–1941* (Lovedale: Lovedale Press, 1941), 152–53.

[19] James Stewart on Lovedale Medical Mission, 18 September 1902, accession 7548 D 80, NLS ; R. H. W. Shepherd, *A South African Health Pioneer* (Lovedale: Lovedale Press, 1952), 81.

[20] The first South African mission hospital was started by the Swiss Mission in the northern Transvaal in 1896 and this was moved to Elim three years later.

[21] Shepherd, *A South African Health Pioneer,* 82–84.

Neil Macvicar (1871–1949) belonged to a later generation of missionaries than James Stewart and Jane Waterston, although like them he came from a Scottish background, and saw medicine as the most powerful tool for helping the African. He had qualified with first class honours in medicine in 1894 at Edinburgh University, and then did six months additional specialist study on eyes and their diseases.[22] Before coming to Victoria Hospital he had worked as a medical missionary for the Church of Scotland at Blantyre in Nyasaland, developing an interest in African diseases and native medicines, as well as in the training of African medical auxiliaries. So closely was Macvicar identified with the hospital that local people called it *Kwa Mavikala* [at Macvicar's].[23] His achievements received public recognition including a 90-bed Neil Macvicar Tuberculosis Hospital built by the government next door to Victoria Hospital.

Victoria Hospital increased from the 20-bed institution of 1902 to 175 beds by 1937. There were six enlargements during Macvicar's time, with notable expansions in 1928 and 1934 to provide specialist maternity, TB and VD facilities. In 1904 the hospital changed its character through ceasing to admit white patients because of the unseemly behaviour of some white male patients to trainee African nurses. Although the Cape Provincial Council matched any funds raised by Victoria/Lovedale, the hospital still experienced periodic financial difficulties. Despite this it was stated that no patient was refused treatment because of inability to pay. Victoria Hospital aimed "to meet the needs of the surrounding native population . . . [and] refuse no class of case . . . admitting all the usual diseases, surgical and medical."[24] The first African patients reacted very positively to its treatments and, for example, after successful minor surgery to extract a needle stuck in a woman's leg, the patient and her friends:

> Gave a startling shout and began to kiss the doctor's hands, his coat, his boots and anything else belonging to him that they could reach . . . and

[22] MB, CM (1894, Edinburgh), MD (1907, Edinburgh), DPH and RCPS (Edinburgh and Glasgow)

[23] "Obituary of Dr Macvicar", *Health Magazine* 126, February 1950; Archibald Scott to Dr MacVicar, 17 June 1898, MS 7535, letter 867, NLS.

[24] *South African Outlook,* 1 June 1934.

> departed with profuse thanks and promises to tell their friends about the hospital, and to do them justice they did so, as the number of patients who applied from their district for admission to the hospital proved.[25]

Improved facilities resulted in even more patients seeking treatment. The return in 1928 of the Macvicar's daughter, Shena, now surgically-qualified, led to surgical operations increasing by 160 per cent in a single year, and in-patient numbers by 90 per cent. Figure 7.1 indicates numbers of in- and out-patients. Compared with other mission hospitals Victoria Hospital treated a high proportion of in-patients, with a ratio of 1: 3.8 of those treated in hospital wards relative to those in the out-patients department. On average an out-patient made two visits to the out-patients department, but in 1918–19 during the influenza pandemic and its aftermath, the ratio of in-patients to out-patients fell to 1: 7 while out-patients made as many as three to four visits each.

The disease profile of cases admitted to the hospital showed distinctive features (see table 7.1). Malnutrition cases and those of tuberculosis were important. In the early years syphilis was of little significance but by the 1930s patients presented it more commonly: Macvicar surmised that this was perhaps less a matter of changing incidence than of fashion.[26] Respiratory conditions (influenza and broncho-pneumonia) were very evident, and showed the effect of climatic conditions, so that a wet, cold winter such as that in 1932 led to a rise in cases. Epidemics, such as that of louse typhus in 1920–21, meant that Victoria Hospital became "to a large extent a fever hospital".[27] Over time obstetric and gynaecological cases gradually became more important. Macvicar's expertise in eye diseases also meant that many patients came to seek his help in operations for cataract and trachoma.[28] Dr Macvicar cautiously acknowledged the

[25] Stewart papers, Cory, MS 16, 457, RU.

[26] *South African Outlook,* 1 January 1933, and 1 February 1935.

[27] Ibid., 1 June 1934.

[28] G. B. A. Gerdener, *Recent Developments in the South African Mission Field* (Cape Town and Pretoria: N. G. Kerk-Uitgers, 1958), 70.

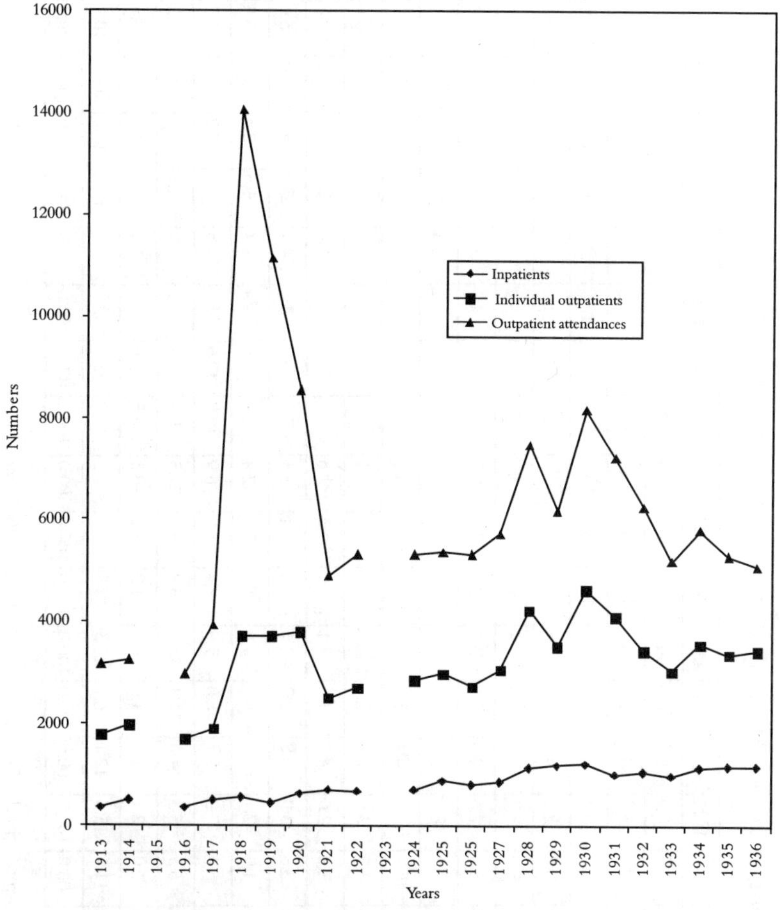

Figure 7.1 Patient numbers at Victoria Hospital, 1913–36

Source: "Annual Reports of Victoria Hospital", in the *Christian Express* and the *South African Outlook*.

impact of the hospital's surgical work. "European surgery especially is a revelation to natives".[29]

[29] N. Macvicar, *Side-lights upon Superstition* (Lovedale: Lovedale Press, 1939), 18–19.

TABLE 7.1: Diseases of in-patients at Victoria Hospital, 1918–36 (%)

	1918	1919	1921	1922	1924	1925	1926	1927	1928	1929	1930	1931	1932	1933	1934	1935	1936
Syphilis	0.0	0.0	0.0	0.0	0.0	0.0	0.0	2.6	3.4	5.6	6.9	5.3	7.7	7.3	5.6	5.8	5.3
TB	22.1	19.7	23.4	24.0	22.5	20.4	19.0	19.1	16.9	17.7	18.0	16.5	14.5	17.7	14.8	18.4	20.7
Flu, broncho-pneumonia	20.0	12.7	9.4	13.8	17.2	10.4	19.8	14.9	10.1	12.9	12.3	13.9	19.5	9.5	11.0	13.9	11.4
Nervous	2.2	3.6	2.7	4.1	2.4	3.8	2.9	3.6	2.3	1.5	1.7	1.5	1.9	1.6	1.9	2.6	3.1
Eye	5.4	5.0	7.7	7.4	7.4	7.4	7.6	6.1	5.7	5.6	5.7	4.8	4.1	5.5	4.9	5.6	4.8
ENT	6.0	5.0	2.6	2.4	1.6	3.6	2.7	2.4	2.6	3.7	4.7	4.3	5.1	4.5	4.1	2.9	3.2
Typhus, enteric fever	1.0	6.8	8.0	2.2	7.3	3.2	4.4	3.4	9.2	6.6	3.5	5.1	5.5	10.9	9.7	2.3	4.1
Enteritis, dysentery	5.0	10.3	4.5	4.4	3.8	7.3	3.4	4.3	5.1	3.3	1.7	2.7	2.5	2.2	2.9	3.4	1.7
Suppurations, septic	2.3	3.9	3.6	2.5	2.6	2.5	1.7	2.0	2.7	4.3	4.2	3.3	2.6	3.6	3.7	4.1	3.6
Skin disease, blood	1.7	2.9	2.0	4.7	1.6	2.1	2.1	1.3	1.6	2.2	1.2	1.8	1.4	2.3	3.3	3.9	2.8
Accident, assault	2.5	3.6	3.9	3.8	2.7	3.1	5.4	4.1	3.1	3.9	5.2	4.3	4.9	5.0	5.6	4.0	5.6
Heart disease, blood	2.5	1.9	2.1	3.3	0.7	1.5	1.9	2.0	2.4	2.0	1.9	4.4	2.4	1.6	2.4	3.5	3.5
Gynaecological, obstetrics	8.9	6.4	7.2	9.7	8.0	7.9	9.4	6.9	6.9	10.0	12.5	11.7	10.5	11.6	12.7	12.8	13.7
Malnutrition (scurvy, debility)	4.4	6.3	5.3	4.6	14.4	13.9	5.9	16.1	21.5	9.4	6.7	6.2	5.4	4.1	2.4	4.0	5.2
Cancer	1.2	1.0	2.1	1.1	1.3	0.6	1.2	1.2	0.3	0.5	1.0	1.1	1.2	1.1	1.0	0.9	0.6
Miscellaneous	14.8	11.1	15.5	12.1	6.7	12.3	12.5	9.9	6.2	10.9	13.0	13.1	10.9	11.5	13.8	11.9	10.7
Total	100.0	100.0	100.0	100.0	100.0	100.0	100.0	100.0	100.0	100.0	100.0	100.0	100.0	100.0	100.0	100.0	100.0

Source: "Annual Reports of Victoria Hospital", in the *Christian Express* and the *South African Outlook*.

Macvicar was one of the first doctors in South Africa to produce sufficient data to elicit scientific conclusions. In the *Journal of Tropical Medicine* in June 1904 he gave an account of 2739 patients treated over a fourteen month period for a variety of diseases. And in November 1932 he published an article in the *South African Medical Journal* on "The Prevalence of Certain Diseases Among the Natives of the Ciskei." This used data quantified from 1913 to show trends in disease among in-patients in Victoria Hospital including that in enteric fever (varied incidence), malnutrition or diet deficiency diseases (drought-related frequency), typhus fever (epidemic flare ups that burnt themselves out), and pulmonary TB (a steady prevalence). See figure 7.2.

Dr Macvicar had a particular interest in tuberculosis, writing his MD thesis on the subject in 1907 and publishing the thesis as *Tuberculosis Among the South African Natives.* In 1935 Macvicar wrote an article on "Tuberculosis of Bones and Joints in Native Patients in the Ciskei" based on an analysis of patients from 1927 to 1935. These patients formed one-fifth of the TB cases in the hospital, but only 3.5 per cent of the total in-patients. Macvicar described innovative treatment, in that patients were moved on to open air verandas and balconies to obtain sunshine, and also benefited from a nourishing diet and a liberal ration of milk. He admitted that he had also wanted to publish the after results of treatment but had been disappointed at the results of a postal survey to former patients and their families, which had produced only a few responses. [30] Victoria Hospital developed specialist expertise in tuberculosis, more particularly for child sufferers, which was one of the particular interests of Sheena Ross (formerly Macvicar).

> Tuberculosis cripple children are being brought in increasing numbers. They spend all their time on their frames in the open air. . . . They improve wonderfully and are very lively. The row of little girls form a choir, always happy to sing to visitors. The little boys play at being a band. . . . It is fair to say that they also do lessons. [31]

[30] N. Macvicar, "Tuberculosis of Bones and Joints in Native Patients in the Ciskei", *South African Medical Journal*, 28 September 1935, 643–45.

[31] *South African Outlook*, 2 February 1931.

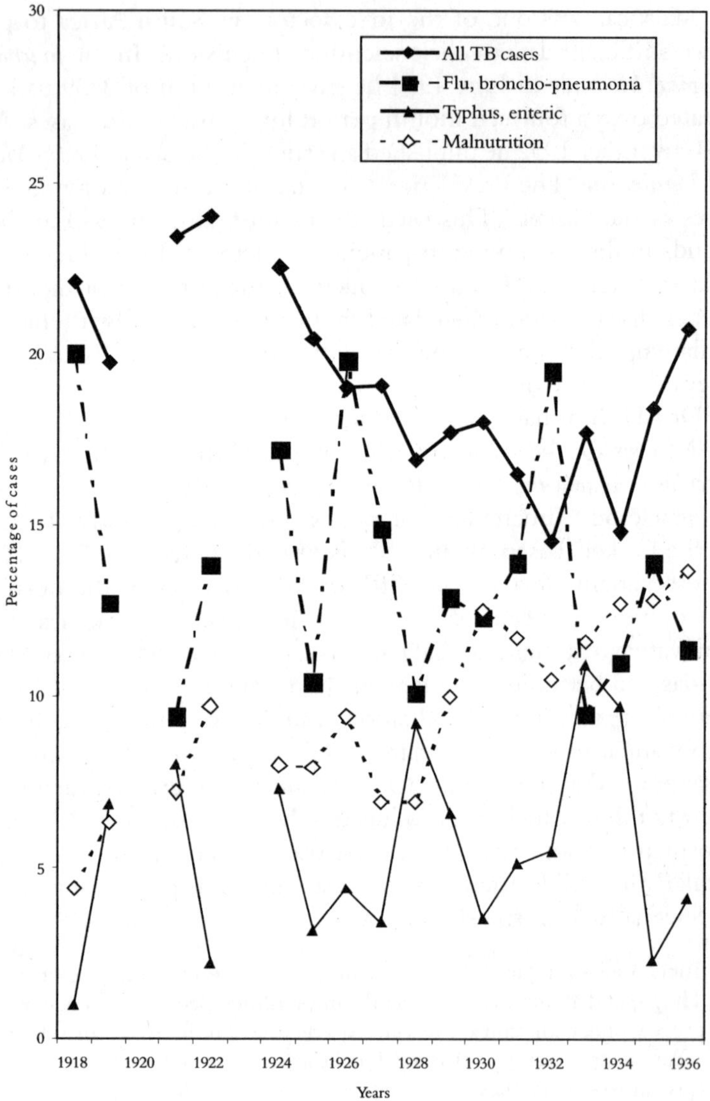

Figure 7.2 Selected diseases among in-patients at Victoria Hospital

Source: N. Macvicar, "The Prevalence of Certain Diseases Among the Natives of the Ciskei", *South African Medical Journal* 25, 26 November 1932, 721–23; "Annual Reports of Victoria Hospital", in the *Christian Express* and the *South African Outlook*.

Most cases spent three years at the hospital, benefiting from the specialist care and good nutrition with lots of fresh air. Even some apparently hopeless cases went home well. New accommodation was opened in 1934 for those

> suffering from tuberculous spinal disease, hip disease and other forms of chronic surgical tuberculosis. The whole of the two new central first floor wards with their wide balcony is already occupied by about seventy children. Most of these little cripples lie on Bradford frames mounted on short legs. With open air, sunshine and an abundance of milk, the majority make good progress and ultimately go home cured.[32]

It was thought that the "heavy hand" of tuberculosis on the local people would not improve until their housing conditions were improved.[33]

Macvicar considered that "A people's diseases reflect their social condition. The prevalence of tuberculosis is a sure sign of poor nutrition."[34] Indeed, the diseases at the hospital, particularly the high incidence of scurvy and debility, signalled the socio-economic distress of the Ciskei. These malnutrition cases were perceived to be related to the drought conditions, which tipped already precarious household budgets into near destitution so that people lived solely on maize. Serious droughts afflicted the area in 1905, 1915–16, 1924 and 1936 but the 'great drought' was during 1926–28. Figure 7.3 indicates the upswing of malnutrition cases following the drought years (marked with an asterisk.) In 1906 in the pages of the *South African Medical Record,* Macvicar had analysed thirty-five cases of what Africans called *umtshetsha*, which had been treated at Victoria Hospital between January and October 1905, during a severe drought. He showed that these were cases of scurvy produced by insufficient fresh food and argued that patients recovered with an anti-scorbutic dietary regimen of lemons and oranges, together with some use of opium for the alleviation of pain.[35] Ten years

[32] *South African Outlook*, 1 June 1934.

[33] *Christian Express*, 2 February 1920.

[34] *South African Outlook*, 1 February 1935.

[35] N. Macvicar, "Notes on Scurvy", *South African Medical Record*, 25 April 1906, 101–3.

later Dr Macvicar concluded that in many families there had been a deficiency in quantity of food consumed but that the chief trouble came from its inferior quality, and the want of fresh food—especially milk—unobtainable because cattle had died for lack of grass. But he warned that "scurvy is a painful reality never very far away from them."[36] In the previous year, 1915, he observed the effects of the drought on the hospital's patients:

> When the fresh food famine reached its most acute stage, many women came . . . some with swollen legs hardly able to walk, with bleeding gums and loose teeth. . . . Besides such cases of definite scurvy, there has been noticeable a general lowering of vitality. Anaemia and debility have been prevalent. . . . Another serious aspect of the poor food problem is the influence exercised by malnutrition upon the course of other diseases. This has been a bad year for consumptives. . . . Influenza has been if anything more troublesome than usual, while dysentery has not failed to follow its usual practice of attacking the victims of scurvy and general debility.[37]

The hospital again had unprecedented numbers of malnutrition cases in 1927. "Men and women were brought to the hospital and crept painfully into the waiting room, their legs swollen with the haemorrhages of scurvy." Nurses gave patients lemons, oranges and sweet potatoes, and managed to save lives, particularly of children.[38] Opportunistic infections then preyed on malnourished bodies. Sheena Ross analysed 208 patients admitted with scurvy, who were treated with lemon and orange juice, but whose condition was complicated by bronchitis and broncho-pneumonia. She showed how little children suffered the worst effects of malnutrition, with 8 out of the 9 deaths being of children under three years old.[39] In 1928 enteric fever followed the drought, while in addition there were high numbers of cases of TB. Later, in 1936, not only were there nine deaths from malnutrition, and another nine where

[36] *Christian Express*, 1 January 1916.

[37] Ibid.

[38] *South African Outlook*, 1 March 1928.

[39] S. Ross, "Scurvy in Native Children", *South African Medical Journal*, 26 September 1931, 596–99.

malnutrition was a major factor in the cause of death, but there was also an even larger number of cases of influenza-bronchitis-pneumonia, with 200 admissions and 32 deaths.[40] (See figure 7.2 and table 7.1) Significantly, although drought was highlighted as a cause of under nutrition, the grossly unequal entitlement of Africans to land was not.[41]

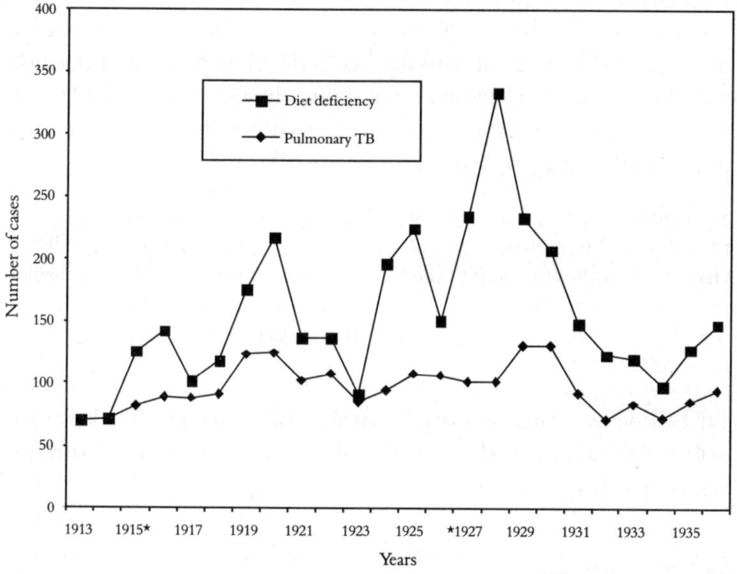

Figure 7.3 Disease and drought, 1913–36

Source: "Annual Reports of Victoria Hospital", in the *Christian Express* and the *South African Outlook*.

In evidence to the Native Economic Commission in 1930–32, however, Macvicar noted the long-term deterioration in condition of the people in the Ciskei, around Lovedale, and its effect on hos-

[40] *South African Outlook,* 1 February 1937.

[41] Diana Wylie, *Starving on a Full Stomach: Hunger and the Triumph of Cultural Racism in Modern South Africa* (Charlottesville: Virginia University Press, 2001) for a fuller treatment of these issues.

pital admissions.[42] One factor was a demographic increase from nearly 245- to almost 335-thousand people between 1911 and 1951, and an ensuing density of population rising from 53 to 72 per square mile.[43] In Middledrift only 20 kilometres from Victoria Hospital, Dr Rosebery Bokwe practised in an extremely poverty-stricken area that had been designated under the Group Areas Act of 1913 for an exclusively black population, and which was dependent for economic survival on the remittances of migrant labour. The area had been described by the commission as "a desolate picture of denudation and erosion."[44] During a prolonged drought in 1945 Dr Bokwe wrote about the intense deprivation suffered by his patients in an article called simply, but dramatically "We are Starving":

> *Siyalamba* [we are starving] is a word one hears often. Nor did one have to hear it said to believe it, it is all too plainly written on those raggedly-clad, sickly bodies brought to me for that bottle of medicine. Few . . . will realise how heart-rending it is to many a medical man to have to dole out 'a bottle' when he knows only too well that all that that poor soul needs is FOOD.[45]

Dr Bokwe was one of a small number of registered black doctors in South Africa, and had been schooled at Lovedale in a distinctive missionary ethos of service.[46]

A Mission Hospital

Beyond its obvious medical rationale the hospital had more subtle objectives, linking 'Western' medicine to the kind of civilising role

42 *Report of Native Economic Commission*, 38, paragraph 62, p. 183, UG22- 1932, South African Union government papers, University of Cape Town Library.

43 "Union Statistics", *Jubilee Issue, 1910–1960* (Pretoria: Government Printer, 1960), table A9.

44 F. Wilson, *Migrant Labour in South Africa* (Johannesburg: South African Council of Churches, 1972), 102–3; *Report of the Native Economic Commission*, 38, UG22-1932, South African Union government papers .

45 Wilson and Perrot, *Outlook on a Century*, 427.

46 Anne Digby, "Early Black Doctors in South Africa", *Journal of African History* 46, 2005, 427–54.

earlier discussed at Grey Hospital. Macvicar assumed that civilisation and hygiene were intimately related when he reflected that "even a short stay is sufficient to introduce the patient to a hygienic mode of life, daily baths, regular meals, fresh air. It is difficult to estimate fully the civilising influence of a hospital. The consumptive patient also learns those simple precautions that are necessary to protect other people from infection."[47] Not that all patients either entered its doors without fear (since initially Africans associated the hospital with death rather than healing), or accepted treatment in the 'white man's' hospital comfortably. Sick children were particularly problematic. Despite earlier optimistic views that resistance to hospital treatment had abated, parents were either reluctant or opposed to their children staying in Victoria Hospital for treatment. Hence in 1946 a doctor noted that Annette Jawie "was sent to hospital in May but at that time mother would not allow child to remain [for] hos[pital] observation. Child now appears worse and mother agrees that it is necessary child may remain at hospital." This little girl had pulmonary TB and was put on the waiting list for the Macvicar TB Hospital. And, in the following year, Sipelo Zozi had acute broncho-pneumonia but Dr Letele (one of the early cohort of black doctors educated within South Africa), noted with concern that "The father is unwilling to have the child treated in hospital, and it [*sic*] is therefore in grave danger at the moment."[48]

Culturally and geographically, Victoria Hospital was sited on a border between modernity and tradition:

> It is a mission hospital: the atmosphere is definitely Christian. Morning and evening prayers are held in the wards daily. Sunday services are conducted by the doctors, and native evangelists pay regular visits to the patients. Each year over 1,300 patients, many of them from heathen homes where they have little contact with Christian teaching and life, spend varying periods in the hospital and are frequently visited by their relatives and friends. There is no doubt that the religious influence of the hospital is felt in a wide circle of native homes and is broadcast over the land by our trained nurses.[49]

[47] *South African Outlook*, 1 February 1923.

[48] Medical reports, 29 July 1946, and 22 January 1947, Cory 16,458 RU.

[49] Stewart papers, Cory, MS 16, 457, RU.

Victoria Hospital called itself "the pioneer mission hospital in the country", and considered its missionary character "the mainspring of its success." [50] At first the hospital was much more successful in winning the confidence of Christian than heathen patients, so that in 1914, for example, only 8 per cent of its in-patients were non-Christian. [51] Two decades later, it was different and Dr Macvicar reflected that

> each year over a thousand persons, many of them from heathen homes who otherwise have little or no contact with Christian teaching or life, spend periods of varying length as members of what is really a big Christian family, and [as] . . . they are frequently visited by their near relatives, one cannot doubt that the religious influence of the hospital is felt in a very wide circle of native homes. [52]

Between 1928 and 1935 the hospital had the evangelising assistance of Mrs Bokwe as an African Bible woman who chose to highlight heathen people in her reports. [53] "One old heathen woman with an incurable disease when taken back to her heathen kraal told her husband it was not her wish to have heathen practices done on her as she had now received the word of God at the hospital." [54] Mrs Bokwe was convinced that in-patients had "thankful hearts" for the doctors' work, and that "with God's help the medicine given them would help their ailing bodies." [55] Macvicar described how in his work as a medical missionary:

> Daily contact with the people led . . . to a deepening sense of the mental and spiritual distress that in many cases complicated or underlay their physical ills. Two convictions were formed. One that it was the duty of the doctor, the medical missionary, to speak to the people and pray with them. . . . The other conviction was that at this stage . . . when . . . the backward stress and pull of their old faith are still strong, their supreme

[50] *South African Outlook*, 1 February 1929, and 1 February 1938.

[51] *Christian Express*, 1 February 1915.

[52] *South African Outlook*, 1 February 1935.

[53] Mrs Bokwe was the mother of Dr Rosebery Bokwe.

[54] *South African Outlook*, 1 February 1933.

[55] Ibid., 1 February 1930.

> need is to gain a secure consciousness of God. It was with this specially in mind that passages were selected for the daily ward prayers.[56]

Religious activity paralleled the hospital's biomedicine and was intended to give it personal meaning. And this may have been welcome to African patients, who customarily sought an individual rationale for their illness from indigenous healers, and who usually found 'Western' medicine deficient in not providing one.

The hospital increasingly directed its efforts at outreach. In 1928 a system of branch dispensaries was set up in outlying villages, with a motor ambulance provided for urgent cases needing to be brought into hospital. Four years later a clinic was opened for out-patients at a neighbouring village, where ante-natal and child welfare clinics were held by the hospital matron and senior nurses.[57] By the 1940s "Ante-natal clinics and a district maternity service are run in connection with the Maternity Training School, and country clinics are conducted by one of the medical staff. At these clinics which are held twice a week, the attendance sometimes exceeds 100, and arrangements have been made for the daily supply of milk to sick children."[58] Out-patients at the hospital's dispensary far outnumbered in-patients, and thus offered a greater opportunity for evangelism. Some came from the 'Red people' [*ababomvu*]; Africans who used a mixture of red ochre and animal fat on their bodies (to protect against the cold and sunburn) and who retained their traditional culture, in contrast to the 'School' or Christian African, who may well have outnumbered them at the clinic.[59] Much of the hospital's evangelistic effort was devoted to these 'Red people'.[60]

Outreach also took the form of health education linking 'unhygienic' cultural practices to superstition. Macvicar had founded a

56 Macvicar, *Side-lights upon Superstition*, 57–58.

57 *South African Outlook,* 1 February 1933, and 1 February 1934.

58 Stewart papers, Cory, MS 16, 457 [post 1940] RU.

59 L. Bank, "Beyond Red and School: Gender, Tradition and Identity in the Rural Eastern Cape", *Journal of Southern African Studies* 28, no. 3, 2002, 631–49.

60 *South African Outlook,* 1 February 1929, 1 February 1931, and 1 February 1933.

Native Health Society in 1909, became its first President and provided the dynamism behind it. The society issued twelve pamphlets or leaflets. Most were in one—or more—of four African languages, featuring diseases such as scurvy, consumption, syphilis and malaria (brought by migrant workers from Natal sugar plantations); as well as health advice on the spread of TB, facts about alcohol, housing and health. These were sent out to all schools with African pupils in the Cape Province, but apparently attracted little interest elsewhere, except from the Native Affairs Department.[61] Later, the Health Society published a trilingual, quarterly *Health Magazine* to replace the leaflets, and which it was hoped would produce "apostles of health."[62] In addition, Macvicar wrote a *Health Reader* for Standard III pupils, where he attempted to make the lessons "simple and practical", and this was used "throughout a great part of South Africa".[63] In addition a health class was begun for senior Lovedale pupils where over the years Macvicar gave instruction to hundreds. In these activities the doctor came to understand the need for him to act as a cultural intermediary. "My chief difficulty has been to understand the native standpoint on many of the subjects touched. In putting forward new European ideas one must bring them into relation with the already existing native ideas, as without this no change in the opinions or habits of the people can be looked for."[64] This insight would have been invaluable in the hospital's pioneering work of training African nurses.

Training African Nurses

Those at Victoria Hospital intended to do more than give nurses a technical training in 'Western' medicine in aiming to turn out nurse missionaries who would work in African communities.[65] Neil

[61] *Christian Express*, 1 October 1912, and 2 February 1914.

[62] Shepherd, *A South African Health Pioneer*, 128.

[63] N. Macvicar, Preface to *Health Reader for Standard Three* (Lovedale: Lovedale Press, 1911).

[64] Macvicar, Preface to *Health Reader*.

[65] Anne Digby, *Diversity and Division in Medicine: Health Care in South Africa from the 1800s* (Oxford and Bern: Peter Lang, 2006), 239–44.

Macvicar argued that "the influence of trained nurses was out of all proportion to their numbers . . . in dealing with superstition, as in dealing with infectious and contagious diseases, the native nurse's close contact with, and her intimate understanding of, the people gives her a position of unique influence."[66] The doctor thought that nurses did "Christ-like work."[67] The strategic role of Lovedale trained nurses was envisaged in these terms:

> Women who can deal intelligently and authoritatively with witchcraft and other superstitious ideas of disease are a new thing in native society. Other educated natives may personally disbelieve—many of them do—but when it comes to giving their reasons they lack data. Only doctors and nurses have the facts at their finger ends. And, as is well known, the belief in witchcraft as a cause of disease is one of the grossest and cruellest things in heathenism. Apart from what they each can do to mitigate suffering and save life, the service native nurses render to their people in the way of enlightenment is of first class importance. The influence of trained nurses is out of all proportion to their numbers.[68]

Macvicar gave two-hour lectures to the nurses in a classroom equipped for practical work with microscopes, a bacteriological incubator and anatomical aids. He believed that in showing the scientific nature of disease to nurses he could undercut belief in witchcraft as a cause of illness.[69] He acknowledged that African nurses needed more teaching than was usual, but was prepared to give this, as well as writing a textbook and a dictionary to help them.[70] The fact that nurses were recruited from 'Cape Coloureds', Xhosa, Zulu, Tswana, and Sotho maximised their subsequent influence as some

66 Macvicar, *Side-lights upon Superstition*, 55.

67 N. Macvicar, "The Training of the Native Hospital Nurse", *Christian Express*, 1 February 1919.

68 *South African Outlook,* 1 January 1936.

69 M. Gelfand, *Christian Doctor and Nurse: The History of Medical Missions in South Africa from 1799–1976* (Sandton: Mariannhill Mission Press, 1984), 77.

70 N. Macvicar, *Africa Tomorrow*? (Johannesburg: SAIRR, 1947), 91; N. Macvicar, *Outlines of Anatomy and Physiology for Nurses* (Lovedale: Lovedale Press, 1927); N. Macvicar, *English/Xhosa Nurses' Dictionary* (Lovedale: Lovedale Press, n.d.).

went back to work in—or near—their communities.[71] Employers' testimony on their Lovedale trained nurses included the observation that one was a keen missionary, while another commented on the nurse's role as cultural diplomat. "The growth of confidence in the [mission] hospital . . . was due in no small measure to the efficiency of her work . . . and particularly her sympathy and tact in dealing with the fears and difficulties of people to whom hospital treatment was a novelty."[72]

Victoria Hospital's first external success in nurse training came in January 1908 when Cecelia Makiwane, a former Lovedale pupil and Victoria Hospital trainee, became the first black nurse in South Africa to be admitted to the Cape nursing register. Numbers in training at Victoria Hospital grew from an annual total of 4 in 1908, to 10 in 1921, and 58 by 1939. By 1935 a total of 68 had been trained. During the early years trainees worked for the institution's own Hospital Certificate, although increasingly taking first the South African Medical Council's Junior Certificate in anatomy and physiology, and then the Nursing Certificate itself, which conferred registration by the medical council. The council recognised the worth of its enhanced training (now with a surgical component), and the hospital became a Class 1 Training School for Nurses in 1930. Up to 1930 only a small minority—7 out of 42—had become doubly qualified through taking a midwifery course at St Monica's, Cape Town. But more nurses wanted to achieve a double qualification, and so took midwifery courses at St Monica's, the Bridgman (Johannesburg), or McCord Zulu Mission Hospital (Durban), so that by 1936 twenty of them had gained a midwifery certificate.[73] The Victoria Hospital course also increased in length: first from three to three and a half years in 1928 (as a result of midwifery courses being added), and then to four years in 1933 (because of the desirability of giving trainees more practical experience in theatre duty, village clinics, out-patient duty, maternity cases, VD cases, and

71 *South African Outlook*, 1 February 1937.

72 Ibid., 1 February 1936.

73 Ibid.

dispensing).[74] This changing profile suggests that aspiration, ambition and a growing self-confidence became mutually supportive resulting in enhanced achievement. To some extent this was also helped by better entry qualifications, as more able girls competed to enter nurse training.[75]

Recruitment of able young women from the African (and in a few instances the mixed race 'Cape Coloured') communities, and accomplishment in vocational training, led to subsequent ability to find nursing employment. At first there had been a strong prejudice against African women training as nurses, both within their own community, and in the wider medical and nursing world, but gradually, "fully trained native nurses are being sent out in ones and twos to work among their people."[76] Dr Macvicar heroically battled prejudice and indifference in attempting to achieve employment for these nurses.[77] Of the 49 African nurses trained by 1931, 3 were employed in missionary institutions, 13 operated as district nurses in locations, 10 worked in hospitals, while 9 held posts in both hospitals and / or African locations.[78]

The nurse-training course gave a high priority to socialisation in which the trainee had to accept a rigorous discipline:

> Character training is the backbone of the nursing course, and it has been the task and privilege of the hospital to turn out good nurses who are at the same time good women, conscientious and skilful, liberated in mind from superstitious ideas of disease, and armed in soul to fight for and with people against the evils that degrade their personal and community life. Heathen people who at first were afraid to enter hospital, are now coming in increasing numbers.[79]

[74] Ibid.

[75] Ibid., 1 December 1932.

[76] Ibid., 1 February 1922.

[77] R. W. Shepherd, "Tribute to Neil Macvicar", *South African Outlook*, 1 January 1950; Gelfand, *Christian Doctor and Nurse*, 278.

[78] T. D. M. Skota, *The African Yearly Register* (Johannesburg: R. L. Esson, 1931), 83, 153, 219, and 281.

[79] N. Macvicar, "Retiring Address", *South African Outlook*, 1 February 1938.

The severe regime imposed by European staff on black nurses could provoke direct action against what might be seen—within the changed context of general black militancy of the late forties—as discriminatory, paternalistic and patriarchal. Strikes by nurses at the hospital occurred in 1949 and 1958 with unrest continuing during the early sixties. Strict discipline at Victoria Hospital and its associated institution of Lovedale had produced unanticipated results within a changing South Africa, where some nurses related an oppressive national government to a socially-conservative missionary regime.[80]

Training Medical Aids / Auxiliaries

As early as 1878 a report by an aide to the Cape Governor, Sir H. B. Frere, commended a medical course for African students at Lovedale in "Giving at once a legitimate career for the aspirations of the educated and ambitious native student, and at the same time striking a deadly blow at that symbol of all that is most detestable and cruel in the native economy, the witch doctor and his pretended services."[81] Educated Africans—such as D.D.T. Jabavu, Professor of Bantu Languages at Fort Hare—grew impatient at the very slow progress in providing trained African doctors for African needs through overseas training. "There are thousands of natives who live beyond the reach of white doctors in our country villages. . . . We need hundreds for many of the white ones no longer care to deal with natives."[82] But only a limited number of Africans managed to achieve full medical qualification abroad, amongst them the Lovedale educated William Soga, James Moroka, Silas Modiri Molema, and Rosebery Bokwe.

80 Mager, *Gender and the Making of a South African Bantustan*, 202; Marks, *Divided Sisterhood*, 110.

81 *Further Correspondence respecting the Affairs of South Africa: Report by Hon'ble Cecil Ashley,* C 2000, 1878, LV, no. 12, British Parliamentary Papers, Bodleian Library, Oxford.

82 D. D. T. Jabavu, *The Black Problem: Papers and Addresses on Various Native Problems* (Lovedale: Lovedale Press, 1920), 165–66.

The medical aids scheme won through after half a century of debate. Initially a three-year training was envisaged for medical aids although, given the disadvantaged educational background of the applicants, this was increased first to four and then to five years.[83] Medical aids were to be trained in sanitary science and preventive medicine, as well as being able to deal with cases of leprosy or malaria. Intake was envisaged as about twelve to fifteen per year, with a graduating cohort of ten. The programme was developed along similar lines to a full medical programme with sciences in the pre-medical first year, a further two years studying sciences with an emphasis on applied techniques such as the preparation of material for analysis in government laboratories. Some experience in out-patient clinics was also envisaged. The final two years provided clinical training: the fourth year was to be spent in the Victoria Hospital studying medical, surgical, midwifery and gynaecological cases, and the fifth year in training at McCord Hospital, Durban.[84] Once qualified and in possession of a government certificate the medical aid was compelled to enter the public medical service.[85] Ultimately the state envisaged that there would be 200-trained medical aids.

Whilst there were individual success stories the general history of medical aids was problematic. In April 1937 the newly-appointed course director, George Gale, resigned because he thought students were being misled, and were being trained as sanitary inspectors when they had enrolled to study medicine.[86] A central ambiguity of the scheme was whether medical aids were intended to do preventive work like a health assistant, or whether they would do curative work like a doctor. Dr Gale recorded that during their training they had been "taught to use stethoscopes, perform minor operations, give anaesthetics, [and] conduct confinements", but that in their

[83] WHO, *Apartheid and Health* (Geneva: WHO, 1983), 95.

[84] Macvicar papers, MS notes on medical aids scheme, February–March 1937, Cory, PR 3085, RU.

[85] WHO, *Apartheid and Health*, 95.

[86] Robert R. Edgar, ed., *An African American in South Africa* (Athens and Johannesburg: Ohio University Press, 1992), 127–28; Shula Marks, "Doctors and the State", in *Science and Society in Southern Africa*, ed. S. Dubow (Manchester: Manchester University Press, 2000), 195.

employment the Department of Public Health forbade such activities because they would have been illegal under the Medical Dental and Pharmacy Act of 1928.[87] Recruitment levels were disappointing, not least because the scheme demanded much but promised little. After five years tuition (only one year less than a full medical training), medical aids did not have the status and prospects of doctors.[88] The opening of full training to black students at the medical schools at the Universities of Cape Town and the Witwatersrand in the early 1940s signalled that the medical aids scheme was becoming obsolete, so that it was formally abandoned in 1943.[89]

Conclusion

Lovedale had sought to bring Africans into the 'civilised' world through the medium of education, and Victoria Hospital had aimed to elevate their health status through 'clinical Christianity.'[90] The missionary medicine at the hospital differed from ordinary 'Western' medicine, because it involved a religious currency signalled by the inscription above the entrance—*Egameni lika-Yesu* [In the name of Jesus]. The implicit cultural contract for patients was that they would receive the treatment of 'Western' medicine but within an evangelising Christian context, and this was especially evident for in-patients whose exposure to 'civilised' values was lengthier and more concentrated. Victoria Hospital had benefited from the prestige and experience of its founding institution of Lovedale, its privileged financial position in receiving early government grants (unlike other mission hospitals), and its well-qualified, dedicated staff. The

87 Gale, "Notes on Medical Aid Scheme" quoted in I. S. Monamodi, "Medical Doctors under Segregation and Apartheid" (unpublished PhD thesis, Indiana University, 1996), 262.

88 MS notes on medical aids scheme, Cory, PR 3085, RU.

89 For a longer discussion of the medical aids scheme, see Digby, *Diversity and Division in Medicine*, 191–98; K. Shapiro, "Doctors or Medical Aids: The Debate over the Training of Black Medical Personnel for the Rural Black Population in South Africa in the 1920s and 1930s", *Journal of Southern African Studies* 13, no. 2, 1987, 234–55.

90 Wells, *Stewart of Lovedale* , 228.

hospital aimed to educate a new generation of students, nurses, and medical aids to spearhead enlightenment in civilised values centred on 'Western' medicine and Christian belief. Unlike so many other missions it did not suffer from geographical and intellectual isolation but instead demonstrated the potential for a powerful missionary medicine. The Free Church of Scotland had a line of hospitals stretching from Sulenkama, in the Transkei, to Tugela Ferry in Natal, and Sibasa in the northern Transvaal; all looking to the senior institution of Victoria Hospital for advice. Nurses trained by Victoria Hospital worked in every part of South Africa—from Cape Town north-east to Durban, and from Johannesburg north to Elim—thus providing an influential professional network.

Victoria Hospital targeted the 'heathen' way of life of African patients, and expected to weaken their loyalty to indigenous medicine. Macvicar envisaged the "witchcraft delusion" being vanquished by the "assured knowledge" of medical science, where "to pass on the light and overcome the darkness . . . is the work and privilege . . . of the medical missionary."[91] The figure of the witch doctor was frequently mentioned but was viewed less as an individual than as a broad symbol of undesirable beliefs and lifestyle, encompassing both the darkness of unbelief and deficiencies of unhygienic living. Although the hospital reports supplied no accounts of direct encounters with 'witch doctors', there was plentiful indirect evidence of staff members' awareness of their powerful influence. It was admitted that 'red' or heathen Africans were reluctant to seek the help of 'Western' medicine. Dr Macvicar acknowledged that "Native patients are accustomed to put their own interpretations upon the words and actions of European doctors, and to make liberal allowances for the white doctor's presumed ignorance of the true inwardness of their, the natives' diseases."[92] This 'inwardness' encompassed the psychological aspects of illness—the effect of the unseen (whether of witches or ancestors) on disease. Even when hospital staff judged that recovery had been effected, for many

[91] N. Macvicar, "Native Health, General Survey and Hospitals", in *Native Health*, ed. N. Macvicar, D. Ryan and H. M. Bennett (Lovedale: Lovedale Press, 1940), 2.

[92] Macvicar, *Side-lights upon Superstition*, 18–19.

African patients a cure still waited upon the diviner who would explain why the sickness had struck, and give complementary therapies to ensure that adverse, causal influences were properly addressed. Consciousness of this hidden dimension was also strong amongst early African doctors educated at Lovedale / Victoria—such as William Soga and S. M. Molema. During the 1880s and 1890s William Soga worked as a medical missionary at Elliotdale in the Transkei, where he referred to Africans as the "unsuspecting dupes" of "wily" healers, and thought it his mission to show his patients "new methods of treatment" in order to deal "a deadly blow at superstition and witchcraft."[93] And writing a quarter century later, Dr Molema thought that "superstition and witchcraft were [still] perhaps, the two greatest curses among the Bantu."[94]

[93] W. Soga, "The Ethnology of the Bomvanas of Bomvanaland" (unpublished MD thesis, University of Glasgow, 1894), 31–32.

[94] S. M. Molema, *The Bantu Past and Present* (Edinburgh: W. Green and Co., 1920), 165, 170.

8

Hospitals and Development of Medicine in Nineteenth-Century Iran

Hormoz Ebrahimnejad

According to an anonymous manuscript written in the 1860s, while "there are more than fifty thousand hospitals across the world, none of them is in Iran."[1] We cannot ascertain to what extent this assertion of absolute absence of hospital in the first part of the nineteenth century in Iran holds true, but relying on our research so far, we have not found any archival record bearing witness to the existence or construction of hospitals in that period. European missions, who returned to Iran after several decades of civil war throughout the eighteenth century, testify that they did not see any hospital there.[2] However, in the first part of the nineteenth century we find medical care in form of camp hospitals accompanying the army and the *dār al-shafâ* (house of healing) funded by the Shiite shrines. None of these forms equate to modern Western standards of the hospital.

The first "modern" hospital in nineteenth-century Iran, called the *marizkhâneh-ye dowlati* (state hospital), was built in 1852. Similar institutions were also built during the second part of the century but the details concerning their number, date of construction and location are scarce and unclear. There have been some recent studies of

1 Anonymous manuscript, untitled, Tehran, the Library of Majles, no. 505, p. 8. For an edition of this manuscript, with English translation, see Hormoz Ebrahimnejad, *Medicine, Public Health and the Qâjâr State* (Leiden, Boston: Brill, 2004), 149.

2 See, for example, General Gardan, *Ma'muriyat-e General Gardan dar Iran,* Persian translation from French by Abbas Eqbâl Âshtiyâni, 2nd ed. (Tehran: Enteshârât-e negâh, 1362/ 1983 AD), 74.

these hospitals,[3] but they have failed to examine them in relation to local medical systems and the development of modern medicine. The aim of this chapter is firstly to give a general picture of hospital institutions in the nineteenth century in the light of their historical roots and background, and secondly, through a critical examination of the information and records of the contemporary sources, to study the impact of the new state hospitals on the development of medicine in Qâjâr Iran.

Military Camp Hospitals

The author of the above-mentioned manuscript on the creation of military hospitals traced back the history of mobile hospitals in Iran to the pre-historic dynasty of the Pishdâdiyân (ca. 1700–550 BC), a practice that continued under the Achaemenid (550–330 BC) and Sasanid (240–650 AD) dynasties. Although no reference is provided for this statement, it does not seem untrue as an army in campaign needs some kind of medical care. This system was thus naturally at work throughout the Islamic period.[4] Perhaps the most enduring form of hospital that existed in Iran from antiquity until modern times was the mobile or "camp" hospital. While fixed hospitals were created by charitable endowments and then disappeared when funding came to an end, mobile hospitals were created whenever an army set out on campaign. As such, they had no permanent base or institution and their creation maintenance and funding were limited to the duration of the campaign.

During the first part of the nineteenth century, Iran was continuously at war, either within its borders against local rebellions, or with Russia over the semi-independent Caucasian provinces. In all these military campaigns camp hospitals accompanied the army.

[3] Hasan Tâjbakhsh, *Târikh-e bimârestânhâ-ye Iran az âghâz tâ 'asr-e hazer* [History of Hospitals in Iran from Beginning to the Present] (Tehran: *Pajuheshgâh-e 'olum-e ensâni,* 1379/2000); Willem Floor, *Public Health in Qajar Iran* (Washington D.C.: Mage Publishers, 2004); Sâdeq Sajjâdi, "Bimarestan", in *Encyclopaedia Iranica*, ed. Ehsan Yarshater (Costa Mesa: Mazda Publishers, 1993).

[4] Al-Qifti, *Târikh al-hokamâ,* Persian translation of 1688, ed. Bahman Dârâ'I (Tehran: Tehran University Press, 1371/ 1992), 545.

Although contemporary sources in the first part of the nineteenth century do not provide precise information about camp or mobile hospitals, they do provide information about physicians and surgeons in each regiment, which suggests the existence of medical care in the army and, by extension, some form of camp hospital. In addition to the military campaigns, the Qâjâr Shahs were usually in movement during the hot seasons; they set out of the capital for a better climate, to flee epidemics or sometimes to compel local governors to pay taxes in arrears. The royal *ordu* (camp) was accompanied by medical facilities under the supervision of chief surgeon or chief physician. In 1813, while Fath 'Ali-Shah was himself heading a campaign against Russians, his son Mohammad-Vali-Mirzâ, governor of Khorâsân, was fighting with the Turcomans in north-east of the country. Upon the victory of this prince, the Shah commissioned the chief surgeon of his army to take a prize to the prince of Khorâsân as a reward for his victory.[5] Such a mission for the chief surgeon, indicating his high position in the state, suggests that he had a number of medical staff under his supervision in the military campaign. This is best confirmed by payroll documents in the first part of the century. In one of these, dated 1252/1836, for instance, a salary is established by the chief physician for the "new surgeons" (*jarrâhân-e jadid*) of the army. In another document the price of drugs spent by one of the physicians of the army is precised.[6] Each regiment (*fowj*) had its own physicians and surgeons.

Many surgeons or practitioners in the regiments claimed to be physicians and they were acknowledged as such because of the need of the army. According to the anonymous MS 505 mentioned above, by the mid-nineteenth century, of two hundred physicians or practitioners working in the regiments stationed in Tehran, only seven or eight deserved the title of doctor.[7] In order to legalise the activity of these rank and file physicians, the government made a

5 Hedâyat, Reza Qoli Khan, *Rowzat al-safâ-ye nâseri* (Tehran: Lith., 1959–60), 9: 491.

6 Archives of the *sâzmân-e asnâd,* no. 295000455, dated 1252/1836, National Library, Tehran.

7 MS 505, 32–33, Majles Library, Tehran; for English translation of this document, see Ebrahimnejad, *Medicine, Public Health, and the Qâjâr State,* 165–66.

rule in 1851 that they should register in the office of the chief physician of the army Dr Kazullani, one of the European doctors hired by the Qâjâr state to train physicians in modern medicine. From now on, the regimental doctors were to practice in the army by the permission of Dr Kazullani.[8] With the modernisation of the army especially in the second part of the nineteenth century, the camp or mobile hospitals were better organised and staffed by modern educated physicians. After the establishment of the Polytechnic School (the *Dār al-Fonun*) in 1851, the medical graduates of this school were usually sent to the regiments of the provinces. In 1856, during the short-lived war between Iran and Great Britain over the isles of the Persian Gulf, one of the medical instructors of the Dār al-Fonun, Mirzâ Seyyed Ali Tabib, probably a traditional physician, was sent to Khorramshar, the port city to serve as chief physician of the army.[9] Writing in 1888, E'temâd al-Saltaneh informs us that there were 106 physicians and surgeons belonging to the army in Tehran and the provinces.[10]

Although there are no specific descriptions of the camp hospitals in extant sources, some evidences show that the main component of these hospitals was their pharmacy. The archival sources as well as the details given in the above-mentioned MS 505 provide evidence that before the modernisation of the army each physician was given either the price of the drug or a ration in drugs that he carried on his transport animal. There were also tents allocated to the surgeons of the army. The same system continued in the second part of the century, when, during the military campaigns, there were separate tents for the storage of drugs and for physicians and surgeons to receive sick or injured soldiers.[11] These provisions must have been impressive, for on 18 September 1897, when twelve thousand troops

[8] E'temâd al-Saltaneh, *Târikh-e Montazam* (Tehran: Lith., 1880–82), 3: 1724; Floor, *Public Health in Qajar Iran,* 189.

[9] Hedâyat, *Rowzat al-safâ-ye nâseri,* 10: 757.

[10] E'temâd al-Saltaneh, al-*Ma'â ser v'al-âsâr* (Tehran: Lith., 1880–82), see the supplementary section on military and state organisation, 8.

[11] For the photograph of one of these camp pharmacies in 1310/1892, see Barjesteh and Eskandari-Qajar, eds., *Qajar Era Health, Hygiene and Beauty* (Rotterdam, Santa Barbara and Tehran: Barjesteh & Co., 2003), 75.

were reviewed by Mozaffar al-Din-Shah close to his summer villa north of Tehran, the Shah rewarded Mirzâ Mohammad Nezâm al-Hokamâ, the chief physician of the army, for his endeavours in organising the pharmacies of the army.[12]

The Dār al-shafâ

Besides camp hospitals, the only fixed hospital establishment recorded in contemporary sources in the first part of the Qâjâr period (1797–1925) were the dār al-shafâs (houses of healing). In the second part of the nineteenth century, however, the usual term for hospital was *mariz-khâneh* (the house of the ill). The better known dār al-shafâ, as hospice or hospital, during the Qâjâr period belonged to the shrine of the eighth Shiite Imam, 'Ali b. Mosâ al-Rezâ (died in c. 819 AD) in Mashhad, presently the capital city of Khorasan province. The date of the creation of this dār al-shafâ is not clear but it is possible that it was operative in 1576 when 'Emâd al-Din Mahmud Shirâzi lived in Mashad and treated the sick amongst the pilgrims of the mausoleum of Ali b. Musa al-Rezâ.[13] Since, in nineteenth-century Iran, the dār al-shafâs were the only surviving form of the fixed medieval hospitals, the study of their main function and financial organisation can help us to assess the state of hospitals in mid-nineteenth-century Iran.

The term dār al-shafâ was most commonly used name for hospital establishments in the Timurid period (1370–1506), but at times, it was also used in the medieval Islamic countries along with other terms, such as *mârestân*, *bimârestân* and *dār al-morzâ*. A careful examination of the dār al-shafâ reveals that some of them at least were not

[12] Afzal al-Molk, *Afzal al-Tavârikh,* eds., Mansureh Etehâdiyeh and Sirus Sa'dvandiyân (Tehran: Nashr-e Târikh, 1361/1982), 139.

[13] Emâd al-Din Mahmud Shirâzi, *Atashak* [Treaty of Syphilis], Persian manuscript, copy dated 984 (1576 AD), the Library of Majles, no. 6307, 2, Tehran. However, since Emâd al-Din Mahmud does not refer to any Dār al-shafâ or hospital there, we do not share the certitude with which some assert that he was working at the dār al-shafâ. See Abdul Bari and Arshad Hussain, "Hakim 'Imâd al-Dîn Mahmûd Shirâzi and Risâla Bîkh-I Chini", *Studies in History of Medicine & Science* 17, no. 1–2, new series, 2001, 73–78; and Tâjbakhsh, *Târikh-e bimârestânhâ,* 185–86.

hospitals in proper term but rather what was called at that period *bayt al-adviya* (drugstore). Pharmacy seems to be the major part of the dār al-shafâs in Tabriz and Hamadân built by Rashid al-Din Fazlollâh, the minister of Ghazan (1343–46) in the fourteenth century. In one of his letters, Rashid al-Din Fazlollâh, warns that the dār al-shafâ of Tabriz had been deteriorating due to the lack of drugs, and that endeavours should be employed to supply it with the drugs as he had ruled (in his *waqf-nâmeh,* or endowment deed).[14] The deterioration of the dār al-shafâ in Tabriz due to lack of drugs can be an indication of this establishment operating more as a drugstore than as a proper hospital where in-patient treatment was provided by regular activity of physicians.

Sometimes, under the Timurids, dār al-shafâ, in its sense of bayt al-adviya (drugstore) was the name of the school. One of the great scholars, Mowlânâ Seyyed Rokn al-Haq (died in 1332), built a *madrasa*, an observatory (with two *minarahs*) across the madrasa, a mosque and a bayt al-adviya (or dār al-shafâ) in 1327.[15] It seems that this bayt al-adviya was in fact a school (of higher education) because another chronicle on Yazd mentioning the constructions of Mowlânâ, indicates that "at the side of the madrasa, he built a 'high school'" (*madrasa-ye 'âli*) that he called it bayt al-adviya.[16] Another madrasa or school built by Shâh Shojâ' (1359–1385) of the Mozaffarid dynasty (1314–1393) in Shirâz was also called dār al-shafâ.[17] Another example was Fâteh dâr al-shafâ in 1470 and Suleymânieh dār al-shafâ in 1557 in the Ottoman Empire, in which medicine

[14] *Savâneh al-afkâr,* pp. 188–90, and 65–67, cited in Tajbakhsh, *Târikh-e bimârestânhâ,* 143–45.

[15] Ja'far b. Mohammad b. Hasan Ja'fari, *Târikh-e Yazd,* ed. Iraj Afshar (Tehran: Bongâh-e tarjomeh va nashr-e ketâb, 1960), 81–83.

[16] *Târikh-e jaded-e Yazd,* p. 125, cited in Tâjbakhsh, *Târikh-e bimârestânhâ,* 130.

[17] Mir seyyed Mohammad b. Seyyed Borhân al-Din Khwavand-Shah (Mirkhond), *Rowzat al-safâ* (Tehran: enteshârâte markazi), 4: 556. See also the entry *Dār al-shafâ* by A. A. Dehkhodâ, *Loghatnâmeh* [Dehkhodâ Encyclopaedia], ed. M. Moin and J. Shahidi (Tehran: Dehkhoda Foundation, 1377/1998), 7: 10270.

was taught together with non-medical and especially religious sciences.[18]

It seems that the term *madrasa-ye dār al-shafâ* (the school belonging to the hospital) that became common in nineteenth-century Iran takes its origin from Timurid dār al-shafâ in its school sense. However, the combination of school and hospital implied in this term has led some historians to conclude that madrasa-ye dār al-shafâ was a medical school.[19] They go further in their comments on madrasa-ye dār al-shafâ by maintaining that this term entails the existence of a hospital nearby,[20] even though there is no mention of a hospital in the document discussing these madrasas. Nonetheless, while in some cases madrasa-ye dār al-shafâ was a medical school, in other cases it was only religious school or a compound that can be called "mosque-school".

Another decisive factor in the history of hospital institutions relates to financial and economic resources for their creation and maintenance. The main source of hospital institutions in early Islam consisted of endowments established by princes or wealthy individuals. Nevertheless, hospitals were not the main beneficiary of charitable endowments. They were far behind other institutions of public interests and especially those with a religious character, such as mosques, *makatb* (primary school), mardrasa (Islamic college), *khânqâh* and *tekyeh* (houses where Sufis and dervish gathered). The author of *Târikh-e Yazd* (c. mid-1441), describes all buildings constructed in Yazd under the Mongols and the Timurids, including hospitals, houses of nobles, etc. While his list counts dozens of madrasas (also used by the founders as their burial place), caravanserais, khânqâh, *hammâm* (baths) and especially mosques, only

18 Arslan Terziuglu, "The History of Istanbul Medical Faculty", *Istanbul tip fakültesi mecmuasi,* University of Istanbul 63, 2000, 81.

19 In his study on medieval schooling in Iran, Arjomand, referring to Rashid al-Din's medical establishments employs the term 'teaching hospitals' which should be the translation of *madrasa-ye dâr al-shafâ.* S. Amir Arjomand, "The Law, Agency, and Policy in Medieval Islamic Society", *Comparative Studies in Societies and History* 41, no. 2, 1999, 263–93.

20 See, for example, Tajbakhsh, *Târikh-e bâmârestânhâ,* 148, 217; Floor, *Public Health in Qajar Iran,* 190.

four establishments of a medical nature called dār al-shafâ or *bayt al-adviyah* are mentioned. One dār al-shafâ in 1268, another in 1320, another in 1327, and the dār al-shafâ of Walchi-Khan that was built on an unknown date (before 1346).[21] In 747/1346, Mohammad b. Mozaffar (1314–58) took over the buildings, including the Madrasa of Atabek-Sâm and the Dār al-shafâ named after Walchi-Khan outside of Yazd. He built then a hammam and a khânqâh and two minarets at the gate of the Atabek madrasa.[22]

Although charitable endowments (*owqâf*) were principally motivated by pious intentions, they became means of acquiring prestige and power in a contest of rivalry between members of "aristocracy". In imitation of the Shah who had his own madrasa and mosques, and rivalling one another, nobles established owqâf for the construction of madrasas, to an extent that, as Kaempfer noted in 1685, in Espahan there existed about one hundred endowed madrasas.[23] Another reason for the increase of the owqâf seems to be rooted in the insecurity of private property in a country, such as Iran, self-assigned and had right to life and property of his subjects. In such a context property established as waqf made it less vulnerable. Principally, waqf, in Arabic means "to protect a thing, to prevent it from becoming the property of a third person (*tamlik* [= appropriation])".[24] Once a property was established in waqf, it could not be transferred as a private property but its administration (*towliyat*) was transmitted by inheritance or by testament. In this case, part of the usufruct of the waqf was allocated to charitable purposes and part of it for the expenses of the administrator (*motawalli*). However, despite the elements of the shari'a that provided some protection for

21 Ja'far b. Mohammad b. Hasan Ja'fari, *Târikh-e Yazd,* for the dâr al-shafâ, see 33, 83, 91, 93. See also 'Abd al-Hoseyn Ayati, *Târikh-e Yazd* (Yazd: Chapkhaneh-ye golbahar, 1317/1938), 138 ff.

22 Ja'fari, *Tarikh-e Yazd,* 33.

23 Engelbert Kaempfer, *Dar darbâr-e Shâhashâh-e Iran,* Persian translation by Kaykavus Jahandari (Tehran: *Enteshârât-e anjoman-e âsâr-e melli,* 1971), 139. For the original version, see Walther Hinz, ed., *Am Hofe des persischen Grossknigs,* 1684–1685 (Germany: Tübingen, Horst Erdmann, 1977).

24 Heffening, "Wakf", in *Encyclopaedia of Islam,* vol. 4, ed. E. van Donzel (Boston: Brill, 1998).

waqf property, there were various ways of circumventing them. The discussion of this matter falls beyond the scope of this chapter but one example can illustrate it: under the Safavids, the position of *Sadr* in the government was in charge of the control of the owqâf (pl. of waqf). But after his death the Safavid Shahs gave this responsibility to a minister of *mowqufât* (endowments) so that they could appropriate the usufruct of the owqâf properties as much as possible.[25] During wars or occupations, no masking procedure was employed to take over the owqâf as it did happen under the occupation of Tabriz by the Ottomans at the beginning of the eighteenth century as well as under the reign of Nâder-Shah Afshâr (1726–37).[26]

The fact that, in medieval Islamic societies, endowing religious establishment conferred more authority, legitimacy or security than endowing hospitals played an important role in the decrease of fund for dār al-shafâs. At the same time, especially in the case of Iran, it also explains the increase in the number of mosques and madrasas during the same period. Not only were charitable endowments for the establishment of hospitals rare, but also funds allocated to them were more easily subject to misappropriation. Already in the seventeenth century, the picture of hospitals given by Western travellers was extremely negative. Raphael du Mans in the 1660s stated that in Persia there was no charitable hospital or institution for the poor, orphans or widows.[27] In September 1684, Kaempfer reported that Espahan, the capital of the Safavids had one hospital, more than one hundred mosques and madrasa and innumerable hammams and caravanserais. But according to Chardin who visited Iran between 1665 and 1680, half of the budget of the hospital that was working with the revenue of an endowment was misappropriated.[28] The situation worsened in Iran in the eighteenth century. To be sure, the

[25] Kaempfer, *Dar darbâr,* 122.

[26] Christoph Werner, *An Iranian Town in Transition: A Social and Economic History of the Elites of Tabriz, 1747–1848* (Wiesbaden: Harassowitz Verlag, 2000), 102.

[27] Francis Richard, ed. *Raphaël du Mans: missionnaire en Perse au XVIIe s.*, (Paris: L'Harmattan, 1995), 2: 31.

[28] Jean Chardin, *Voyages du chevalier Chardin, en Perse, et autres lieux de 'orient* (Rouen : Fernand, 1723), 297–98.

anarchy that prevailed in this period during which the most stable power—that of Karim-Khân-e Zand (1759–79)—did not last more than nineteen years, can partly explain this lack of hospitals at the turn of the century.[29] But what was more determining in the decline of the hospitals was the sustained trend of the adverse political, financial as well as socio-cultural factors over the centuries.

We have mentioned the Timurid origin of the etymology of dār al-shafâ as a school rather than a hospital. The relationship between school and hospital, implicit in the term madrasa-ye dār al-shafâ, can also be explained in the light of the decline of the dār al-shafâ, to the benefit of religious school. The madrasa-ye dār al-shafâ might have been originally a medical school attached to a dār al-shafâ. This is also echoed by the observation of Cabanis, writing at the end of the eighteenth century, that colleges in the Islamic countries 'had always a hospital in their neighbourhood.'[30] When the latter declined due to the lack of funding, for the reasons explained above, their madrasas survived. We can also speculate that, after the decline of a dār al-shafâ, instead of another hospital that would face a similar fate, a madrasa was built at its place and for this reason was called madrasa-ye dār al-shafâ. One or a combination of the above suggestions would explain the history of three schools called madrasa-ye dār al-shafâ, in Tehran, Qom and Shirâz in the nineteenth century. All of these establishments were madrasas only and, despite received opinion, they had no medical function. The old *sahn* (courtyard) of the mausoleum of Ma'sumah (died in 201/816), sister of Emam Rezâ (died in 203/818) in Qom, has an establishment called the *madrasa-ye dār al-shafâ.* The old sahn was first built by a vizier of Shah Abbâs III Safavid in 1645; Fath'Ali-Shah Qâjâr (1798–1834) renovated and expanded it and built the present dār al-shafâ,

[29] For the change in political and social structure of Iran in the eighteenth century, see A. K. S. Lambton, "The Tribal Resurgence and the Decline of Bureaucracy in the Eighteenth Century," in *Studies in Eighteenth-Century Islamic History*, ed. Thomas Naff and Rogen Owen (Carbondale & Edwardsville: Southern Illinois University Press, 1977).

[30] P. J. G. Cabanis, *Sketch of the Revolutions of Medical Science, and Views Relating to Its Reform,* French translation with notes by A. Henderson (M. D. London: Printed for J. Johnson [etc.] by Bye and Law, 1806), 324.

which is in fact a religious school. It was only later, in 1304/1886, that prince Kâmrân-Mirzâ constructed in the dār al-shafâ a marizkhâneh (hospital) and appointed a physician as its director, together with several practitioners and nurses, and allocated some funding for drugs and meals for the patients. But this marizkhâneh disappeared and it was transformed into a residence for students of religion in 1337/1919.[31]

Other institutions that superseded hospitals in attracting charitable endowments were khânqâh, *tekyeh* and *zâwia* and, the caravanserai, or inn for travellers. It is worth mentioning these because they were a sort of hospice, with religious characteristics and were found throughout Islamic civilisation in India, Iran, Turkey, and North Africa, as well as in some other African countries. The khânqâh, a Persian word composed of *khâneh* (house) and *gâh* (site or position) was a place where the Sufis gathered. They were normally permanent residence for the Sufis, however they also housed Sufi travellers. The newcomers were offered food and sleep but the guests were meant to respect certain protocols and rules, such as arriving at about sunset, and staying inside the khânqâh for three days before visiting the city or town in which the khânqâh was located.

The tekyeh (place where one leans to repose) was also a place where the Sufis and dervish lived. In *takâyâ* (pl. of tekyeh), poor people, who were recommended by a dervish, could also be housed and provided with food and/or beds.[32] Nevertheless, these Islamic institutions did not provide medical care to the sick poor. The tekyeh, such as that built in Tehran by Naser al-Din-Shâh, was principally a theatre for commemoration of the tragic death of Imam Hoseyn in 680 AD in Kerbela (Iraq). These takâyâ, which still exist throughout Iran, are also places of prayer and almsgiving. Some tekyehs have established dispensaries out of the charitable donations and the revenue of their owqâf. As far as we know, only two small hospital-like institutions were created by the Qâjârs, one by Kâmrân Mirzâ

[31] Dehkhodâ, *Loghatnâmeh,* 7: 10270; Afzal al-Molk Kermâni, *Târikh va joghrâfiyâ-ye Qom,* ed. Hoseyn Modarresi tabâtabâ'i (Qom: enteshârât-e Vahid, 1976), 60–61.

[32] About these institutions, see Mohsen Kiyâni, *Târikh-e khânqâh dar Iran* [History of khânqâh in Iran] (Tehran: Tahuri, 1369/1990), 106–7.

in Qom (see above) in 1886 and the other by Anushirvân-Mirzâ Ziyâ'al-Saltaneh in 1884 in Semnân.[33] But they created several tekyehs and khânqâhs in the Shiite religious cities in Iraq, Najaf, Kerbela and Kazemayn, some of which are still functioning.

Modern Military or State Hospitals

These historical and socio-political factors partly explain the fact that, despite the unprecedented spread of epidemics and the increasing number of troops, only two or three hospitals were built with a limited capacity in the second part of the nineteenth century in Iran. There were also few hospitals created by the foreign missions in Tehran and other major cities such as in Espahan, but we focus mainly on those established by the Iranian themselves because the hospitals of the foreign missions were created by foreign funds for charitable or political purposes quite different from those that informed the creation of state hospitals in Iran.

As mentioned earlier, the records on hospitals in the second half of the nineteenth century are extremely confusing, to the extent that it is hard to construct a clear chronological account of their creation and development. Before the mid-nineteenth century, there was no fixed military hospital in Iran; barracks sometimes provided rudimentary medical care for soldiers. The military modernisation that began under 'Abbas Mirzâ, the heir apparent and governor of Azarbaijan, did not take a serious form before the mid-nineteenth century. In this period, Mirzâ Taqi-Khân, who became the first prime-minister of Nâser al-Din Shah, began a series of reforms, including the creation of a modern school and a hospital for the use of the army. The school was intended to train skilled officers educated in modern sciences (engineering, infantry, cavalry, artillery, mathematics, medicine, pharmacy and natural sciences), with 62 per cent of the students studying military sciences as well as engineering and mathematics that had direct military applications.[34]

[33] E'temâd al-Saltaneh, *al-ma'âser al-âsâr,* 79.

[34] Monica Ringer, *Education, Religion, and the Discourse of Cultural Reform in Qajar Iran* (Costa Mesa, California: Mazda Publishers, 2001), 79.

The major source of information about the hospital is the weekly journal, *Ruznâmeh-ye Vaqâye'-e Ettefâqiyyeh* (*RVE*), that was first published in 1851, as part of the prime-minister's modernisation projects. According to this journal, the hospital had accommodation for four hundred in-patients and, in the first year of its operation, received 1,238 such patients.[35] Most patients were soldiers of various regiments from the provinces but the homeless and sick poor were also admitted. The chief physician of the army, accompanied by two or three medical students, worked in the hospital every day and sometimes during the night. Although we should be circumspect about the account provided by the state journal *RVE* marked by its panegyric tone, its information is unique and provides important indications of the nature of Iran's first state hospital. The information from this journal, that the first year of the activity of the hospital was during 1852, is confirmed by E'temâd al-Saltaneh who, talking about the events taking place between March and July 1852, noted that the construction of a (military) hospital between the barracks of Dowlat and Qazvin gates of Tehran, with four hundred beds, a house for the physicians, kitchen, etc., was ordered.[36]

Dr Jakob Polak the instructor of anatomy at the medical school, who had worked in the first state hospital, does not mention it but he claimed that he had persuaded the government to build a hospital in 1855. Polak's claim can be substantiated by a contemporary chronicler who informs us that a hospital for the army was built upon the order of the shah in *tanguze'il* and *sichqâne'il* (Turkish years corresponding to 1272–73 /1855–56) and Dr Polak took his student there for training.[37] It is not, however, clear why this chronicler does not mention the first hospital built in 1269/1852. We cannot ascertain if the above sources refer to two different hospitals or to one and the same. If the latter is correct, the credit should go to the *RVE* because it mentions and gives information about it in its sev-

35 *Ruznâmeh-ye Vaqâye'-e Ettefâqiyyeh,* no. 102 (14 January 1583). In the following issue (no. 103, 22 January), however, the number of the patients treated in this hospital is recorded 2238.

36 E'temâd al-Saltaneh, *Târikh-e Montazam-e nâseri,* vol. 3, ed. Rezvâni (Tehran: Donyâye ketâb, 1733).

37 Hedayat, *Rowzat al-safâ,* 10: 813.

eral issues. In other words, the hospital was probably built in 1852 rather than 1855.

Other sources talk about a hospital built around 1867–68. Without mentioning his references, Cyril Elgood maintains that "in pursuance of modernising the country a new hospital was founded in Tehran that was opened in 1868. This corroborates other information from a Persian source, according to which, in 1867, the walls of the city were enlarged: from the north 1800 *zar'* (≈1,8 km) and from the three other sides 1000 *zar'* (≈1 km) in order to respond to the growing population of Tehran, and at the same time a new hospital was constructed.[38] This hospital was also called marizkhâneh-ye dowlati (state hospital). It was probably this hospital that Nâser al-Din-Shâh visited, together with the Dâr al-Fonun School, on 11 October 1873, just after his return from his tour in Europe that lasted from May to September 1873. During his stay in London, he made a visit to St Thomas's Hospital on 4 July. Some secondary sources claims that Nâser al-Din-Shah, inspired by hospitals he had visited in Europe, ordered the construction of a modern hospital on European model. Accordingly a civilian hospital, called also marizkhâneh-ye dowlati was built in 1874.[39] There is, however, no contemporary source that confirms this account. Presuming that such a hospital was created, there were, so far, at least three state (or military) hospitals built in Tehran in 1852, 1868 and 1874. When mentioning the construction of the military hospital in 1868, Elgood maintains that twelve years later (i.e., 1880) a new military hospital was built and the old one (i.e., 1868) was assigned to civilians. We cannot ascertain whether his report on the construction of 1880 hospital is accurate, as no other source mentions it. Only E'temâd al-Saltaneh, writing in 1888, refers to a modern artillery hospital (*dār al-shafâ-ye jadid-e tupkhâneh*) without giving its date of construction. In this hospital two physicians, one surgeon, one pharmacist,

[38] E'temâd al-Saltaneh, *Târikh-e Montazam-e nâseri,* 3: 1898; E'temâd al-Saltaneh, *al-Ma'âser al-âsâr*, 73.

[39] Mohammad Hasanbeigi, *Tehrân-e qadim* [Old Tehran] (Tehran: Enteshârât-e qoqnus, 1366/1987), 209–10.

and four nurses were employed together with administrative and security staff.[40]

Although these hospitals were sometimes built specifically for the military, the categorisation of civil and military hospitals for this period, as it is made by Elgood, does not necessarily reflect the reality, because the hospital system was not so much developed so that the military and the civilians could have their own hospitals. As the anonymous booklet on the establishment of the first state hospital underlined, the military hospitals, called at times "military", "state", or "royal" hospitals, were not so much discriminatory and were also used by the civilians, particularly the sick poor.[41]

Modern hospitals were constructed on Western model with the aim of providing in-patient treatments for the military as well as clinical training for the students of the Dār al-Fonun. However, their construction, organisation and administration were strongly marked by local factors. Although there are records of both medical treatment and clinical training in these hospitals,[42] these functions were scarcely fulfilled according to the modern Western medical system, as, for example, the absence of dissection for anatomy lectures indicate.

The director of the first hospital in 1852 was Mirzâ Mohammad-Vali-ye Tabib, a traditional court physician. Additionally, the court physician was commissioned to write plans for the restoration of the hospital, which, according to him, had been deteriorating due to the "carelessness of the officials". These guidelines for the organisation and administration of the hospital were prepared principally by referring to medieval hospitals and the medical students were advised to read the sources that were used during the medieval period.[43] In the case of the hospital built in 1868, Elgood initially maintains that Polak and Schlimmer were its first directors but later in his book he

40 E'temâd al-Slataneh, *al-Ma'âser al-âsâr,* 16 (annex).

41 MS 505, edited by Ebrahimnejad in *Medicine, Public Health and the Qâjâr State*.

42 See MS: *On Diseases Commonly Affecting Soldiers in the Barracks,* MS 506, c. 1857; and MS 505.

43 Ebrahimnejad, *Medicine, Public Health and the Qâjâr State,* see especially part 1, chapter 3.

contradicts or rather corrects himself by stating that the graduates of the Dār al-Fonun directed it in the first twelve years of its activity.[44] The state hospital constructed supposedly in 1874, for the first five years was directed by Mirzâ 'Ali-Akbar-Khân Nâzem al-Atebbâ and after him by Dr Mohammad-Khân Kermânshâhi, both educated in modern as well as in traditional medicine. Moreover, the marizkhâneh-ye dowlati, together with the Dār al-Fonun, were both under the responsibility of the ministry of education. After the death of prince E'tezâd al-Saltaneh, the director of the Dār al-Fonun and minister of education—a post that was also called at times "ministry of science", *vazir-e 'olum*—on 13 December 1880, Shah appointed 'Aliqoli-Khân Mokhber al-Dowleh, minister of Telegraph, as director of the Dār al-Fonun and the marizkhâneh-ye dowlati. A few months later, on the occasion of *Nowruz,* the new Iranian year (21 March 1881), Mokhber al-Dowleh was named minister of science.[45]

The role played by the Iranian physicians in the establishment of "modern" hospitals went hand in hand with the presence of traditional sciences in the modern school of the Dār al-Fonun. This came from the fact that the Persian traditional physicians at the court were involved in the development of medicine sponsored by the patrimonial Qâjâr state. From an educational and scientific aspect, this implied a mixture of modern and traditional methods in both Dār al-Fonun and the hospital. Dr Treacher Collins, visiting Espahan in 1894, reports that he met native doctors who were anxious to watch his operations with their own eyes in his dispensary, some of whom "had acquired a smattering of Western science and methods at the Medical College in Tehran".[46]

The administration and organisation of the hospitals were marked by the same problems that characterised other institutions in the country, and there is evidence of mismanagement or misappropria-

[44] Cyril Elgood, *A Medical Hitory of Persia and the Eastern Caliphate,* repr. (Amsterdam: APA-Pjilo Press, 1979), 511–12 and 545.

[45] E'temâd al-Saltaneh, *Târikh-e Montazam-e nâseri,* vol. 3, 1948, pp. 2017, 2021.

[46] Treacher Collins, *In the Kingdom of the Shah* (London: T. Fisher Unwin, 1896), 167.

tion of funds allocated by the government for the hospital. Carla Serena, for example, recounts an episode where Prince E'tezâd al-Saltaneh, minister of education, embezzled the money paid by the Shah for the military hospital. As a result the only residents of the hospital were the guards, and when the Shah made a surprise visit, the soldiers were ordered to feign illness, but the Shah was not taken in and cancelled the hospital's allocation. Nevertheless, the minister managed to provide some justification for what had happened and continued to receive the money for the hospital.[47] The mismanagement or lack of expertise in administration and organisation was so great that, in 1889, Dr Albo was named as the head of the state hospital and, in 1896, Mozaffar al-Din-Shâh appointed a committee of German physicians to administer and modernise its equipment. In 1914, Dr Ilberg was at the head of the state hospital and when he left Iran at the outbreak of the First World War, Dr Loqmân al-Molk, the personal physician to Ahmad-Shâh Qâjâr was named its director. From then on, the administration of the marizkhâneh-ye dowlati was subject to political vicissitudes, and French, German, English and Iranians were, in turn, placed in control of the hospital, according to circumstances.

The State Hospitals and Development of Modern Medicine

Although the state hospitals built during the second half of the nineteenth century were insufficient for the army, let alone for whole country, they played an important role in the modernisation of medicine because, together with the school of Dār al-Fonun, were the only doors through which medical reforms took place under the state patronage. We have earlier underlined the traditional features of the state hospitals, but on the other hand, they possessed characteristics that differentiated them from their medieval ancestors. The establishment of state hospitals was part of the modernisation of the army and medical education and not for charitable purposes. Their creation was usually decided by the reformist ministers; the first hospital in 1852 was initiated by the prime-minister, Mirzâ

47 Carla Serena, *Hommes et choses en Perse* (Paris: G. Charpentier et Cie Editeurs, 1883), 143–44.

Taqi-Khân Amir-Kabir, while Mirzâ Hoseyn-Khân-e Sepahsâlâr, the fourth prime-minister of the Shah was the instigator of the hospital built in 1874.[48] Unfortunately there is no clear indication of how the state/military hospitals were financed but from scarce data it appears that unlike the medieval period, when the expenses of the hospitals were paid by the revenues of the owqâf, under the Qâjârs the state hospitals were directly created out of the royal treasury and sometime wealthy members of the government also made some donations. Other sources were also used including the revenue of some provinces, donations from some ministers, as well as the royal waqf. Nâser al-Din-Shah had endowed 48 hours per week of the water supply of a newly created *qanât* (subterranean water irrigation) in Tehran for the needs of the inhabitants of the Royal Ark, the royal garden as well as the state hospital.[49]

Since the creation of modern hospitals was part of the process of state-building in which were involved statesmen of both traditional and modern outlooks, a major characteristics of the state hospitals was the active participation of traditional physicians in their medical or administrative activities. The institutional involvement of traditional physicians in hospitals was intertwined with, and at the same time further awakened their medical and scientific curiosity. As the professional integration of physicians increased with new institutions, especially military hospitals, modern medical schools and sanitary councils, they became more dynamic intellectually. Furthermore, the shocking effects of unremitting epidemics of plague and cholera brought them to apply their old humoral theories in order to heal the disease if not to explain it. Writing in 1863, one of these physicians, Fakhr al-Atebbâ, provided several reasons why in his time they paid more attention to epidemics than in the earlier centuries. One of the reasons was that in the past centuries epidemics did not occur as often as they did in the nineteenth century and their duration was from forty days to two, three or maximum seven months and that in any case, a choleric patient succumbed

[48] Floor, *Public Health and the Qâjâr State,* 193.

[49] See Mirzâ Mohammad Taqi Sepehr, *Nâsekh al-Tavârikh,* ed. Jamshid Kiyanfar (Tehran: entesharate Asâtir, 1377/1998), 3: 1516.

within two or three days. This fact did not allow physicians to undertake thorough experimentation and treatment on patients. The other reason was that in the past physicians believed that cholera was contagious (*mosri*) and therefore did not approach patients out of fear of being contaminated. This further prevented physicians from experimentation and systematic examination of cholera.[50] What is significant in this statement is the crucial importance that a traditional physician attached to clinical examination and bedside medicine. Bedside medicine did exist in previous centuries in Islamic countries but Fakhr al-Attebbâ was implying that traditional physicians now placed more emphasis on clinical medicine and systematic experimentation. It was mainly due to the new institutional environment, coupled with the unprecedented spread of epidemics, that the millenary bedside practice in Galenico-Islamic medicine was reinvigorated.

Some historians have claimed that clinical medicine and the first genuine hospitals (sites of medical experimentation and education) were born with Râzi in the tenth century.[51] No doubt Râzi's method and writing were marked by bedside medicine, but throughout the history of Islamic medicine there is more than one case to which one can refer as an example of clinical practice. Bahâ' al-Dowleh's work in the seventeenth century was also characterised by genuine clinical knowledge.[52] There was, nevertheless, no systematic and institutional trend in clinical method or practice in medieval Islam. The principle of working at the hospital for medical training was accepted in medieval Islam and, for example, was recommended by Nezâmi-ye 'Aruzi, the contemporary of Avicenna, in the eleventh

50 Mohammad Râzi Kani Fakhr al-Attebbâ, *Meftâh al-amân* [Key of Safety], 1279/1863, MS 2822, National Library, Tehran, folios, 3–4.

51 Françoise Cloarec, *Bîmâristâns, lieux de folie et de sagesse: La folie et ses traitements dans les hôpitaux médiévaux au Moyen-Orient* (Paris, Monréal: L'Harmattan, 1998), 72.

52 See Kholâsat al-tajârob, gist of experiences, Istanbul, Suleimanie Library, MS 1131 HKm. See also Cyril Elgood, "Bahá-ul-Douleh and His Quintessence of Experience", *Annals of Medical History,* new series 10, 1938, 261–65; this article was also reproduced as a chapter in Elgood, *Safavid Medical Practice: Or, the Practice of Medicine, Surgery and Gynaecology in Persia Between 1500 AD and 1750 AD* (London: Luzac, 1970).

century.[53] However, this should—to use the expression of Frantz Rosenthal—"be considered as the expression of someone's thinking as to what the ideal medical situation ought to be" rather than an expression of reality.[54]

The nineteenth-century traditional medical literature, however, displays a more sustained interest in clinical observation, despite the fact that the concept of disease remained essentially humoral. Modern theories of contagion were refuted by many traditional physicians in the nineteenth century because they prevented physicians from visiting or treating patients.[55] It was within this general context that the author of MS 505, on the establishment of state hospitals, urged physicians of the army to visit patients at the hospital in order to put into practice their theoretical knowledge, or to increase their skill. These local factors in favour of hospital practice worked to the benefit of the influence of Western medicine. By the 1850s and 1860s, when European instructors came to Iran and became committed to the reform of medical education, there was growing interest in hospital-based medical schools throughout Europe.[56] It seems that state or military hospitals and medical school established with the development of the Qâjâr state, followed closely European precedents and examples from India, Ceylon and Turkey. Moreover, these new institutions were received favourably by the Iranian physicians because they offered them a greater opportunity to consoli-

[53] Nezâmi 'Aruzi, *Chahar maqâla* [trans. E. G. Browne, *The "Four Discourses" of Nidhami-i-Arudi-Samarqandi*] (London : Luzac & Co., 1900).

[54] Frantz Rosenthal, "The Physician in Medieval Muslim Society", in *Science and Medicine in Islam: A Collection of Essays,* ed. Frantz Rosenthal (Great Yarmouth, Norfolk: Variorum, 1991).

[55] See, for example, Mirzâ Mohammad-Taqi Shirâzi Malek al-Atebbâ, *Tâ'uniya* [Treatise on Plague], lithograph edition (Tehran: Library of Majels, c. 1247/1831); Astarâbâdi, *Safineh-ye nuh,* c. 1892 (for the English translation of this manuscript, see Hormoz Ebrahimnejad, "Religion and Medicine in Qâjâr Iran", in *Religion and Society in Qâjâr Iran,* ed. Robert Gleave (London: Routledge-Curzon, 2004), 401–28 (see appendix); MS 505.

[56] Lindsay Granshaw, "Fame and Fortune by Means of Bricks and Mortar? The Medical Profession and Specialist Hospitals in Britain, 1800–1948", in *The Hospital in History,* ed. Lindsay Granshaw and Roy Porter (London: Routledge, 1989), 208.

date and enhance their professional and institutional identity. As is apparent from a pamphlet written by a traditional physician, against the lectures of Dr Polak at the Dār al-Fonun, many traditional physicians of the army attended the medical school and worked at the hospital.[57] Therefore the first state hospital was not only built for medical treatment but also, and primarily, for the purposes of medical education. One of the chief aims of Dr Polak, as professor of anatomy at the Dār al-Fonun, was to find a hospital where he could take his students for clinical practice.

Both European doctors and their Persian colleagues promoted the cause of public hospitals, despite their differences of opinion on theoretical matters. For the chief physician of the army, the author of the above mentioned MS 505, the marizkhâneh-ye dowlati was to be the centre for medical education, an instrument of reuniting surgery and medicine, a site of observing diseases systematically. In other words, in order to understand the nature of modern hospitals in nineteenth-century Iran one should examine how the institutional, epidemiological, cultural and socio-political contexts related to the expansion of the army and the spread of the epidemics informed both the intervention of Western countries and the involvement of traditional physicians in medical reform.

The Qâjâr government was also anxious to bring medical education and practice under state control. This is illustrated very clearly in the above-mentioned document (MS 505), the main purpose of which was twofold: a) to promote practical medical knowledge versus theoretical medicine; b) to centralise the medical service in the base hospitals, or marizkhâneh-ye dowlati (state hospitals). According to the author of this source, Iranian physicians had ignored surgery and devoted themselves only to the treatment of humoral diseases. Surgery had become the profession of the third-hand practitioners, although it was important not only for injuries inflicted in battle, but for the extraction of tumours, stone bladders, etc. Moreover, by practising at the hospital, physicians could consult one another in case of a difficult diagnosis or treatment and there-

[57] "On Diseases Commonly Affecting Soldiers in the Barracks", c. 1857, MS 506, Library of Majles, Tehran.

fore could provide better service. The base hospitals were most appropriate to Iran because, although every regiment had several doctors, most were unskilled. The few experienced and knowledgeable physicians of the empire could not serve in all regiments, whereas at the state hospital they could provide quality treatment to soldiers of all regiments. The other reason for the necessity of a state hospital was that, in the regiments, it was difficult to check or to prevent the activities of the unskilled practitioners that were numerous in the army. Having little trust in the physicians of their own regiments, soldiers often consulted the doctors of other units who were seldom better and sometimes even worse. Finally, in the absence of a hospital, the drugs were distributed among regimental doctors who either misappropriated them or had no suitable place for their safe storage, whereas in a hospital they could be safely stored and distributed among ill soldiers upon prescription.[58] In sum, the centralisation of medical service was a key factor in the improvement of medical knowledge and practice.

All learned traditional physicians knew theoretical anatomy, which they called *tashrih* (explanation). According to 'Aqili, writing in the eighteenth century, good anatomical knowledge was required not only for surgical operations but also for accurate application of drugs on various parts and organs of the body.[59] Anatomy was therefore part of the curriculum in traditional medicine and, for this reason, Dr Mirzâ 'Ali, instructor of modern medicine at the Dār al-Fonun, termed one of his courses *tashrih-e jadid* (modern anatomy), versus the "old anatomy" or "descriptive anatomy" of traditional medicine.[60] During the first half of the nineteenth century, some physicians became acquainted with anatomo-pathological medicine, either by studying in European countries or in Iran by the help of foreign physicians. Dr John Cormick, for example, who came to Iran in 1810 and served in the army, educated some physicians about smallpox and his students translated his book on smallpox

58 MS 505, 13–17.

59 Aqili, *Kholâsat al-hekmah* (Bombay: s. n., 1845), 29.

60 Dr Mirzâ 'Ali, *Amrâz-e 'asabâni* [Nervous Maladies] (Tehran: lithograph edition, 1297/1880), 3.

inoculation into Persian. Dr Ernest Cloquet, who had been hired, in 1845, by Mohammad-Shah (1834–48) as his personal physician, also taught anatomy to his students at his home.[61] So far, anatomical knowledge, whether based on traditional or modern medicine, remained mainly theoretical. Dissection could not be practised and this remained the case for the rest of the century. The emphasis of the author of the booklet on the establishment of state hospitals, according to whom "learned physicians avoided practising surgery and only the rabble and ignorant have been inclined to this profession," indicates that the practice of surgery could not go much further than bloodletting and bone-setting; more invasive operations were understandably disastrous.[62] This author therefore insisted that surgeons of the army should not only spend their time studying but also observing and practising "manual operations".

The above-mentioned author believed that although the presence of surgeons at the hospital in peacetime was not indispensable (since most wounds and ulcers were of humoral nature and their treatment was to balance the humors), manual operations such as the extraction of cysts and stones was often necessary. Such operations were not totally absent in Iran; but details in the contemporary newspapers reporting medical news show that they were multiplied by the European physicians. In 1852, Dr Polak operated on twenty-three patients to remove bladder stones and only one of them did not survive.[63] It appears that Polak and other Western physicians focused on surgical practice in order to introduce anatomical medicine, in a country where dissection was avoided. Thanks to their activity, surgery beyond traditional bloodletting gained momentum. In September 1856, the RVE reported that Hâji Mohammad Ali, the surgeon of the army who had studied several years at the Dār al-Fonun and completed medicine as well as theoretical and practical surgery, had been honoured by the Shah as the Chief Surgeon of the army and his salary increased from 100 to 150 toman per

[61] E'temâd al-Saltaneh, *Târikh-e Montazam-e nâseri,* 3: 1728; Hormoz Ebrahimnejad, "L'introduction de la médicine européenne en Iran au XIXe siècle", *Sciences Sociales et Santé* 16, 1998, 69–96.

[62] Ebrahimnejad, *Medicine, Public Health and the Qâjâr State,* 185.

[63] E'temâd al-Saltaneh, *Târikh-e montazam-e nâseri,* 3: 1749.

annum.[64] Three years later, the same journal, reporting the activity of the medical school, underlined the fact that the medical students have now mastered anatomy in both theory and practice and each of them has written treatises on medicine and anatomy, while in the past they did not know anything more than what they could read in the classical books of traditional medicine.[65] More ambitious surgical operations were later performed by the graduates of the Dār al-Fonun. *Dânesh Journal* reported in 1882 that Mirzâ Ali-Akbar-Khan Shirâzi, physician of the sanitary council of Qom, successfully extracted a *Lipoma* (*sal 'eh-ye shahmi*) from the thigh of an old man. In another issue this journal reported that thanks to modern medical education, Mirzâ Mohammad Tafreshi, physician of the sanitary council of Sâri and graduate of the Dār al-Fonun, extracted bladder calculi from a father and his son.[66] By the early twentieth century, when the issue of certificates (*ejazeh-nameh*) allowing practice of medicine became the norm, all medical authorities who wrote these certificates underlined the fact that their candidate had mastered modern medicine in addition to traditional medicine. The components of modern medicine, were, according to Mirzâ Seyyed 'Ali- Boqrât al-Molk, one of the graduates of the Dār al-Fonun, physics, chemistry, anatomy, physiology, pathology and therapeutic. In these documents modern medicine was usually synonymous with *tebb-e 'amali* (practical or manual medicine).[67]

The main development in the nineteenth century was thus the emergence of what was called "manual" (*tebb-e yadi*) or "practical" medicine (*tebb-e 'amali*), as opposed to literary or bookish medicine.

Although the introduction of modern Western medicine played a crucial role, the more fundamental factor in this development, was that the local traditional medicine in the context of compelling social and medical realities came to perceive and recognise the ne-

[64] RVE, no. 294, 17 Moharram 1273/ 17 September 1856.

[65] RVE, no. 456, 14 December 1859. See also no. 458, 13 January 1860.

[66] Dânesh, no. 5, 16 August 1882, and no. 14, 27 December 1882.

[67] Archives of Sâzmân-e asnâd of the National Library, Tehran, nos. 297028920, (1907–1912), and 297000166 (1910).

cessity and effectiveness of 'manual medicine'. It was largely due to this 'recognition' that the development of modern medicine found a firm footing in Iran. This phenomenon is illustrated in the role that the above mentioned author of MS 505 attributed to the hospital "in pulling medicine and surgery together after thousands of years of divorce and restoring to surgery and surgeons the place they deserved within the medical profession." [68]

[68] MS 505, 63–64 ; Ebrahimnejad, *Medicine, Public Health and the Qâjâr State,* 184–86.

9

Pride and Prejudice: Hospitals, Medical Authority and Public Voice in Late Ottoman Southern bilâd al-Shâm

Philippe Bourmaud

On Monday, 12 April 1909, a delegation of Christian notables of Bethlehem brought to Jerusalem a petition for the French General Consul, stating that:

> For almost 20 years, the inhabitants of Bethlehem have grown accustomed to getting treatment at the French Hospital of our town.
>
> They got free healthcare that made them grateful toward France.
>
> This year, we were very sorry to note that a great many of our poor patients find it hard to go there and are compelled to attend the German Hospital [in Jerusalem].
>
> This lamentable change is due to the presence, in recent times, of an Italian physician from Jerusalem, who imposes on us very expensive fees for operations. He has not been afraid to undertake even very dangerous operations, that resulted in hastening the death of the sick. Furthermore, an Austrian monk, physician at Tantour [half-way between Jerusalem and Bethlehem], is also present in the hospital, where he managed to get admission to a certain patient for whom he had particular interest.
>
> We are surprised, and even angered to see two foreign physicians interfering in the life of the hospital, when they are very far from enjoying public esteem, as we are very satisfied with the official physician of the hospital, whom we have come to appreciate after his four years' stay among us. [1]

[1] ministère des Affaires éstrangères Quai d'Orsay, Correspondance Politique et Consulaire (henceforth CPC), Nouvelle Série, Turquie (henceforth NS Turquie), 430; as well as ministère des Affaires éstrangères Nantes, Consulate in Jerusalem, A (henceforth MAE Nantes, Jerusalem, A),108: Petition

Four days earlier, Dr Arab, the official physician of the Hôpital de la Sainte Famille (HSF) of Bethlehem, had been dismissed by Mère Mayaud, Superior of the hospital. In course of the six-odd months that followed before he finally relinquished his position, at least four more petitions, expressing contradicting views, were submitted regarding this affair. The case, as recorded in great detail in the French Diplomatic Archives, raises suspicion of manipulation. Yet the contents of the petitions, and the very fact that they represent public voice, might be a rare hint at indigenous perceptions of the practice of medicine in the Western hospitals of southern bilâd al-Shâm (present-day Jordan and Israel-Palestine).

I would like to suggest three approaches in support of this view. The first one is to understand the contents of petitions, gossip and rumours, as an affirmation of norms, by reversing the accusations they formulated. Second, what kind of public acceptance, or rejection of the rules and principles of hospital medicine is there to be found? Third, what were the patients' expectations regarding deontology? News about internal conflicts over hospital rules, which spread outside the hospital, thus shows that medical institutions never ceased to be public institutions, even though their rules could be exceptional, sometimes objectionable, in the eyes of the public. Yet hospitals worked, not only as institutions with specific set of rules but sometimes with arbitrary derogations to these rules. Those derogations showed a certain degree of arbitrariness in the supervision of hospitals, which was enhanced by interferences from foreigners (consulates, religious bodies, etc.). Does this amount to what Giorgio Agamben describes as a "state of exception",[2] which in those circumstances would mean that the heads of the hospital could possess some kind of sovereignty, exerted over the hospital and the life of patients? To what extent were the relationships

---

addressed to Gueyraud (French Consul in Jerusalem) on 12 April 1909. Of these two versions of the same petition, the one in the Quai d'Orsay claims to be a translation from Arabic, while the original in Nantes (with the seals of the signatories) is in French. As we shall see later, language was deemed a rather good indicator of the significance of such document.

[2] Giorgio Agamben, *Homo Sacer* (Torino: Giulio Einaudi editore, 1995).

within the hospital of a political nature? And how did the Ottoman administration react to it?

The definition of hospital as a place, both open and exceptional, suggests that relationships within the hospital were not of a man-to-man nature. At the same time, hospitals worked as institutions and as fields of influence. There was a chain of authority, and the distribution of power created affinities and preferential treatments. In spite of the effects of power due to the concentration of medical knowledge and skill, people from outside wanted to voice their opinions on hospitals. For sure, petitions were not a simple expression of opinion; from their instigation to their reception, they involved active influence. Though it is interesting to discover who the signatories were, the point is to determine who wrote the petition and on whose behalf it was signed. In short, how far were the petitions able to influence the balance of power? And what gave popularity to the manner in which hospitals functioned?

To a certain extent, hospitals did not need publicity. They were very visible, and their physicians were endowed with social status. Nevertheless, public image was as socially construed as it could be socially tarnished. Professionalism, career, beneficence, prestige of the institution, were all socially elaborated notions as was the image of Western medicine as radically different from, and superior to, indigenous medicine. They depended on how the practitioners themselves fashioned their professional activity, on how they oriented their career, and on the reputation they strove to acquire. Petitions worked at the same time for and against physicians, but according to pretty much the same set of categories. What part did medical systems, technology, national interest or personality play in the shaping of representations?

The HSF, an institution described with a wealth of detail, provides a good insight into these questions; but since it is definitely documented from a partisan source—the French Consulate in Jerusalem—I have deemed it necessary to consider other petitions, from the archives of the Church Missionary Society (CMS), an Anglican society with an active Palestine mission. Together, and biased though these sources are, they allow comparisons and help define patterns of behaviour at the hospital and ways of reading the petitions; they give contents to hospital rules, public voice and public image; but the first thing to do now is to put them into context.

Western Medicine in Late Ottoman Context

Judging from statistical data only, there was an accelerated movement of hospital foundations in southern bilâd al-Shâm between the 1870s and the First World War. Four hospitals had been created from the 1840s to the 1860s. By 1914, about thirty such institutions were unevenly dispersed in the main population centres and on both sides of Jordan.[3] The significance of this growth is yet to be qualified, in the face of obviously contrasted opinions about hospital treatment.

The historical conditions of this development are easy enough to describe: they indicate, not a response to a specific medical or epidemiological challenge, but a mix of normative reformism, imported conflicts of interest, and cultural or religious imagination. Of this, Bethlehem is quite characteristic.

In February 1886, shortly before its arrival in Jerusalem, on 3 May 1886, of the Roman Catholic nursing and schooling congregation of the Filles de la Charité,[4] the French Consulate in Jerusalem received a petition of worthies from Bethlehem, demanding that the Consulate should found and fund a physician and a dispensary for the Catholic community of Bethlehem.[5] The authors of the document argued that the distance was too great, and the expense of a car too high, to go to Jerusalem or to the (Austrian) hospital at Tantour, in case of an emergency at night. The delegation led by a *mukhtâr* (responsible for a local religious community or a village in their relationship with the Ottoman authorities), received assur-

[3] Norbert Schwake, *Die Entwicklung des Krankenhauswesens der Stadt Jerusalem vom Ende des 18. bis zum Beginn des 20. Jahrhunderts*, 2 vols. (Altroggen: Herzogentrath, 1983).

[4] "Les Sœurs de Saint-Vincent de Paul en Terre Sainte", *La Terre Sainte*, no. 325, 1 February 1889, 34.

[5] MAE, Nantes, Jerusalem, A, 108: Petition addressed by residents of Bethlehem to the French Consul in Jerusalem on 23 February 1886 (in Arabic, with French translation).

ances from the consul that their demands would be met; and in a second petition, a wider group of Catholic inhabitants of Bethlehem thanked the Consul for his munificence, arguing that the same request, presented first to prelates of the Catholic Church, then to other consulates had not met with any success.[6]

The Tantour institution was Catholic Austrian,[7] and the apparently grateful citizens of Bethlehem found it convenient to remind the French that other powers courted them. In the aftermath of the French-Prussian war in 1870–71, national competition between the main European powers was exported to the Middle East, and religious or charitable institutions were founded on these grounds. Bethlehem, with its Biblical background, was a place of choice. By 1909, no less than three hospitals[8] as well as schools, orphanages and monasteries had been opened there. A balance between the geography of religious symbols and the medical needs of more populous areas was late in coming, so that by 1914, Bethlehem was indisputably over-medicalised.

The timing of both petitions is suspicious. Indeed, the French Foreign Ministry had been trying for decades to get the Filles de la Charité to settle in Jerusalem, so as to counter the influence of the other main nursing congregation in Palestine, the Sisters of Saint Joseph de l'Apparition, who were seen as close to the Jesuits and hence obedient only to the Pope. The Sisters of Saint Joseph were not entirely and faithfully French as the diplomats wanted,[9] and

6 MAE, Nantes, Jerusalem, A, 108: Petition addressed by residents of Bethlehem to the French Consul in Jerusalem on 8 March 1886 (in Arabic, with French translation).

7 Thomas F. Stransky, "The Austrian Hospital at Tantur, 1869–1918", in *Austrian Presence in the Holy Land in the 19th and Early 20th Century: Proceedings of the Symposium in the Austrian Hospice in Jerusalem on March 1–2, 1995,* ed. Marian Wrba (Tel Aviv: Publication of the Austrian Embassy in Tel Aviv, 1996), 98–121.

8 MAE, Nantes, Jerusalem, A, 108: Report of Dr Henry (physician of the HSF) to Gueyraud, 11 June 1910.

9 MAE Nantes, Jerusalem, A, 103: Despatch from Edmond de Barrère (French Consul in Jerusalem) to the French Ambassador at Constantinople, Jerusalem, 20 December 1859; MAE Nantes, Jerusalem, A, 103: Barrère to the French Foreign Minister, Jerusalem, 15 February 1865.

the main means of pressure for French diplomats was by casting threats over the continuation of governmental subsidies.[10] The issue was a matter of temporal discipline and sovereignty. The sovereignty dispute was to be partly settled by compromises over the choice of the religious congregation in charge, and the nationality of the physician. Furthermore, the rules of hospitals separated, in theory, responsibilities between physicians and nursing staff, so as to avoid the subordination of one interest to another. This meant that no power was supreme—again, in theory—within the hospital, and that the setting and application of hospital rules determined who would really have the power.

The contribution of consulates in the development of hospitals was not only confined to financial matters. The 1867 reform of the Code of Foreigner's Property in the Ottoman Empire allowed foreigners to acquire land in full property and to build on it; yet at the same time, it made it compulsory to get a *firman* (authorisation from the Sultan) for any new building.[11] This firman had to be strenuously negotiated through the Embassy at Constantinople, who received applications through several consulates of the Empire. This in turn gave power and centrality to the consuls. At the HSF, the first superior of the institution, Mère Marmier, was nearly at open war with Mère Sion, and sided against her with Ledoulx, the French consul.[12] In spite of this close relationship, the needed firman was only granted in 1892, five years after the beginning of the building of the HSF, which had proceeded against the demands of the

[10] MAE Nantes, Jerusalem, A, 108: Gueyraud to Pichon (French Foreign Minister), Jerusalem, 14 June 1909.

[11] "Protocole en vertu duquel les étrangers peuvent être admis à la jouissance du droit de propriété", in *Législation Ottomane ou: Recueil des Lois, Règlements, Ordonnances, Traités, Capitulations et Autres Documents Officiels de l'Empire Ottoman,* ed. Grégoire Aristarchi Bey (Constantinople: Imprimerie Frères Nicolaïdes, 1873–1888), 1: 22–25.

[12] MAE Nantes, Jerusalem, A, 108: Mère Marmier (Superior of the HSF) to Ledoulx (French Consul in Jerusalem), Bethlehem, 26 May 1889.

Ottoman authorities in Bethlehem.[13] In fact the role of the Consul in the construction of the hospital evolved into that of a patron.

Another motivation for promoting European hospitals lay in cultural and religious conceptions of the "Holy Land" during the last decades of Ottoman rule. Along with the development of Biblical critical science, came new forms of piety focused on the actual geographical content of the Bible. This brought to southern bilâd al-Shâm pilgrims and missionaries who view the region as a destitute zone in sharp contrast to descriptions taken from the Scriptures; a land at the root of culture, yet crippled by tradition, both religious and medical.[14] Such notions would be re-used by the indigenous population, such as the signatories of the petition of 8 March 1886, who lament their "foresaken hometown", due to lack of a physician.[15] Yet Bethlehem, far from being a destitute town, had known a steady economic and demographic growth since the 1850s at least, in keeping with the building of European Church institutions and the emergence of religious tourism.[16]

By 1909, besides international beneficence, the notables who dominated the municipality had taken it upon themselves to assume responsibility for public health and medicine for the poor. Municipalisation of the Ottoman Empire, however patchy, was part of the process of Ottoman reform from 1839 onwards. Starting from the 1860s, municipalities were founded in the region, and the empowerment of local worthies meant first and foremost devolution of

[13] MAE, Nantes, Jerusalem, A, 108: Governor of Jerusalem to Ledoulx, Jerusalem, 8 May 1890; telegram of the French Ambassador in Constantinople to Ledoulx, Constantinople, 17 February 1892.

[14] Alex Carmel, "A Note on the Christian Contribution to Palestine's Development in the 19th Century", in *Palestine in the Late Ottoman Period: Political, Social and Economic Transformation,* ed. David Kushner (Jerusalem / Leyden: Yad Izhak ben-Zvi / E. J. Brill, 1986), 302–8.

[15] MAE, Nantes, Jerusalem, A, 108: Bethlehem Petition, 8 March 1886.

[16] Alexander Schölch, "European Penetration and the Economic Development of Palestine, 1856–1882", in *Studies in the Economic and Social History of Palestine in the Nineteenth and Twentieth Centuries,* ed. Roger Owen (Oxford: St Antony's College / McMillan Press, 1982), 10–87.

expense.[17] Evergetism was promoted through national legislation, for instance, through the Health Regulation of 1 January 1871. The municipalities had to pay the wage of municipal physicians and hospitals.[18] This meant that the appointment of municipal physicians—such as Dr Arab in Bethlehem[19]—was a testimony of local wealth and civic pride. Only the richer or more proactive communities could afford it.

Elsewhere, local evergetism took special significance. In Nablus, men of clout, including the municipality, united in 1901 in the decision to found a municipal hospital, in protest against the missionary purpose of the hospital of the CMS there and the arrogance of the hospital's head physician.[20] There was obvious resentment, and not only on the part of the Muslim majority, against the religious and political interferences of European powers in the life of the Empire. Beyond the religious aspect, such municipal mobilisation was a sign of loyalty to the Sultan against foreign influence at all levels of Ottoman public life. The foundation of a municipal hospital was an assertion of scientific and technical autonomy from Europe. They worked as a symbol of sovereignty. However, ironically enough, these hospitals could not work without nurses, and the only ones available in Nablus belonged to the French congregation of the Sisters of Saint Joseph.[21] Nursing implied a relationship with other bodies, and often itinerating work, which made it disreputable for Syrian women. Western hospitals needed nursing staff, which Middle Eastern societies would only provide in very short supply.

[17] Ruth Kark, "The Contribution of the Ottoman Regime to the Development of Jerusalem and Jaffa, 1840–1917", in *Palestinie in the Late Ottoman Period: Political, Social and Economic Transformation,* ed. David Kushner (Jerusalem / Leyden: Yad Izhak ben-Zvi / E. J. Brill, 1986), 46–58.

[18] *Annuaire oriental de médecine et de pharmacie* (Istanbul: s. n., 1892).

[19] MAE Nantes, Jerusalem, A, 108: Gueyraud to Pichon, Jerusalem, 9 August 1909.

[20] Dr Habib Salim to the Reverend Baylis, Nablus, 25 May 1908, Group III (henceforth G3), Mediterranean Mission, Personal papers (P/O), 1908/64, Birmingham University Library, Church Missionary Archives (henceforth CMA).

[21] Jules-Antonin Jaussen, *Coutumes Palestiniennes: Naplouse et son District* (Paris: Librairie orientaliste Geuthner, 1927), 251–52.

At another level, such display of sovereignty was largely based on an importation of science and training methods. From the 1890s until 1909, the official physician of the HSF was a graduate of the medical faculty of the Université Saint-Joseph, founded by the Jesuits in Beirut in 1882. Together with the medical faculty of the Syrian Protestant College (founded in 1867 by American missionaries),[22] it provided Arabic-speaking medical staff for hospitals and dispensaries, while the only option for a medical training so far was as distant as Cairo or Constantinople. The Faculty at the Université Saint-Joseph as well as most hospitals kept by French congregations in the Middle East, were all financed by French Government, even after the wave of radical secularisation in the years 1902–5. Dr Arab and his predecessor Dr Philippe Barakat, both Ottoman citizens, took their medical degrees at the Université Saint-Joseph and looked to the French government for job and protection.[23]

To sum up, asking whether the development of hospitals in late-Ottoman Syria was endogenous or exogenous is of limited relevance. Of course, certain institutions would be identified as foreign, and others not; yet the dynamics at work in the affirmation of Ottoman sovereignty in the medical sphere were part of the dialectics of competing national interests. Through legal procedure, medical training, and control of the profession or even through reactions against foreign intrusion, Ottoman authorities contributed to make medicine an increasingly extraneous practice, even as they tried to nationalise it. Ironically, hospital medicine was a widely nationalised, yet hardly Ottoman field.

Hospital Norms at Variance

Extraneous norms can create tensions and defiance wherever they are exported. In the case of southern bilâd al-Shâm, "prejudices

[22] Ghada Yusuf Khoury, ed., *The Founding Fathers of the American University of Beirut: Biographies* (Beirut: AUB Press, 1992).

[23] MAE Quai d'Orsay, CPC, NS Turquie, 430: Dr Barakat (physician of the HSF) to the French Foreign Ministry, Bethlehem, 8 September 1897; MAE Nantes, Jerusalem, A, 108: Report on the HSF by Dr Emile Arab to Gueyraud, Bethlehem, 25 May 1909.

against the hospitals,[24] as physicians called it with a positivistic undertone, implied that it was the internal order of hospitals which created anthropological hindrance. But the petition quoted above suggests just the contrary. Was it the rule, or the arbitrary derogation to the rule of the hospital, which fostered "prejudice"? What kind of medical deontology did people expect within hospitals, if one reverses the complaints? As to the HSF, the petitions suggest that patient attendance was reduced by conflict around hospital rules.

The origins of the affair are not clear. Rumours spread as the conflict became more intense;[25] yet as Consul Gueyraud insisted that right from the start, Mère Mayaud had assured him that her decision had no professional or moral origin, it is best to stick to what she claimed.[26] Officially, the declining statistics of the HSF had persuaded her that Dr Arab had lost the confidence of most patients. Dr Arab, on his part, was prone to interpret his dismissal as a plot to get rid of him by Brother Hoenigman (the physician at the Tantour Hospital) and Dr Claudio Mancini, an Italian physician in Jerusalem who operated on an irregular basis at the HSF.[27] Mancini wanted nothing but Arab's job. So far, there is nothing more in the story than sneaky competition for a position. The problem thickened as the issue gave a chance to complain about certain physicians and to assert certain ideas about medical care.

If we follow Dr Arab's defence of his professional skills, and his attacks against Dr Mancini, Brother Hoenigman and Mère Mayaud, the internal problems of the HSF affected the patients in several ways. First of all irregularities in the chain of command and the application of prerogatives created confusion. According to the native physician, Dr Mancini had gradually taken greater liberties with Dr Arab's service. After doing an interim job at the HSF between Dr Barakat's and Dr Arab's tenures in 1905, the Italian doctor had been allowed to come to the hospital for surgical operations, for which

24 MAE Nantes, Jerusalem, A, 108: Arab to Gueyraud, 25 May 1909.

25 MAE Nantes, Jerusalem, A, 108: Note by Gueyraud, "Démarche à Bethléem le 2 août 1909".

26 MAE Nantes, Jerusalem, A, 108: Gueyraud to Pichon, Jerusalem, 14 June 1909.

27 MAE Nantes, Jerusalem, A, 108: Arab to Gueyraud, 25 May 1909.

Dr Arab lacked skill.[28] By 1908, Mère Mayaud had allowed Mancini to bring his patients to the hospital and treat them there. Dr Arab went on to complain that by the spring of 1909, Mère Mayaud would decide which patients under the care of the official physician needed surgical operation, lock Mancini's patients in single rooms at the time of Dr Arab's visits, and claim that they had already received their treatment through the Italian physician.[29] During the summer, the nurses under Mère Mayaud's orders would simply ignore Dr Arab, thus turning his medical service into a joke.[30] Part of Dr Arab's defence is aimed mainly at arousing the anger of the French diplomats, whose government subsidised the HSF, by claiming that, Mancini's—and to a lesser degree, Hoenigman's—invasion is a deliberate effort to make the French hospital "international and cosmopolitan":

> The interference of two foreign physicians in the French Hospital in Jerusalem has caused enormous gossip among the people here. They could not figure out who was the real physician of the hospital in the end, and therefore whom one should go to in order to get admission for a patient or organise an operation. This led the indigenous population to stay away from the hospital or to attend, albeit with heart pangs, the Swedish hospital in Bethlehem or the German Hospital in Jerusalem. The statistics of the hospital went down during the elapsed year: clearly, the official physician is not responsible for this![31]

Clashes between physicians, either mutually or with the staff responsible for the upkeep of the hospital, were quite common. Hence the very same accusation of plotting had been levelled at Mancini by Dr Tissot, the physician of the French Hôpital Saint-Louis in Jerusalem, the year before.[32] Yet at that time, the discussion had

[28] MAE Nantes, Jerusalem, A, 108: Arab to Gueyraud, 25 May 1909.

[29] Ibid.

[30] MAE Nantes, Jerusalem, A, 108: Gueyraud to Pichon, Jerusalem, 3 August 1909.

[31] MAE Nantes, Jerusalem, A, 108: Arab to Gueyraud, 25 May 1909.

[32] MAE Quai d'Orsay, CPC, NS Turquie, 430: "Projet de règlement de l'Hôpital Français de Jérusalem fait par M. Outrey, Consul Général de France à Jérusalem et annoté par le Docteur Tissot" (1908); Dr Tissot to Pichon, from Jerusalem, 12 Febraury 1908.

been limited to the rather theoretical question of framing new rules for the French hospital in Jerusalem, whereas in Bethlehem, disruptions in the service of the HSF could not be hidden. Whether one has to believe Dr Arab or not is immaterial; the existence of a precedent makes his contentions plausible. Obviously, the normal work of the hospital appears to have been linked with the authority of its physician. For admissions, personal relationships with him or with Mère Mayaud mattered most.

At the HSF, the Filles de la Charité had the advantage to be constantly present by the side of the patients. It gave them more power, and so they could either choose to ignore Dr Arab and his orders, so as to push him out[33] or to assist him normally, once his dismissal had been ensured as Mère Mayaud wanted to make up with him.[34] Though the theoretical hierarchy within hospitals gave medical power and responsibility to the physician, and organisational power to the Sisters, Dr Arab's reliance on nursing Sisters who would stay in charge in the hospital much longer than himself, meant that Mère Mayaud was fully in charge of organisation and of medical affairs.

The native physician pushed his point further with the case of Jamilah Dabdoub, suffering from liver cancer, who had been treated for two months by Hoenigman. The Austrian physician decided when she was nearing death, to have her admitted at the HSF, without Arab's knowledge. The patient died before she could even be operated, and the morning after, Arab was surprised to see her coffin taken out of the HSF, as he was not aware that she had been admitted to the hospital in the first place. Obviously, the only reason for the admission of Jamilah Dabdoub in the HSF was to keep Hoenigman's reputation clean.[35] Whoever saw the coffin coming out of the hospital would infer that one of Dr Arab's patients had died, which would be supported by hospital statistics. As the HSF was identified with the personality of its official physician, the events of the hospital tended to translate into recognition or a denial of competence on the part of Dr Arab.

33 MAE Nantes, Jerusalem, A, 108: Gueyraud to Pichon, 3 August 1909.

34 Ibid., 30 August 1909.

35 MAE Nantes, Jerusalem, A, 108: Arab to Gueyraud, 25 May 1909.

From the Ottoman administration's point of view, only the official physician was in charge of the hospital; yet confusion created by the special permission given to Mancini and Hoenigman to practise within the hospital created complications on that level too, until the very end of Dr Arab's service at the HSF. When a man from Bethlehem was treated thereafter being the victim of an aggression, and died there, Dr Mancini, who was on the premises, took care of him, and left after he died. When a delegation of the *mudîriyyah* (local governorate) of Bethlehem came to check what had happened to him, they enquired about the case with Dr Arab, who had known nothing of it. Much to the grief of the family of the deceased, the body was kept for examination. A delegation of three, including Dr Arab, was appointed for that purpose. Since Dr Mancini had not given any information, the report could only be superficial. On top of that, Dr Arab complained that in his functions of physician of the municipality, he would have been able to deal with the case speedily, had his prerogatives of physician of the HSF been respected. As the matter stood, he had to admit to the authorities that his position at the hospital was at best precarious, and that he could not really fulfil his responsibilities as head physician.[36] Thus, the situation at the HSF looked, in the eyes of the local administration, like the emperor's new clothes.

Part of the reluctance of patients regarding hospitalisation was due to that personalised perception of medical treatment. The hospitalised patients' stress due to their own state was reinforced by a latent notion that they are in the hands of the physician, who has sovereign power over their life, and of virtual impunity due to the closed framework of the hospital and its nearly-foreign status. In theory, deontology and hospital rules were supposed to calm down such fears, yet they were not easily shrugged off. As it was customary to keep the family away as much as possible, in the name of hygiene, air circulation or what not, hospitalisation was in itself a sharp break away from the day-to-day life of most patients. Hospital wards were beyond the immediate reach of family solidarity and protection, as

[36] MAE Nantes, Jerusalem, A, 108: Arab to Gueyraud, Bethlehem, 25 October 1909.

depicted in the case of a Bethlehemite, Elias Ijha, brought to the HSF by Mancini and Hoenigman for an operation. They invited Dr Arab to join them as the operation had begun; yet it became directly clear that the man was in extreme agony, and the operation was unnecessary. The following day, a German-speaking neighbour of Elias Ijha asked Hoenigman why they had operated the man if they knew he was going to die. The Austrian physician answered that they wanted to check their diagnosis, which, according to Dr Arab, gave birth to the idea that the HSF conducted medical experiments at the expense of its patients' lives.[37] Either Hoenigman simply neglected medical secrecy and the feelings of Ijha's next of kin, or he intentionally instrumentalised the body of a sick man, in the name of the rights of science, to discredit the HSF and, along with it, Dr Arab. In both cases, he gave credit to the intuition that rules and deontology were no sufficient protections for patients. As underlined by Dr Arab's reference to the questioning by a German-speaker, linguistic difference reinforced the estrangement that patients might feel, since most of the time the physician could hardly speak Arabic. This gave an advantage to the physicians, who would hardly ever have to answer for their medical acts.

No less scandalous was the allegation, expressed in a petition attacking Mancini and Hoenigman and supported by the French Consul, that one of the patients of the Austrian physician, treated in a single room, was a woman known to be his lover.[38] Again, hospitals could easily be seen as a school for scandal. A derogation granted by Mère Mayaud to Mancini and Hoenigman, allowing them to have their private patients at the hospital, was interpreted as an act of near-sovereignty. Ironically, single rooms were exceptional, and the normal display of several beds in each hospital ward met public expectations of morality. While such a display was meant to spare space and time, it also allowed control of behaviour. Every patient would be a witness to the actions of each of his room-mates, which would guarantee family honour, a value which was no less important than individual life.

[37] Ibid., Bethlehem, 25 May 1909.

[38] MAE Nantes, Jerusalem, A, 108: Bethlehem Petition, 12 April 1909.

Petitions often dealt with financial matters: petitioners usually claimed a right to free medicine and treatment, or conversely, express their reprobation for the venality of medical staff. Most denominational hospitals were free for their religious community, except the protestant ones,[39] either a symbolic contribution for admission was asked[40] or free treatment was reserved only to poor patients. Yet free health care on a denominational basis had been turned into a norm by various missionaries, especially the Catholics. Mancini was against this practice while at the HSF and in the words of Consul Gueyraud, his greed was notorious. Yet if he asked an already expensive fee of 50 francs for his intervention of the dying Elias Ijha—whose wife was compelled to mortgage their house to pay,[41]—he claimed 300 francs from a French missionary to remove his appendix.[42] These casuistic fees were not what seemed scandalous in his venality: he was mainly criticised for his ostensible exploitation of poverty. The rules of the HSF were perceived as subject to ample derogations, so that the norm progressively lost its meaning.

Hospitals were understood to be a service and a manner of beneficence, and not an innovation on a non-existent medical market. If a hospital failed to respect this principle, patients would go away to another hospital, regardless of national influence and of denomination. As a result, free health care, which was at first a provision for poor patients, would become universal; a provision designed to ensure medical service for the indigent would become a norm, as though Bethlehem as a whole was an indigent society. However, an increasing affluence touched the upper stratum of its population

[39] J. R. L. Hall (secretary of the Palestine Mission of the CMA) to Reverend Baylis (secretary of the Parent Committee of the Palestine Mission), Jerusalem, 18 September 1900, G 3 P/O 1900/149, CMA; Petition of the Jerusalem Protestant Congregation to the CMA, 28 August 1900.

[40] MAE Nantes, Jerusalem, A, 108: Gueyraud to Mère Marie Kieffer, General Superior of the Filles de la Charité, Jerusalem, 28 May 1909.

[41] MAE Nantes, Jerusalem, A, 108: Arab to Gueyraud, 25 May 1909.

[42] MAE Nantes, Jerusalem, A, 108: Gueyraud to Mère Vincent Sion, Superior of the Jerusalem House of the Filles de la Charité, Jerusalem, 7 July 1909.

as the people of Bethlehem became more and more dependent on Europe.

Hospitals may well have been, in the end, a space of near-sovereignty; yet in the petitions, the notion of what is "foreign" is unclear, as shown by the declarations of allegiance which come up in each petition addressed to French diplomats; then, it seems to mean any foreigner in the Ottoman Empire, except the French. Thus, foreign near-sovereignty in the hospitals was disguised as legitimate authority. Those who drafted the petitions had learned to walk the walk and talk the talk of French diplomacy in the Middle East.

The Fiction of Public Mobilisation

Taken at face value, petitions seem to reflect the image of a society driven by public opinion and bent on transparency, where what goes on within hospitals is worthy of debate in the name of public interest. It would be a mistake, however, to consider the signing of a petition as a transparent act, producing a representative sample of local society.

There is verisimilitude in the way petitioners make their point, even though one might contend that their arguments are contrived to fit with the notion that diplomats and missionaries have of local *mores*. The protagonists of the affair fashioned petitions so that these would answer the recipients' anticipations of what local rationality is, and mirror an exotically enthusiastic image of France, Austria, Italy, the Latin Patriarchate, and what not. This was also clear to their recipients.

The French Foreign Ministry entertained doubts about the veracity of those petitions: it took unusually good care to check its information. To make sure that Mère Mayaud indeed bore ill-will to Dr Arab, the Ministry ordered Consul Gueyraud to dispatch a mission of inspection. Dr Drouillard, the physician of the French government in Jerusalem—who was also the physician of the French Hospital in Jerusalem, the Hôpital Saint-Louis, and a man whose record shows deep integrity—was officially sent on 19 May 1909 to help Dr Arab on two urgent operations. Yet Mère Mayaud did not even allow him into the hospital, in spite of a letter of recommendation from the Consul, on account of Dr Drouillard's being attached to another hospital.[43] Gueyraud negotiated with Mère Mayaud, the Superior of the Palestine mission of the Filles de la Charité, and when Drouillard came back on the following day, he was allowed to see the two patients treated earlier by Dr Arab, but not a third patient in similar need.[44] From Gueyraud's testimony, it appears that Mère Mayaud was enraged about Drouillard's intervention as he was the physician of the Hôpital Saint-Louis. Mère Mayaud was identified with the rivals of the Filles de la Charité, the congregation of the Sisters of Saint-Joseph de l'Apparition, who worked at the hospital.[45] Gueyraud's insistence on the two French hospitals working together was unlikely to allay her anger.[46] She may also have resented Drouillard's inspection in principle.

Such scepticism stemmed from linguistic realism, as long as it fitted French interests. Gueyraud debunked a petition from the same camp addressed in July 1909 to the Latin Patriarch and "written in excellent Italian, which no native is able to do."[47] Another petition attacking Dr Arab and defending Dr Mancini, Brother Hoenigman and Mère Mayaud was addressed to the French Foreign Ministry in September 1909; and a reader from the Ministry annotated it:

> The Catholics of Bethlehem write darn good French for people who only sign with their murour [Arabic seal]. One wonders whether the signatories simply understood the meaning of their request.[48]

This is hypercritical: the *murûr* is indeed an alternative to signature (in Arabic or, as for the signature of a man called Antoine Mansour, in Latin alphabet), yet it is not a definite sign of illiteracy. Some of the seals are apparently shaped as a trademark; designed according to European stamping fashion. One seal says: "Michel

[43] MAE, Nantes, Jerusalem, A, 108: Dr Drouillard to Gueyraud, 19 May 1909.

[44] Ibid., 21 May 1909.

[45] MAE Nantes, Jerusalem, A, 108: Gueyraud to Pichon, 3 August 1909.

[46] Ibid.

[47] Ibid., 9 August 1909.

[48] MAE Nantes, Jerusalem, A, 108: Petition addressed to the French Foreign Minister by the Latins of Bethlehem, 20 September 1909.

J. Dabdoub—Bethléem (Palestine)" in French and Arabic; other mentions "H. Mansour—Bethléem Palestine", in French only.

A sociological analysis of signatures and seals indicates that petitions expressed a highly hierarchical idea of public voice. In the HSF case, all petitions bore, on the top line of signatures, the seal of at least one mukhtâr. Mostly, the mukhtâr-s who signed were Latin Catholics, yet the names of Armenian and Greek Christian religious representatives, such as the Armenian Suleiman Musa, also appear.[49] In one of the petitions, the title of the signatories is detailed: notably, a "mukhtâr of the central quarter"; a "mukhtâr of the Greek (melkite) rite" and a "chief of the Armenian rite"; the engineers of the municipalities of Jerusalem and Bethlehem; the representative of the Imperial Ottoman Bank; a few tradesmen and craftsmen; one *rentier*; and five men linked with tourism (the correspondent of the Cook touring company and four mother-of-pearl craftsmen, whose production of religious souvenirs were the traditional industry of Bethlehem).[50] Eminence is defined within geographical, religious and professional frameworks; yet tourism also creates relations of dependence, as shown by Gueyraud's commentary that the signatories of a petition supporting Hoenigman are mostly owners of souvenir shops attending Austrian clients, and therefore clients of the Austrian physician.[51] Anyway, it is unlikely that in a tourist town such as Bethlehem, the most influential men would not be unwilling to give a hand to the protectors of their European partners.

The elusive understatement of power and legitimacy is sought through the claim for unanimity, or at least mass and majority. In the latter phase of the affair, the number of signatories is much higher than in the earlier part: 18 signatories on the 12th of April[52] but no less than 88 on the 7th of August. The growth is not linear, but it signals gradual mobilisation. In the last petition, the

[49] MAE Nantes, Jerusalem, A, 108: Petition addressed by residents of Bethlehem to Gueyraud, Bethlehem, 30 May 1909.

[50] Ibid.

[51] MAE Nantes, Jerusalem, A, 108: Note by Gueyraud, appended to the petition of the "latin rite of Bethlehem" addressed to him on 7 August 1909.

[52] MAE Nantes, Jerusalem, A, 108: Gueyraud to Pichon, Jerusalem, 14 June 1909.

signatories claim to represent three-fourth of the Catholics of Bethlehem, whereas Gueyraud more soberly thinks that they represent three-fifth of the Catholic population, which was quite divided as a result. [53] There is little to say about the recipients, except that those mentioned were either diplomats or religious heads. Though the investigators are likely to be the physicians themselves, and though the content of the petition may refer to satisfaction or dissatisfaction with medical service, petitioning about the hospital took its course completely outside the place.

Petitioners followed closely the course of events. In a matter of days after Dr Arab's dismissal was announced, the first petition was written. [54] A second wave of petitions took place by the end of July, after the announcement that an agreement was reached about the HSF: Dr Arab would stay in his position until a successor could be found, and neither Mancini nor Hoenigman would be allowed at the HSF. Petitions attacking Dr Arab, or Dr Mancini and Brother Hoenigman, arrived at the Latin Patriarchate of Jerusalem and the French Foreign Ministry. The reaction of the Latin Patriarch, who answered the complaints of Mancini and Hoenigman by giving them certificates of good behaviour, is not so much a sign of partisanship, as that of the contents of the petitions, which cast a slur on the physician's personal honesty and sleazy charges against him. The matter became radicalised by straying away from its medical origin.

On 7 August 1909, another petition was addressed to the Latin Patriarch, right after the decision had been taken by the direction of the Custody of the Holy Land—the Franciscan society holding the trusteeship of most Catholic holy places in the Holy Land and Syria in general, and an important landlord and tour operator in the region—to prohibit the delivery, at the pharmacy of the Custody in Bethlehem, of prescriptions made by Dr Arab. From the point of view of the Custody, it was just upholding the claims of Mancini and Hoenigman, physicians of the Custody in Jerusalem and Bethlehem respectively. As the pharmacy was the only one in Bethlehem

[53] MAE Nantes, Jerusalem, A, 108: Gueyraud, 7 August 1909.

[54] MAE Nantes, Jerusalem, A, 108: Bethlehem Petition, 12 April 1909.

to deliver medicines for free, the reaction was immediate and radical. If one takes Gueyraud's word on it, Catholics had stopped attending the church of the Latin parish (held by the Custody), postponed their children's baptism, and threatened to stop asking for confession—from members of the Custody—for their death. Furthermore, they professed an intention to attend the Greek or German Lutheran hospitals and, implicitly, to convert to Greek orthodoxy or Protestantism.[55] This of course sounds extreme, yet most conversions from one church to another in the Ottoman Empire, were based on such internal conflicts. Unsurprisingly, the Custody backed down since it could not take lightly the case, which involved too many men of credit and religious authority in Bethlehem. The accelerated production of petitions and charges indicate that the conflict fostered a new balance of power within the Catholic institutions. This corroborates the conclusion drawn from the growing number of signatures.

By the end of August 1909, the matter was independent of Dr Arab and whatever had been going on at the hospital so far. The events had gone too far to be considered as the product of any kind of manipulation by European actors. However, it clearly shows whose interests had been satisfied. Of the initial actors of this affair, only Mère Mayaud continued with her job, and had the satisfaction of working with a French physician, as she had declared that she did not want to ever work again with physicians from the Université Saint-Joseph.[56] The French consulate had to give up its *protégé* and the project of a synergy between the two French hospitals in the area, yet the solution was satisfactory in the eyes of French diplomats, since the HSF retained its French character. The congregation of the Filles de la Charité exercised its power and thus managed to maintain its full control over the HSF without clashing head on with French diplomacy. On the contrary, the Custody had chosen to intervene and had alienated part of the Catholic community; it had to let down the ambitions of Mancini and Hoenigman. The chain of successive petitions became effective when it ceased to concern

[55] MAE, Nantes, Jerusalem, A, 108: Bethlehem Petition, 7 August 1909.

[56] Ibid.

an individual and threatened the institutional unity of the Roman Catholic Church in Bethlehem.

Petitions were representative in a twisted way: that is, representative of status and authority within institutional groups, and of economic interests which, in the special case of Bethlehem, commended loyalty to well-defined foreign interests. It is altogether clear that the main protagonists in the case of the HSF were themselves the agents of conflicting national interests, which defined their sphere of action and their career prospects.

Medical Career and Professional Reputation

Medical authority was not based only on charisma; it needed funding and institutional support. Hospital physicians were bound by loyalty to the national powers that protected them; however, changes of allegiance happened, though religious allegiances were only exceptionally reversed. In any case, the influence that physicians enjoyed was based on their reputation. How did they use their national and political loyalties in their career plans? How did these plans influence their public image? Again, the case of Dr Arab vs Dr Mancini is an interesting study.

Mancini charged notoriously high fees, and tried as he might to get a stable job in a hospital, so as to use the premises for his private *clientèle*. Gueyraud, who used to be on friendly terms with him, clearly revealed Mancini's ambition of going back to Europe after a few years. In the meanwhile, all that Mancini wanted was to gather "certain capital", with which he could settle down somewhere.[57] At the HSF,[58] as in the Hôpital Saint-Louis the previous year,[59] he had endeared himself with the religious personnel of the hospital. Interestingly, French protection was perceived with mixed feelings by religious institutions after the Secularisation Law of 1905. By contrast, the Italians became increasingly friendly to Church interests abroad. At the beginning, Mère Mayaud said she feared that

[57] MAE Nantes, Jerusalem, A, 108: Gueyraud to Pichon, 14 June 1909.

[58] MAE Nantes, Jerusalem, A, 108: Arab to Gueyraud, 25 May 1909.

[59] MAE Nantes, Jerusalem, A, 108: Outrey (then French Consul at Jerusalem) to Pichon, Jerusalem, 25 February 1908.

Consul Gueyraud wanted to make her hospital secular. This was a strategy to gather support from her congregation against Gueyraud, and a way to stave off any degree of integration of the HSF and the Hôpital Saint-Louis under the aegis of the French Consulate.[60] Against French interventions, missionary congregations could balance French protection with both influences from Rome—the Holy See and the new kingdom of Italy.

Mancini was not a pawn in the game of national competition, he understood it fully, and would play it in a determined manner. He married the daughter of former French Consul Georges Outrey,[61] which enabled him to gain the support of the deputy Italian Consul to his cause during the summer of 1909.[62] He even became, for a while, Consul in Jerusalem for the kingdom of Belgium[63] (consuls did not have to be nationals to represent a given country in the Ottoman Empire). A job at the French hospital in Bethlehem, with a wage of 2000 francs a year, was not an end in itself[64] yet he was determined to make as much money as he could out of the job. Furthermore, an official position, such as physician of a foreign hospital, could also help him give expertise in a variety of fields. In a matter of years, he could go back home a richer man, with a good reputation and connection. However, his fine manners did not seem to fool anyone about his real intentions: neither the petitioners who lamented the departure of poorer patients from the HSF, nor the sisters working at the HSF. When asked if he had treated them during the cholera epidemics of 1909, one of them answered: "Oh no! We would all be dead then!"[65] He did not care to play the part of a dedicated and humanitarian physician, since he considered his network within the European circles of Jerusalem and Bethlehem sufficient to make him successful.

[60] MAE Nantes, Jerusalem, A, 108: Arab to Gueyraud, 13 April 1909.

[61] MAE Nantes, Jerusalem, E, 26: Gueyraud to Bompard (French Ambassador in Constantinople), 4 March 1909.

[62] MAE Nantes, Jerusalem, A, 108: Gueyraud to Pichon, 14 June 1909.

[63] MAE Nantes, Jerusalem, E, 26: Gueyraud to Bompard, 4 March 1909.

[64] MAE Nantes, Jerusalem, A, 108: Arab to Gueyraud, 25 May 1909.

[65] MAE Nantes, Jerusalem, A, 108: Gueyraud to Mère Vincent Sion, 7 July 1909.

Future opportunities were probably not much open for Dr Arab, who did not try to cash in on his job in Bethlehem as much as Mancini. Nonetheless, he conceived his tenure as physician at the HSF as a stepping stone in his career. He insisted on both his disinterestedness as a physician in Bethlehem, and on the fact that he intended to use his position there as an experience on which he might be able to earn a reputation for himself at some other place, either Palestine or Beirut. In his eyes at least, there was no contradiction, and he described his dedicated job in Bethlehem as an unpleasant and even dangerous task

> which consists in [of] entering real slums, in bending over patients lying on an earthen floor, in inhaling putrid smells, in making oneself thus in a state of receptivity to contagion and of *minoris resistentiae* [weakened resistance]: none of this encourages a young physician to take such a job.[66]

This is pretty melodramatic and *pro domo*, of course, still it underlines the importance of medical visits at home in his duty, while Mancini only practiced at the hospital. However, Arab thought of his dismissal essentially as a stain to his reputation and future professional hopes.[67] Gueyraud was favourably impressed, and insisted until the end that a solution be found, which would not be detrimental to the physician's career. One may add that French protection was apparently not an empty word. By 1912, Dr Arab was *chef de clinique* (deputy-head of a medical department in a hospital) at the Hospital of the French Medical Faculty in Beirut, and tried to establish his name by publishing articles on popular medicine in Palestine in French medical journals.[68]

Nonetheless, for both physicians, career was directly linked with national interests and with hospitals as an institution; or rather, a job as head physician in a hospital was but a beginning. This was quite a normal path within the framework of Western medicine, yet it came in sharp contrast to the usual practice in the hospitals of

66 MAE Nantes, Jerusalem, A, 108: Arab to Gueyraud, 25 May 1909.

67 Ibid.

68 "La Médecine populaire en Syrie et en Palestine", in *La Presse médicale*, no. 26, 1912, 386 sq.

earlier Ottoman times. Until the late eighteenth or early nineteenth century, there had been one hospital in Jerusalem, *al-bimâristân al-salâhî*, with physicians and surgeons attached to it. Practitioners were organised in a guild, whose delegate was chosen and supervised by the *Qâdî* (chief judge) of the *Harâm al-Sharîf*, the sanctuary of the Dome of the Rock and the Al-Aqsa Mosque; such a job was only for the most experienced physician in town.[69]

A change was noticed with the coming of medical training in the new universities. Foreign hospitals began to recruit much younger physicians, who could not afford a private practice yet, but were looking forward to earn a name for themselves through the institution. Education, rather than experience, commended marks of social respect: one of the petitions designed to defend Dr Arab mentions him first as "Dr Emile Effendi Arab", then simply as "Dr Emile Effendi", an honorary title which refers first and foremost to his academic training.[70] Studies and official positions such as hospital physician and physician of the municipality entailed social status.

The same petition also insisted on the easier cultural access patients found with Dr Arab, who spoke Arabic as a native speaker and knew local traditions and customs, as well as their physical constitution and the "specific diseases of [the] country".[71] Dr Arab, who said he found medical interest in local pathology and medicine, seemed to share this nativistic view of medicine.[72] However, nativism is an ambiguous category, since Arab's argument also fitted with the vision of French consuls, who distinguished between medicine for the indigenous population and medicine for the Europeans. This meant that appointing native physicians was a political decision, aimed at creating influence in spite of France's linguistic policy. Hypothetically, the French Consulate might have come to the conclusion that choosing French-speaking physicians was a counter-productive policy, but in that case, diplomats were most

[69] Amnon Cohen, *The Guilds of Ottoman Jerusalem* (Leyden / Boston / Cologne: Brill, 2001), 82–83.

[70] MAE Nantes, Jerusalem, A, 108: Bethlehem Petition, 30 May 1909.

[71] Ibid.

[72] MAE Nantes, Jerusalem, A, 108: Arab to Gueyraud, 25 May 1909.

discrete about it. However, medical beneficence and the funding of French schools were two very distinct items of national promotion.

There was no coherence in the way French diplomats favoured French or Ottoman physicians alternatively in French hospitals. The French hospital in Bethlehem should have an indigenous physician because Bethlehm was held to be an "indigenous" town; however, Jerusalem, the main focus of French beneficence, was not, because of its small European population. More than ten years before the case related here, Dr Naamé, another physician from the Université Saint-Joseph, had applied for the job of physician to the Hôpital Saint-Louis. Then-French Consul Auzépy advised his superiors against appointing him because, as an "Oriental", he would be disregarded by other physicians in town, and his appointment would be seen as an insult by the French living in Jerusalem, as well as a testimony of weakness in the eyes of the native population of the city. He would be much better fitted for work in a purely indigenous town. Auzépy had his own candidate to defend, of course, yet his words were much more definitive about native physicians than about any European candidate.[73] Ten years later, Gueyraud reports the various compliments he heard from Europeans in Bethlehem about Dr Arab's professionalism.[74] It is hard, though, to infer that everyone got reconciled with, let alone be enthusiastic for, native physicians. In 1910, hardly months after Dr Arab had been replaced by a Frenchman, Dr Henry, statistics had known a sharp increase in the number of patient attendances, which seemed to contradict the nativist approach which had prevailed before.[75] This was probably due to Henry's pleasant character and his popularity,[76] though he attributed it principally to his French nationality.[77] Choosing a French physician or promoting a graduate of the French medical

[73] MAE Nantes, Jerusalem, A, 104: Auzépy (then French Consul to Jerusalem) to Bapst (French *chargé d'affaire* in Constantinople), 19 July 1898.

[74] MAE Nantes, Jerusalem, A, 108: Gueyraud to Pichon, 3 March1909.

[75] MAE Nantes, Jerusalem, A, 108: Henry to Gueyraud, 11 June 1910.

[76] MAE Quai d'Orsay, CPC, NS Turquie, 430 : Gueyraud to the French Foreign Minister, Jerusalem, 16 April1913.

[77] MAE Nantes, Jerusalem, A, 108: Henry to Gueyraud, 11 June 1910.

Faculty in Beirut remained a political choice, and would remain so as long as the French kept their institutions as a political asset in the competition for the spoils of Syria.

There is hardly anything worth mentioning about the way hospitals as institutions and Western medicine in general come out through the petitions: it is stereotypically laudatory and indeed recipients were unlikely to be receptive to other views. For instance, Dr Arab made medical technology one of the conditions to maintain the prestige of the HSF. After Dr Drouillard's visits in May 1909, Mère Mayaud decided that the one patient, whom Drouillard was not allowed to see, needed an operation which could not be performed with the equipment available at the HSF. Dr Arab answered in a vexed manner that for the sake of the reputation of the hospital, she should not make such claims: not only because she did not have a medical degree and was therefore not entitled to giving a medical opinion, but also because the surgical materials there were "nearly complete", and so she should not seem to infer that the hospital's service was not operational. However, Mère Mayaud's behaviour backfired. She asked the municipality of Bethlehem to take the patient to the German hospital in Jerusalem for the operation but the delegates of the municipality decided to hand over the patient to the complete free care of the Hôpital Saint-Louis and in turn to Dr Drouillard.[78] How real, or how potential the loss of reputation of the HSF might have been, cannot be said, though we should take Dr Arab's word with a pinch of salt. There was a definite competition for modernity among the hospitals, and undoubtedly the latest tool used was advertisements. It would be inaccurate to argue that this was a device to create an economic output for national medical technology; such technology, local and symbolic as it was, was hardly significant in spreading Western medical knowhow. Nonetheless, the display of modern medical science was part and parcel of the policy of European nations in the Middle East. In case of France, the key word was influence: of this, the visibility of modernity could be an exponent. Yet it did not replace the interpersonal mediation of

[78] MAE Nantes, Jerusalem, A, 108: Gueyraud to Mère Marie Kieffer, 28 May 1909.

influence which was sought, for instance, through the appointment of native physicians.

The historiography of late Ottoman Middle East tends to present the transformations of the region under the influence of either European actors, or through the general movement of Ottoman Reform launched in the 1840s. As far as medicine is concerned, there is little doubt that most of the investments in health institutions were the result of foreign policy within the Ottoman Empire. The significance of this movement can be very diversely interpreted: historians have underlined the patchy character of European educational institutions and their insignificance, though they were nurturing the future elite.[79] As far as medicine was concerned, this logic is only partly relevant: indeed, the training of physicians was a way of creating a professional class related to European powers, and hospital was a means for this goal. Furthermore, the concentration of medical institutions in certain areas deprived them of significance in terms of medical geography and health service. Yet wherever they existed, hospitals were a significant feature of European networking. Western hospitals were seen by European organisations, as a means to influence a wider circle than the relatively few families whose pupils attended European schools. Indeed, in Bethlehem, medical service was sufficiently engrained by 1909, to cause deep communal tensions.

At the same time, the perceptions of Western hospitals tend to show how paradoxical European policies of influence could be. As the social distribution of signatures in petitions show, medicine helps create networks of clients, patrons and supporters. It works according to implicit and very hierarchical preconceptions of Middle Eastern sociology, yet at the same time hospitals are kept as much at distance as can be from Ottoman officials. In case of the HSF, petitions did not reach the local Governor of Bethlehem, who was taken aback by the situation there in October 1909. Each protagonist had a stake in this—from the point of view of the physicians and

[79] Jacob M. Landau, "The Educational Impact of Western Culture on Tradition Society in Nineteenth-Century Palestine", in *Studies on Palestine During the Ottoman Period,* ed. Moshe Ma'oz (Jerusalem: The Magnes Press / Yad Izhak Ben-Zvi, 1975), 499–506.

especially for Dr Arab, it was a matter of official status and hence, of professional pride. In the eyes of the Catholics of Bethlehem, the whole affair was a communal matter, which they would keep away from the mainly Muslim Ottoman administration. People appeared to consider free health care as a service indeed, yet not as a right: else, the whole matter would probably have taken a more official course, and it would have been brought before an Ottoman court. As far as supervising institutions and consulates were concerned, the administration of hospitals was a question of authority, which is precisely what fostered the widespread notion that those places were a space of foreign near-sovereignty.

Indeed, it is important to underline the link between medical development and sovereignty in the late Ottoman period, as Robert Blecher has done for the northern part of the bilâd al-Shâm.[80] Yet before medicine became one of the means available for the mandatory powers to bargain the admission of their sovereignty over the land with the indigenous population, the status of hospitals fostered foreign sovereignty in a different way. Once the permits for the building of hospitals had been granted, the physicians and staff were given much leeway to practice medicine as they would, sometimes in spite of popular reluctance, and with uncontrolled power over the life and body of their patients. This made them effectively sovereign, as the Ottoman state would very seldom intervene in the hospitals, and especially in legal matters. Even then, they would have to negotiate with the head physician.

The publicity of hospital matters is rather puzzling: public mobilisation about hospitals, such as in the case of the HSF, was socially effective. It worked according to the logic of international politics, but it did not reach the local and national administrative levels. As the Palestinian press was very nascent at the time of the HSF affair, it is also doubtful that it was ever referred to in the newspapers. It is therefore hard to envisage petitions as a representation of "public opinion" on the decisions of foreign institutions. Most likely, petitions and rumour mirrored the need of a show of public debate to

[80] Robert Ian Blecher, *The Medicalization of Sovereignty: Medicine, Public Health, and Political Authority in Syria, 1861–1936* (PhD diss., Stanford University, June 2002).

justify the sovereign decisions of European actors according to their own criteria of common good. Part of what went on at staff level within the hospital was indeed made public, or rather leaked to the population, for institutional reasons. Foreign medical beneficence needed native approbation, especially after the winter of 1908–9, when constitutional government and individual liberties were secured by the deposition of the Sultan Abdul Hamid. These political circumstances gave special significance to petitions and the choice of native vs expatriate physicians, as a nativist streak entered the European discourse about medicine and the Middle East.

10

Mediating Therapeutic Uncertainty: A Mission Hospital in Nepal

Ian Harper

Introduction

> United Mission Hospital Tansen strives to provide high quality medical care that is affordable, effective, efficient and accessible to all who come here, within the limitation of available resources, with love and respect as exemplified in the love and compassion we find in Christ Jesus. [1]

"WE serve, Jesus heals" reads the large sign over the main entrance to the United Mission to Nepal (UMN) hospital, located at Bhusal Danda, a couple of kilometres outside of Tansen, Palpa district, Nepal. Situated some 120 miles south-west of the capital Kathmandu, with over 120 in-patient beds and seeing over one hundred thousand out-patients per year, this hospital remains one of the

I would like to thank all those at the United Mission to Nepal and the people of Tansen who made this research possible. I would also like to thank Dr Christopher Davis, my PhD supervisor, who supported the research throughout; Professor Murray Last who asked me to present an earlier version of this paper at the UCL Medical Anthropology seminar, and the participants at this event for their feedback; Deepak Thapa and Kanak Dixit who asked me to present an earlier draft of this chapter at a public lecture in 2004 in Kathmandu for the Social Science Baha—the feedback here was also invaluable; to Pratyoush Onta for his unfailing criticism of my work and Jeevan Sharma and Emily Cowall Farrell for their insights; finally to the participants of the Hospitals Beyond the West Conference for their feedback and discussion, and the editors of this volume for their comments and suggestions. All mistakes of fact and responsibility for the interpretations rest with me.

[1] United Mission to Nepal (henceforth UMN), *Celebrating 45 Years in Nepal* (Kathmandu: UMN, 1999).

busiest hospitals in Nepal. Missionary medical services in Tansen were started in 1954 and developed over the years—with associated public health, community health and outreach facilities—to its current size. By 2000 it was a local employer with nearly 350 Nepali (and 19 expatriate) staff. Since its inception the Mission Hospital has had a continuous and significant presence both in, and around, Tansen.[2] It has been the epicentre of medical care in the area since the early years of its foundation. Its catchment's area for patients extends beyond Palpa district to other outlying districts often more than a day's travel away.[3] A significant number also attend the hospital from India, many of whom refer to it as the "TB hospital". To visit it on any day involves jostling with the large numbers of people seeking its medical services. Outside the hospital a whole industry has developed catering to patients and their relatives; tea houses, hotels, a couple of new pharmacies, impromptu bazaars, and herbalists. It is quite different to the usually quiet and half-empty public hospital in town. At the same time the Mission Hospital, and having worked there, carries considerable social capital as well as medical prestige. Outside local clinics and pharmacies, a number of signs advertise the credibility of the practitioner in an increasingly competitive marketplace as working in, or having worked in, the Mission Hospital.

This chapter emerges both from my work as a medical doctor, and more latterly from a retraining in anthropology. It is a part of

[2] My use of the "ethnographic present" here relates to the time of my PhD field work between 1998 and 2000, supported by the ESRC: Ian Harper, "Mission, Magic and Medicalisation: An Anthropological Study into Public Health in Contemporary Nepal" (unpublished thesis, University of London, 2003). There have been significant changes in Nepal since this fieldwork was conducted, and the conflict and Maoist insurgency has affected a range of UMN's services, including the shutting of hospitals and the cessation of the Palpa Community Health and Development Programme. As such this paper reflects the period up to 2000, but the situation may now have changed considerably.

[3] To indicate distances does not reflect the time investment that many people put into coming to the hospital. Travel in Nepal, particularly in the hilly and mountainous regions, is extremely arduous and involves long treks and bus rides.

a broader ethnographic project conceived to understand medical practice in Nepal, both in relation to broader political fields and relations between a number of different healers. This has involved questions of how efficacy is understood and interpreted. My main interpretive task then is to understand why so many people attended the Mission Hospital in Tansen, and why they sought to see, in particular, the foreign doctors working there. To do this my argument develops along a number of interrelated strands.

I begin by focusing on the discursive production of Nepal as a closed land and its "opening" up to the world following the revolution of 1951, developed from a reading of early missionary and other texts of Euro-Americans who arrived in Nepal in this early period. The status of the health of the people and their needs within these early discourses is highlighted. I do this not only from the perspective of "clinical Christianity"—that combination of medicine and Christian ideology which since the turn of the twentieth century had become recognised in mission circles as one of the most persuasive ways of spreading their faith to other countries[4]—but to focus on the similarities and close relations with other early development discourses on the needs of the country, and the rationale behind this. This section is followed by one which looks at the foundation and early years of the Mission Hospital in Tansen developed from ethnographic interviews with residents of the town on their perceptions of the hospital and the early missionaries. The main interpretive thrust of the chapter attempts to explain the continued popularity of the Mission Hospital at the turn of the twenty-first century despite the recent mushrooming of availability of many medical services. This, I suggest, derives from a combination of the high standard of effective, efficacious medical care available over the years, and the consequent good reputation of the hospital, but one discursively mediated by the practices and perceptions of development that this emerges from. The capacity for biomedical services to cure certain conditions has come to be seen by many in Palpa as

[4] Rosemary Fitzgerald, "'Clinical Christianity': The Emergence of Medical Work as a Missionary Strategy in Colonial India, 1800–1914", in *Health, Medicine and Empire: Perspectives on Colonial India*, ed. Biswamoy Pati and Mark Harrison (New Delhi: Orient Longman, 2001), 88–136.

being an intrinsic property of the "foreign" doctor and their capacity to heal. This fetishisation of the foreigner as healer is consequent on the geopolitical relations, and vast structural inequalities that exist between Nepal and its developed Euro-American elsewhere.

Mission and Medical Discourse, and the Constitution of Nepal's Health Needs

Uncolonised, Nepal under the autocracy of the Ranas—the hereditary prime-ministers till 1951—maintained a vigorously controlled policy of exclusion of Europeans and their influence from the realm, a strategy necessary for their maintenance of feudal control.[5] One consequence has been a discursive trope that dominates how Nepal is represented in English, that before 1951 it was a "closed" and "isolated" Kingdom that "opened" up to the rest of the world following the overthrow of the hereditary Rana regime. Such a trope, even as the rest of the world was in the process of decolonisation, allowed the sudden and dramatic discursive colonisation of what had previously been seen as little more than an empty cartographic space (excepting a few key texts by European and other visitors, particularly those of the orientalist scholar, Brian Hodgson). A huge amount of wish fulfilment seemed to have been poured into this space as explorers, travellers, scientists, anthropologists, missionaries, developers, those from a Euro-American elsewhere were exposed to the secrets of the closed land for the first time and Nepal was "worlded"; a form of epistemological colonisation of supposedly empty cartographic spaces.[6] One of the reasons this is such a powerful metaphor is that in many ways Nepal continues to be "worlded" by those who have greater discursive force than others, particularly in relation to development or *bikaas*, a point to which I return. This is an important metaphysical point, and one that it is necessary to expand upon to address the rest of the analysis.

[5] Mark Liechty, "Selective Exclusion: Foreigners, Foreign Goods, and Foreignness in Modern Nepali History", *Studies in Nepali History and Society* 2, no. 1, June 1997, 2–68.

[6] Gayatri Chakravorty Spivak, *The Post-Colonial Critic: Interviews, Strategies, Dialogues* (New York and London: Routledge, 1990)

For example, in the biography of the missionary Dr Helen Houston, Hankins introduces us to Nepal in the chapter "The Mysterious Himalayan Kingdom", as

> A country long forbidden to foreigners, Nepal is aptly called 'the last home mystery'. This country, where one can step in and out of centuries many times a day, offers unparalleled adventure.[7]

It was both the geographical conditions and the people that had kept Nepal isolated from rest of the world. The scientist and bird collector, Ripley wrote in 1952:

> Hidden among the ridges, in a gem-like valley of its own, lies Kathmandu, the capital of Nepal, a secluded storied city, out of the world, beyond time, the "Jewel in the lotus". . . . If Nepal's geography conspired to keep it remote, its people have conspired to keep it inaccessible. From the welter of half a hundred tribes, each in its mountain fastness, has arisen a government of the unconquered Ghurkhas, the most warlike of all the people of the hills.[8]

Ripley's visit had been arranged by the American Charge D'Affaires in New Delhi, George Merrell, who had recently been in Nepal to conduct negotiations on the exchange of diplomatic relations between the United States and Nepal.[9] For Ripley

[7] Gerald W. Hankins, *A Heart for Nepal: The Dr. Helen Houston Story* (Winnipeg: Windflower Communications, 1991), 36.

[8] Sydney Dillon Ripley, *Search for the Spiny Babbler: A Naturalist's Adventure in Nepal* (Kathmandu: Ratnar Pusthak Bhandar, 1978), 2.

[9] Ripley had been invited to Nepal as an ornithologist, and had been influenced massively by the Orientalist and Natural Historian Sir Brian Hodgson. "To me and my fellow ornithologists, students of birds around the world, Nepal has always had a particular fascination because of the researches of a single man", wrote Ripley in 1952. Ripley, *Search for the Spiny Babbler*. Hodgson had added no fewer than "one hundred and fifty good new species to the Avi-fauna of the British Asian Empire, and few and far between have been the new species subsequently discovered within the limits he explored". W. W. Hunter, *Life of Brian Houghton Hodgson: British Resident at the Court of Nepal* (New Delhi and Madras: Asian Educational Services, 1991 [1898]), 304.

Apart from this contribution Ripley also trained Indian artists to paint birds with "extreme accuracy from a scientific point of view" and he published no fewer than 127 papers on ornithology and mammology in scholarly

> Such a trip would demonstrate where a lot of rather mysterious bird species described by Hodgson and merely labelled "Nepal" really came from. It would solve a number of evolutionary problems, and incidentally such a trip would also involve exploration of territory unknown to outsiders. [10]

He was backed by the Smithsonian Institution, Yale and the National Geographic Society, and his work required the shooting of many birds as it was necessary to have "fresh specimens", sent back to the Smithsonian.

Amongst these explorers, scientists and missionaries was Dr Bob Fleming, who was later to co-author the book "Birds of Nepal". One of the teachers contributed to the Woodstock school at Missoorie in India by the American Missionary board, he had received permission to travel to Nepal in the winter of 1949–50. With a team that included Dr Bob Taylor they visited Butwal, Tansen, Tukuche, Baglung and Pokhara over a three-month period. In Tansen, elderly residents I spoke to remembered that whilst one of the first missionaries had been ministering to the sick, the other had spent all his time up in the woods of Srinigar hill (above the town) shooting birds!

> During this time we collected 720 bird skins representing 256 species. We discovered a new species of green pigeon which we named *Teron pompadora conoveri* after our sponsor, Dr Covoner of the Chicago natural History Museum. [11]

The naming of new species was not at all concerned with local classificatory practices. As with medical practice and the taxonomy

---

journals of the time, as well as providing 9,512 specimens of bird to the British museum between 1843 and 1858, as well as 1,241 drawings. One of the great orientalist scholars of the nineteenth century, he had lived as resident in Nepal between 1821 and 1843. Like many others at the time, trained to rule in the days of Empire, he had emerged from Hailbury, his mind dominated by the political economic liberalism of Malthus; one of his major intellectual influences, Hunter, *Life of Brian Houghton Hodgson.*

[10] Ripley, *Search for the Spiny Babbler*, 10.

[11] Quoted in Jonathan Lindell, *Nepal and the Gospel of God* (Kathmandu: Pilgrims Book House, 1997), 136.

underlining its epistemology, it seems to float above like the hovering birds over any local historical or cultural considerations.

Apart from these scientific activities, we have a range of mission organisations along the border with Nepal, but in India. Cindy Perry's 1989 thesis, *A Biographical History of the Church in Nepal*, lists forty[12] missions lining the Nepal border, prior to its "opening".[13] Here it was that much hard work went on, "an era of softening, breaking up the hard soil, and planting seeds of the gospel".[14] Mobile clinics also dotted the border and allowed the combination of "medicine and evangelism".[15] Leprosy sufferers, for example, crossed to the mission in Chandag Heights, or Kalimpong, because it was in Nepal that the leper was "buried alive, and treated with cruel inhumanity", as stated by a visitor. Rauxaul had the Duncun Hospital since 1929, and other Indian towns along the border with missions including Jogbani, Nautanuwa, Rupandehi, Tandpur, Pithogwah and Dharchula.[16] From these sites young converts developed the skills as dressers, nurses and compounders. It was from these border posts that particularly women we are told, but also some men, were living, preaching and working and who all had "a tremendous burden for Nepal":

> Missionaries had purposely situated themselves at key points along these borders, waiting for the day Nepal would open up. They established a Christian presence, attracted an audience, built credibility with the Nepalese who streamed across the borders, slowly saw some profess faith in Christ, and they prayed.[17]

Perry describes a continual flow of people across the borders of this (supposedly) closed land—closed, as I have suggested, to an

12 Lindell lists only twenty five missions. Lindell, *Nepal and the Gospel of God*.

13 Cindy Perry, *A Biographical History of the Church in Nepal* (Kathmandu: Nepal Church History Project, 2000), originally submitted as an MA thesis to Wheaton Graduate School, Wheaton, Illinois, 1989.

14 Perry, *A Biographical History of the Church in Nepal*, 63.

15 Ibid., 64.

16 Saubhagya Shah, "The Gospel Comes to the Hindu Kingdom", *Himal,* September–October 1993, 35–40.

17 Perry, *A Biographical History of the Church in Nepal,* 62.

Euro-American epistemological gaze—as they looked for jobs, joined armies, sought medical attention. But missionaries were also slipping into Nepal at any available opportunity, often at the request of the ruling elite. Dr Kitty Harbord, for example, was said to have visited Tansen, spending several months at the Governor's palace in both 1928 and 1930. As Leichty has pointed out, this was one category of foreigners that the Rana's did want to avail themselves to, and one that the missionaries attempted to exploit. [18]

"Lord hear our prayer, so that the doors may be opened for the Gurkhalis to receive salvation", the opening lines of a song composed by Ganga Prasad Pradhan in 1900, became a prayer sung for fifty years, "flung to the heavenlies in earnest petition". [19] And in 1951, as the prayer was answered, missionaries all along the borders "streamed" into Nepal. The Nepal Border Fellowship, as the loose association of border missions had been called, had served its purpose.

Dr Fleming—Christian evangelist, scientist, bird collector, and taxonomist—was part of this wave of missionaries poised on the border. Bird watching has since become central to the myths and stories of the United Mission to Nepal. For example, Jonathon Lindell's 1979 book, *Nepal and the Gospel of God,* has several references to the sketches made by Hem Poudyl: "Dr Bob Fleming's bird expeditions in the mountains of Nepal occasioned the forming of the United Mission", reads one caption. [20] "Bird trips, medicines, letters and meetings went into the mix that made up the United Mission to Nepal", reads another. [21] Grace Fletcher's 1965 biography of the Flemings, *The Fabulous Flemings of Kathmandu*, reports it to us thus: "We Christians waited two thousand years to get into Nepal". Dr Bob is fond of saying, "then when the Lord was ready he sent a bird to show us the way". [22]

[18] Liechty, "Selective Exclusion", 1997.

[19] Perry, *A Biographical History of the Church in Nepal.*

[20] Lindell, *Nepal and the Gospel of God,* 135.

[21] Ibid.,148.

[22] Grace Nies Fletcher, *The Fabulous Flemings of Kathmandu: The Story of Two Doctors in Nepal* (London: Hodder and Stoughton, 1965), 17.

While he was in his "new Eden" collecting bird specimens beneath the Himalayas, the latter standing "aloof, regal, immovable, lost in time, to whom a million years were but a day that is gone" in a "Nepal where few westerners had explored before", his friend was ministering to another need:

> Dr Carl Taylor was equally busy exploring another kind of mountain—the urgent needs of hundreds of sick patients at Tansen. Rumour flies faster than radio waves. When the people of Tansen heard there was a trained doctor of medicine tenting on their village parade grounds, they rushed there in such crowds that Dr Bob Fleming had to place his tin trunks, which held his bird specimens, in a circle around their tent to keep it from being spilled over. Dr Taylor performed operations until his rubber gloves were in ribbons.
>
> "You never saw so many desperately sick people, Bethel" Dr Bob told his wife almost tearfully when he got back to the Woodstock school. "They had tuberculosis, leprosy, worms, goitres as big as Volkswagen rubber tyres around their necks, tumours that must have been building up for years in swollen abdomens. . . . The children were heartbreaking. One baby had been burned over three quarters of his body and the wounds were suppurating into a mud poultice.[23]

In the winter of 1951–52, he and his wife returned with Dr Carl and Anne Fredericks, who also took their children. This was their third trip to Nepal having been previously at the request of Paul Rose, who at the time was setting up the United States Operating Mission (USOM), and was renting a former Rana palace while in Kathmandu. Here the Flemings had got to know many of the leading Kathmandu families as well as the Royals and had put in their request to open a hospital in Nepal.

Permission to open the hospital in Tansen then came on 18 May 1953. A letter written at this time by the Fredericks, reveals the excitement and discursive dimensions of the decision:

> We personally have been granted permission by the Government of Nepal to open a hospital in Tansing where we previously spent six busy and happy weeks treating the sick and making friends. It is thrilling because we are to be pioneers in a land long closed to the gospel, a kingdom with

[23] Fletcher, *Fabulous Flemings of Kathmandu*, 22.

> almost no Christian, and particularly no modern medicine or surgery. It is a nation of unrest, full of communist infiltrators, a flimsy bulwark between Red Tibet and strategic India. It is a land where there is everything to be done by Christians and Americans. We have a Macedonian call—by name—and must answer! [24]

The decision to open the hospital was made, according to Lindell, despite the suspicion of foreigners and the prejudice towards Christians, because of "new attitudes of openness and the desire to get quick, modern medical service for their people". [25] So was born within mission history a remarkable exercise in establishing a Christian Mission on the widest cooperative basis, one which by 1999 had thirty-four Member bodies, and seventeen Affiliated Member Bodies based in the US, the UK (Scotland, England), Australia, India, Germany, Japan, Norway, Canada, Ireland, Denmark, Finland, Sweden, Switzerland, Korea, Philippines, Netherlands, Singapore. [26]

At the same time that missions were establishing their programmes, so too was the US. As Mihaly's political analysis of foreign aid in Nepal demonstrates, aid is mainly about the strategic concerns of the giver and their own domestic concerns. [27] He suggests that the major concern of the American Aid programme was the rising expectations of many people from underdeveloped parts of the world:

> These people of [the underdeveloped areas] have been stirred by a growing awareness of the possibilities of human advancement. . . . By leaving them unable to fulfil their reasonable aspirations, their misery makes

[24] This letter is the first in the UMN archives related to the Hospital at Tansen, held at the University of Edinburgh. There is an extensive collection, and a future project is planned to look more systematically at this invaluable resource to develop a discursive history of health and development in Palpa district.

[25] Lindell, *Nepal and the Gospel of God,* 143.

[26] UMN, *Celebrating 45 Years in Nepal.*

[27] Cf., Narayan Khadka, *Foreign Aid and Foreign Policy: Major Powers and Nepal* (Delhi: Vikas Publishing House Pvt Ltd, 1995).

> them fertile ground for an ideology which will hold out to them the promise, however false, of means towards a better life.[28]

The United States targeted its aid at areas where they perceived the threat of communism, either internal or external, and the greatest threat was the vulnerability of the peasantry. Political stability of countries like Nepal depended on their capacity to improve the productivity and status of the agricultural population, and thus the prevention of Communist incursion, by encouraging political stability. Paul Rose was the "First American", who after arriving in Nepal in January 1952 set up the United States Technical Co-operative Mission to Nepal. Rose was a humanitarian, who was working within the concerns of a political and strategic nature[29]—and it is precisely the boundaries between these points of intersection that interest me here. The "poverty and backwardness" that he came across profoundly affected him. After visiting Pokhara, for example, we are informed in the officially sanctioned history of US Aid to Nepal that he left "with a feeling that time had been moving slowly here for centuries, but people were aching for a change".[30] He decided to target increased food production, elimination of disease, schools for all and basic reform as the programme goals. This culminated in the village development programme, which encompassed projects in agriculture, health and education. But,

> Simply assessing the general state of health in Nepal in 1951 is rendered difficult by the near—absolute lack of statistics. A USOM document written in 1958 noted: reliable health statistics do not exist. This makes the assessment of health conditions and their exact nature and scope very difficult to relate to the specific problem of resource development and utilisation (1962 capital Assistance Programme).[31]

[28] The US, Department of State, Point Four: A Co-operative Program for Aid in the Development of Economically Underdeveloped Areas (1950), quoted in Eugene Bramer Mihaly, *Foreign Aid and Politics in Nepal: A Case Study* (London, New York and Toronto: Oxford University Press, 1965), 29.

[29] Mihaly, *Foreign Aid and Politics in Nepal*, 30.

[30] Christa A. Skerry, Kerry Moran and Kay M. Calavan, *Four Decades of Development: The History of U.S. Assistance to Nepal, 1951–1991* (Kathmandu: USAID Nepal, 1992), 8.

[31] Skerry et al., *Four Decades of Development*, 47.

Nonetheless the document is still able to paint a grim picture of Nepal's overall health status:

> It is estimated that fifty percent of the population lives in highly malarious areas. Surveys seem to verify that the infection rate for malaria runs as high as 100% in some villages. Tuberculosis, smallpox, typhoid, cholera, dysentery, syphilis, kala-azar, filariasis, leprosy, maternal and infant tetanus, hookworm, tapeworm, amoebiasis and other intestinal parasites, kidney stones, rheumatic fever, goitre, and other deficiency diseases are debilitating a large segment of the population.
>
> Infant mortality, always a revealing indicator of a populations overall health status, was 255 per 1,000 in 1951. One-third to one half of children died before reaching adulthood, and this figure contributed to Nepal's exceptionally low life expectancy rate—28 years according to a 1952 estimate.[32]

In the absence of any statistics, startling claims and the evocation of the overwhelming imperative to act justified planned US intervention and aid in the health sector. Skerry and others go on to point out for us an interpretation of the synergistic relationship between health and development—one that repeats itself today—in that the negative impact of such health spreads across all sectors. Some examples of this impact are disease and malnutrition, lower economic productivity, sapping energy that could be better used in farming, road building, studying, teaching. Low school enrolment and resultant low literacy rates, high fertility rates, reduced agricultural productivity—all these result from poor health, and contribute to it as well. A reasonable level of health care services can thus be considered an economic necessity as well as fundamental human need.[33] Here, again, we see how biomedically defined health related issues are productive within broader political and economic frames.

With a backdrop of *dhami-jhankris* (as the local mediums and shamanic practitioners in Nepal are frequently generically referred to) as the only providers of rural health care, and barely any hospitals or health workers, we are informed that there were no injections, no

[32] Skerry et al., *Four Decades of Development*, 48.

[33] Ibid.

nurses, no paramedical workers, no health posts, no service delivery system for the rural populace. Nepal's health sector required "everything": manpower, supplies, institutions, physical infrastructure and an effective service delivery system reaching a widely scattered rural populace.[34] As Tatsuro Fujikura has pointed out in his excavation of American discourses of democracy and community development in Nepal, the country was viewed as a "blank slate", a development "laboratory".[35] Nepal was, he suggests, for many a particularly desirable space for development experimentation, "a small, pure, non-modern country by the beginning of the 1950s".[36]

Remembering the Mission Past

During my anthropological fieldwork many of the older residents of Tansen spoke to me with great affection of the earlier missionaries, particularly how they were prepared to make home visits and the efforts they made to mix with people.[37] As has been noted for elsewhere in Nepal—from the Kunde hospital in Solu Khumbu—the reputation of the foreign doctors was as much related to their

[34] Ibid., 49.

[35] T. Fugikura, "Technologies of Improvement, Locations of Culture: American Discourses of Democracy and 'Community Development' in Nepal", *Studies in Nepali History and Society* 1, no. 2, December 1996, 271–311.

[36] Fugikura, "Technologies of Improvement", 272.

[37] This ethnographic section is developed from a number of interviews and encounters from my fieldwork, conducted between September 1998 to March 2000. Most of the interviews were conducted as part of the broader participant observation fieldwork method, and the data and answers to my questions were noted down in a rough notebook during the encounters, and transferred to my field-note books either that evening or at the first available opportunity. Some of the observations and interpretations are garnered from multiple encounters from a range of people, but where specific individual responses are noted at length I refer these to my field notes with the dates of the interviews. If they are not in quotation marks they were not recorded, but summaries of the conversations. All the respondents here have been anonymised in accordance with the first anthropological ethical principle of the protection of informants' identities.

capacity to integrate locally as to the surgical cures they offered.[38] Sister Ingerborg, for example, had been one of the first to arrive in Tansen in 1955, and was honoured by the Literary Academy, Palpa Tansen with a lifetime's achievement award in 1998. She was widely referred to as the Florence Nightingale of Palpa, and along with Dr Fredericks and the later arrived Dr Iwamura was amongst the most fondly remembered of the missionaries. I heard general complaints that now the hospital is so much bigger, and with attempts at "Nepalisation"—the process wherein middle and higher level management was handed over to Nepali nationals as well as the hiring of more Nepali doctors—it is quite different from how it used to be. One complaint was the difficulty to get past the "sorters", as the mid-level health workers and first point of diagnostic contact with the hospital, were frequently referred to locally. The fact that they had to be got past to get access to the doctors, particularly the foreign ones, and that the waiting time for getting an out-patient appointment (without nepotistic connections) was now much longer was mentioned with some irritation by many. Those elite who could afford it would now go straight to Gorakhpur in India or to Kathmandu. In short, these middle classes were increasingly denied access to this "personalisation" of contact with the bureaucratic health services.[39]

The "Royal preceptor" (the priest to the royal family and exiled to Palpa in 1924), had a key role in inviting the missionaries to come to Tansen to stay and start a hospital. They had run the hospital out of their large house first, and there was, I was assured by one of his descendents, a lot of resistance to it.[40] Without his grandfather's "source and force" then it would have been impossible. The fact that a senior Brahman priest would want to invite a group of foreign Christians to set up a hospital in Tansen seemed odd to me, and his grandson was unsure why he would have wanted to invite them.

[38] Vicanne Adams, *Tigers of the Snow and Other Virtual Sherpas: Ethnography of Himalayan Encounters* (Princeton, New Jersey: Princeton University Press, 1996).

[39] Madhusudan Sharma Subedi, *Medical Anthropology in Nepal* (Kathmandu: Udaya Books, 2001).

[40] Interviews with MP, Tansen, field notes 20 July 1999; 26 December 1999.

It had to do in some way with his own past, and exile, as well as a desire to change some of the prevailing social conditions. He certainly would not have wanted them to proselytise, I was assured, but would have appreciated their desire to serve "the helpless people". There was also the considerable support of Rudra Shamshere Rana, the Chief District Officer (the highest administrative post at district level), and a significant group of elites who were also very helpful. All were powerful and prominent local figures.

There was, however, also considerable opposition to them as well, particularly from one powerful "compounder" I was told. The personal physician to the Ranas, was also well connected and he turned many locals against Dr Fredericks. The answers I received to the question why there was this resistance were along the following lines: The monopoly that he had over medicine sales in Tansen; the anti-Christian feeling; as well as people being against the foreigners as they were perceived to be low castes—the "untouchables"—from foreign countries, perhaps the latter being the main social reason. I heard stories of people purifying their houses with gold water after foreigners had visited them, a point raised when several informants wished to tell me how much Nepali society had changed, as this does not happen now. This point also prevented people from accepting the medicines.

Further more than occasionally contradictory points also arose. Costs to get treatment were minimal from the Mission Hospital at the time, but it was because people were not aware of the low costs that they did not come at first. It also became a little more popular after the surgical operations started. There was at the time another government hospital here as well, now closed, a fifteen bedded public hospital, the P. Chandra hospital (named after Prithvi Narayan and Chandra Shamshere). This was staffed by Bengali doctors who used to come for three-year stints at a time. There was great resistance to the "whites" (the term *kwire* a derogatory and commonly heard term for whites) taking blood—they used to take it to drink that is what people used to say, I was told by one informant![41] It

[41] Interview conducted in Tansen with LD, who worked in the Mission Hospital for over 30 years from 1956. Fieldnotes, 17 March 1999.

wasn't until after the 1960s, two years after moving to its current site that the reputation of the hospital started to improve. Several people linked this to the public health work of Dr Iwamura who walked extensively in the area, particularly with his TB research and free medicines. I was to hear time and again of this doctor and his work, and the reason for his popularity. Interestingly he became a part of the healing stories of one shamanic healer I interviewed; that he had been attacked by the sacred arrows of a shaman, and his own medicines had been unable to cure him of this. Some contrasted his relations with the public to the present ones, and the current hospital policy not to visit patients at their homes. It was also pointed out that Siddhartha Highway, which opened in 1968, helped considerably in allowing people to have greater access to the hospital.

Others preferred to highlight the political issues at the time. There was also the question of the communists in particular and their resistance to *samrajyabad* or (American) imperialism —Dr Fredericks was an American, I was reminded on several occasions. There was the "Yankees go home" demonstration, a time when a group burnt an effigy of Fredericks. For example, one early administrator told me that there were several things that I needed to understand about the time when Dr Fredericks had arrived in Tansen.[42] The world was divided into power blocs, either for or against the US or Russia, the cold war was going on and there was strong anti-American feeling amongst communist groups here as elsewhere. It was also a time of great change within Nepal, he said, of the early days of democracy and into all this Dr Fredericks arrived. It was only because of Dr Fredericks's great diplomatic skills that he, and the hospital, managed to survive. Another administrator highlighted that "the Yankees go home" demonstration, in either 1954 or 1955 had been a political issue, agitated by the communist party and was not so much against the Christians as against "the East India Company". There was a rumour in the town that the "West" was going to take over Nepal. However, the situation changed after the wife of Kamal

[42] Interview with SR, Tansen, who worked in the hospital from its opening till 1978. Fieldnotes, 11 April 1999.

Raj Regmi, the main organiser of the protests, took a job in the hospital!

The Christians I interviewed preferred to highlight the difficulties of and resistance to religious change. One senior Christian nurse from Darjeeling, pointed out that 1960 was the year when the party-less Panchyat system came into being and it seems that not only was this when the first Christians were jailed in Nepal, but also when the Mission Hospital's main critics were also jailed, including Kamal Raj Regmi. [43] The resistance was mainly related to the idea of Christians coming, in her opinion. And so, I asked, how did change come about then and how did it become the popular hospital of today? Firstly, the nurse reckoned it was the road arriving in 1968 that allowed large numbers of people from the Tarai (the flatlands bordering with India) and Butwal easier access. Secondly, she considered that the service genuinely focused on the poor and needy. Thirdly, not only people's "awareness" of the benefits of allopathic medicine grew, but also the attitude of the missionaries changed, like female doctors for female patients.

Another retired senior sister, given a lifetime service to the people of Tansen award by the town council, said that the people of Gairegau were against the opening of the hospital by them. [44] A major resistance to the uptake of medical ideas was that houses had to be purified after a foreigner had left—she had seen people bringing cows along with them to purify their homes after they left. Her own feeling was that Dr Iwamura had a major contribution to the acceptance of medical ideas locally. This was after he brought a small portable X-ray machine from Japan and had introduced mass screening for tuberculosis. It was only then that the hospital had become really popular. He started this in 1965 and would have been gathering pace as the road came in. The nurse was reluctant, though, to talk of resistance and politics and preferred instead to talk of work still to be done. She cited huge changes, like how the fear of leprosy had

[43] Interview with LR, Tansen. She had started work in the Mission Hospital from 1960. Fieldnotes 21 April 1999. The jailing of Christians in 1960 was pointed out by several informants, including SR.

[44] Interview with SM, Tansen, who arrived in 1968 from Darjeeling to work in the hospital. Field notes, 26 April 1999.

diminished—only rarely do we hear the terrible curse of the past "May leprosy befall you" (Nepali—*kor lagos, talai*!) with its intimations of great sin having been committed. Today leprosy patients share ward space with others. She told me of a young boy in her flat, indicative of the work yet to be done, who had constipation but had been rushed off to see a shamanic practitioner, then been taken to a clinic, where the family had put their hope in Vitamin A capsules.[45]

For others, whether Christians or not, they preferred to tell me of the missionaries' character and strengths. Dr Fredericks always laughed at all this I was told, by one senior and prominent local figure. Never before had he met anyone like Dr Fredericks. He had typhoid once, and with a temperature of 103 he had gone out to the dispensary to work. It was to his strength of character he referred, for he had never met anyone like this before, and had offered to help in dispensing the free medicines from the clinic. The senior person reckoned that it was only the few "compounders" who caused the problems, and indeed his second eldest son who called in and sat with us for a while, said the same thing. Here there was no talk of politics, only fond memories, a sea of them, as he reminisced for several hours.[46]

I have never met Dr Fredericks, but I did have the opportunity to see some film footages of him, that had been shot the year before I arrived. When he had returned to Tansen he was interviewed for the local cable TV channel.[47] In answer to the interviewer's direct question about resistance and the Mission Hospital's presence, he

[45] For an analysis and ethnography of this programme see Ian Harper "Capsular Promise as Public Health: A Critique of the Nepal National Vitamin A Programme", *Studies in Nepali History and Society* 7, no. 1, 2002, 137–73.

[46] Interview with PP, Tansen, 30 December 1999.

[47] This has been extensively researched by Michael Wilmore. See Michael Wilmore "Local Media and Development Culture in Nepal: A Case Study of Ratna Cable Television and Communication for Development, Palpa in Tansen", *Studies in Nepali History and Society* 6, no. 2, December 2001, 347–87; and Michael Wilmore, "Indigenous Media and the Anthropology of Development in Nepal: A Case Study of Local Media Use in Tansen, Palpa District, Nepal" (PhD dissertation, University of London, 2002).

laughed and said that there were a few problems but he treated some of their family and friends and soon the problems were resolved. Many of the staff they turned to communism and the communists were against him, he said, and so there was a small demonstration. Kamal Raj Regmi was a communist, but later he became a friend. Now, though, after treating many people there is friendship. And look at the hospital now, there is a city there! The land had cost the mission only Rs 4 at the time and was given to them by the central government. Even through the television screen it was easy to warm up to this now elderly man, who used the interview as an opportunity to say that he hoped all his old friends were well, and that he had not forgotten them. [48]

Medical Efficacy and the Space of the "backwards"

For this section I return to the discursive production of health related needs, and how to deal with them. Grace Fletcher's 1965 biography of the Flemings is interesting for the way in which it sets up, in striking prose, the idea of the modern coming into contact with its pre-modern predecessor. It is

> The fantastic story of two space age missionaries, Dr Robert and Dr Bethel Fleming, who trekked happily together over the high Himalayas and slid down a mountain of mud to bring modern medicine to the fabled valley of Kathmandu. They found nine million people fighting a losing battle with almost every known disease from cholera to worms. [49]

Nepal is "a disease riddled country" in which, "trying to cure and educate its almost entirely illiterate people, to make the jump from the Middle Ages to the present in one great leap" is not an easy task. [50] Some, perhaps most, of the assumptions shared with the USAID picture merge here. American man was soon to walk on the moon and the limits to what could happen in this space age

[48] Shown to me during an interview with RU, Tansen. Field notes: 31 December 1999.

[49] Fletcher, *Fabulous Flemings of Kathmandu*, 15.

[50] Ibid., 88.

seem boundless, and yet the Middle Ages still cling to earth in some places.

The trace of this imagery, of Nepal living in the past of an imaginary Euro-American elsewhere, is still present and powerfully created and re-created through the idiom of "development" or bikaas. It has become the dominant frame for attempts at unifying the citizens of the nation state, through the idioms and continuum of "underdeveloped" and "developed".[51] Adhikary has written on the unification of Nepal under the rubric of development, and that it acts as a means of furthering both the symbols of the dominant group, and their values.[52] Pigg has suggested that the idiom has come to define and shape the identity of village-dwellers and city-dwellers alike as people and places are arranged around the idiom of development.[53] In the media, at seminars and conferences I tried to talk with people locally in Palpa (both ex-pats and Nepalese), which is an extraordinarily powerful organising metaphor that displaces a temporal difference cartographically across space. Nepal is like England in the sixteenth century, one friend in a small village outside Tansen confided in me. After a long discussion with one missionary friend over these issues he conceded, that it may not be the Middle Ages, but Nepal is certainly hundred years behind. This imagining of Nepal into the past is supported by a massive global development apparatus, buoyant on the very idea of this displacement. Medical discourse is similarly buoyant on this displacement and much of medicine's efficacy may be related to this metaphysics, combined with the spectacular success of a few key therapeutic interventions.

From what does the efficacy of medicine arise? Wherein lies its extraordinary power, aside from its political authority in relation to the state and aside from its moral authority linked to a missionary presence? The medical practice with which the Flemings and Dr

[51] Mary Des Chene, Editorial, "In the Name of *Bikās*", *Studies in Nepali History and Society* 1, no. 2, December 1996, 259–70.

[52] Kamal Adhikary, "Naming Ceremonies as Rituals of Development", *Studies in Nepali History and Society* 1, no. 2, December 1996, 345–64.

[53] Stacy L. Pigg, "Inventing Social Categories Through Place: Social Representations and Development in Nepal", *Comparative Studies in Society and History* 34, 1992, 491–513.

Fredericks arrived in Nepal was riding the wave of perhaps the only truly revolutionary moment in the history of medicine, that of the discovery, industrial production and beginnings of wider availability of antibiotics.[54] Surgery and anaesthesia were also advanced to the degree that painless operations were possible. At some extra-discursive level, then, the consumption of an antibiotic, if you had an infection, was likely to cure you. We are not in an era, for example, described by David Arnold in the introduction to allopathic practices in India in the eighteenth and nineteenth centuries, a time when the internal logic and capabilities of medical science itself were so fundamentally different.[55] No one in the 1950s was speculating on possible miasmic causes of illness predisposed to particular conditions. All that has been worked out and we have a medical science much more certain of its capabilities; namely, the capacity to delineate a disease and, crucially, to effectively intervene. The mission hospital made such services considerably more widely available to people in the area.

In part, then, the efficacy of medicine arises from the metaphysics of the space created by the banishment of the pathological from the idealised norm.[56] Michel Foucault's introduction to Canguilhem's thought suggests that the potential form of this history of science does not stop recounting the battles against "prejudices", "resistances" and "obstacles".[57] But this form of knowledge of biomedically defined pathological existence in another place, during this sudden epistemological colonisation, does not allow in other ways of knowing (Hobart's claim that the growth of knowledge is also

54 Roy Porter, *The Greatest Benefit to Mankind: A Medical History of Humanity from Antiquity to the Present* (London: Fontana Press, 1997).

55 David Arnold, *Colonizing the Body: State Medicine and Epidemic Disease in Nineteenth-Century India* (Berkeley, Los Angeles and London: University of California Press, 1995).

56 Gorges Canguilhem, *The Normal and the Pathological* (New York: Zone Books, 1991).

57 Michel Foucault, Introduction to *The Normal and the Pathological,* by G. Canguilhem (New York: Zone Books, 1991), 14.

the concurrent growth of ignorance resonates here).[58] The high prevalence of the diseased condition of Nepal's people is continually, and incessantly, juxtaposed against the total inability of existing local practitioners to do anything about it. The battle was already lost, absolutely, without medical sciences' intervention—regardless, perhaps, of whoever brings it. And yet it was the foreign Christian missionary who did bring it to Palpa in a form that made it more widely available.

As a boy in the early 1950s in Pokhara, Nanda R. Shrestha recalls the Christians bringing not just their religion but medical facilities. He reflects that "while some would declare that the missionary hospital spawned a new, modern era of Western medicines and medical miracles, it undermined the local medical knowledge and practices".[59] These services were provided free or with minimal charge, and usually with a mockery of local medical and religious practices.[60] What occurred was a rapid change in the perception of whites, who became the *sahibs*, he suggests, a term that has a dominant-subordination class element to it, as whites were placed at the highest pedestal. From here they were able to rationalise their sense of superiority and their treatment of Nepalese as inferiors who needed to be saved. Shrestha believes that in the existing caste hierarchy the whites had a higher position than the Brahmins. So it was the Shining Hospital in Pokhara that came to symbolise development, and it was brought in by the whites, who knew the language of science and the technology of development. They *were* "development" and consequently mimicry of their ways became the way to progress. From this narrative position, Shrestha then sets up the conditions

[58] Mark Hobart, Introduction to *An Anthropological Critique of Development: The Growth of Ignorance*, ed. Mark Hobart (New York and London: Routledge, 1993).

[59] Nanda Shrestha, *In the Name of Development: A Reflection on Nepal* (Kathmandu: Educational Enterprise (P) Ltd, 1999), 51.

[60] It is interesting and perhaps instructive to note here that for Shrestha this is mainly Ayurveda and not shamanic practice. Ayurveda, the scriptural and textually based, mainly urban form of medical practice is used by few Nepalese when compared to the ritual and shamanic healing (or *dhami-jhankris*, as referred to earlier).

for the emergence of a band of Nepali "elites", who only needed to replace terms like "boy" with "poor" and "underdevelopment", for the colonial civilising mission to be resurrected as the mission of development.

Yet I wonder if it is not this very hierarchy he describes, with the foreigner paradoxically poised at the top of the pile that in no small part is responsible for the *magical* attraction of allopathic practice in contemporary Nepal. To conclude the chapter I will expand on this idea.

Conclusion: Dialectical Magic and the Sweet Smell of Gold

In his essay on "foreignness" in modern Nepali history Mark Liechty explored the power invested in this and how it is tied to local political projects.[61] He focuses on the time up to 1951 and notes that there was considerable flow of "foreign" goods and ideas, particularly to Kathmandu, tightly controlled by the Ranas. He observes that of the very limited number of foreigners who visited Nepal as guests of the state, 40 per cent were doctors or dentists invited to treat the Aristocracy. It was these visitors who carried the—quoting Helm—"authority of distant knowledge".[62] These healers in Nepal could thus be transformed into potentially useful people, and given privileges other than "missionaries, foreigners and infidels".[63] He suggests that the massive changes seen in the Kathmandu valley (and I would add elsewhere) since 1950 is due to the relatively unrestrained access to foreignness and its powers since 1950. Similarly Hoftun, Reaper and Welpton suggest that the real change of 1950–51 was the full, unrestrained exposure of Nepal to "outside" ideas and influences.[64]

[61] Liechty, "Selective Exclusion", 1997

[62] Ibid., 18.

[63] Ibid., 19.

[64] Martin Hoftun, William Raeper and John Welpton, *People, Politics and Ideology: Democracy and Social Change in Nepal* (Kathmandu: Mandala Book Point, 1999), 45. This period of political history has also been written on by, amongst others, by Rishikesh Shaha, *Modern Nepal: A Political History, 1769–1955* (Kathmandu: Manohar, 1996); John Welpton, *A History of Nepal*

During my research it soon became apparent that the Mission Hospital is associated, still, with the presence of the "foreign", "American" or "white" doctor. For many this was the single most important reason stated for their coming to the hospital. Here are a couple of examples amongst many. JP had a diagnosis of tuberculosis and had travelled over four hours on the bus from the Tarai (the flatlands to the south). I asked why she had come all this way to buy her medicines and she replied "in the hope that they would cure me, I have heard this is a good hospital". And who says this, I asked. "Local villagers. They say there are white people there, and they examine you and give you good medicines. That is what people in the village say, and they all come here".[65] And to Bimal I asked, from Palpa, who also had tuberculosis: Why did you go to the Mission Hospital and not to one of the many other clinics around? "Because there foreigners would examine me, find the cause, and treat me accordingly, and with this hope I went there".[66]

In the hospital this demand to see the foreign doctor is anticipated. In one of the rooms I was using to interview people was a large sign in Nepali stating that attendance at the hospital did not mean that the patient would necessarily be seen by the foreign doctor. In one casual conversation I had at a bus stop six hours from Tansen, a woman said she had heard that there were five hundred American doctors working there, and was that true? Once as I was walking around in the west of the district, an old woman stopped me on the path and said, "Look at this body, old and wasted, give me some

---

(Cambridge: Cambridge University Press, 2005); Hoftun et al., *People, Politics and Ideology*. Political biographies covering the period include those of Tanka Prasad Acharya—James F. Fisher, *Living Martyrs: Individuals and Revolution in Nepal* (Delhi: Oxford University Press, 1997)—and BP Koirala; Kiran Misra, *BP Koirala: Life and Times* (New Delhi: Wishwa Prakashan, 1994). Locally, and locating Palpa's role in these events are works by B. Pangeni. *Palpama Prajatantraka andolanka say din* (Kathmandu: United Graphic Pra. Li, 2049); and a collection of essays edited under the auspices of a local intellectual club, the Saturday Club and published locally in Tansen: Palpama 2007 sālko andolan—the revolution of 2007 in Palpa.

65 Taped interview with JP, Tansen, 23 March 1999.

66 Taped interview with B, Tansen, 23 March 1999.

medicines to make me better"! At one medical camp I attended in a neighbouring district, as a further example, a discussion sprang up around the medicines being more powerful at the mission, because they came from *bidesh* or foreign countries. "It's the sweet smell of gold" [67] was the reply I received on asking at this medical camp why they had needed one of the missionary doctors there? In my opinion, all the trained health assistants were more than capable of diagnosing and treating most of the conditions they encountered. Yet I was told that the people in the area wanted a foreign doctor and this was the main reason, even though those running the camp agreed that they could have managed it on their own. [68]

"The holy man in your own home is a vulture, the one in the forest a saint" (Nepali—*Gharko yogi gidda, banko yogi siddha*) was the saying used by one Tansen resident I interviewed. We were talking about the sense amongst some of the more wealthy local elite that the only people who saw you these days at the mission were the "sorters". [69] As the hospital had got busier, so many people in Tansen felt they were being denied direct access to the foreign doctors. What does that saying mean I asked? People need to be seen by "white skin" he suggested, completely unprompted. The saying indicates that people from outside must know something, but here, inside, people know nothing, he continued. Nepalese denigrate their own knowledge, he said. It may have been in some of the old books but Nepalese only realised the value of something after being told by the missionaries. I searched for signs of resentment and anger at this but couldn't detect any. One senior nurse in the hospital told me that many Nepalese want to be examined by the foreign doctor and it doesn't even matter that it isn't by a doctor as long as they are foreigners. She recounted, laughing, a story of some-

[67] Nepali—*sunma sughanda*. While "it's the sweet smell of gold" is the literal translation, "it's the icing on the cake" is perhaps a more appropriate less literal translation. Thanks to Rod Chalmers for pointing this out to me.

[68] One aspect of a range of conversations with staff at camp on their work and practices, field notes, 8 January 2000. I attended this camp as part of the research which was held in Allam Than, Sanjya district, a six-hour walk from Tansen, on 7 and 8 January 2000.

[69] Conversation with MP, Tansen, 26 April 1999.

one pleading with an engineer at the hospital as they demanded to be examined. People believe that they are all good doctors, all well read, up to date and know a lot and they have a strong faith / belief in them she told me.[70]

For many, then, this attraction was as much magical as based in therapeutic efficacy. At the end of *Madness and Civilisation* Foucault is led to ponder on the paradoxical evolution of a magic of medical practice that emerges at the same time as mental illness moves towards a knowledge immersed in positivism.[71] For Foucault it is the asylum, and the doctor-patient couple, which forms a microcosm, symbolising the massive structures of bourgeoisie society and its values. In brilliant enigmatic prose, Foucault suggests that it is from this very alienation that the doctor derives the power to cure. "It was thought, *by the patient first of all* that it was the very esotericism of the doctors knowledge, accepting all the doctors knowledge, accepting self-surrender to the doctor, accepting all the doctor's prestige in advance, that allowed cure to occur . . . submitting from the very first to a will he experienced as magic, and to a science he regarded as prescience and divination, a reification of a magical nature, which could only be accomplished with the complicity of the patient himself".[72] While we are not here dealing with theoretically notorious epistemological ruptures in history, the magical reification to which Foucault refers seems even more valid in a situation into which a new epistemological order is introduced then associated with a foreign presence.

This is testament, perhaps, to a magical reification in which the mission (with its American, foreign, or white, rarely, if ever, Christian doctors) is invested, symbolically, with the power to cure. This is however a magic determined by a structural inequality, a dialectical relationship, that exists between Nepal and its Euro-American elsewhere; a hierarchy, both economic and technical, invested symbolically in the white skin of those who made the antibiotic, and set

[70] Interview with LR, 21 April 1999.

[71] Michel Foucault, *Madness and Civilisation: A History of Insanity in the Age of Reason* (New York: Vintage Books, 1988).

[72] Foucault, *Madness and Civilisation*, 275–76.

of very effective diagnostic procedures and healing practices within biomedicine, more widely available within this area of Nepal from the 1950s to the present day.

11

Expectations, Encounters and Ecclesiastics: Mission Medicine in Zululand, South Africa

Helen Sweet

In South Africa, Black Africans were severely medically disadvantaged as a result of racial divisions long before apartheid was formally introduced in 1948. In 1911 only one in seven doctors lived in rural areas[1] largely because the more lucrative practices which would finance their medical livings were to be found in 'white' urban areas. Anne Digby shows that this disparity did not improve significantly over the next seventy years with the doctor: patient ratio falling as low as 1:19,000 in black 'homeland' areas such as Qwaqwa in 1982.[2] In 1993 South African rural communities were 'almost entirely Black African with 50 per cent of the thirty million African, but only one per cent of the coloured, Indian and white populations, living in rural areas'.[3] However, in contrast with much of South Africa, the area now known as KwaZulu Natal had a very substantial number of Lutheran missions as well as many of other denominations. Most of these provided some form of medical support although this varied considerably both according to the individual mission (and also according to the inclination towards or

I would like to thank the Wellcome Trust for funding the research for this paper.

[1] Union of South Africa Official Reports and Papers: UG32 Census of 1912, Part V Occupations, 706–7.

[2] Anne Digby, *Diversity and Division in Medicine: Health Care in South Africa from the 1800s* (Oxford, New York: Peter Lang Publishing, 2006), 420–25.

[3] D. Cooper, R. Hamilton and H. Mashaba, *Race Relations Survey, 1992/1993* (Johannesburg: SAIRR, 1993).

away from medicine as part of evangelism, of those staffing them). They were almost invariably located in the poorer, rural areas and came from Sweden, Norway, America and Germany,[4] but in addition there were Anglican, Catholic and Church of Scotland missions also located within the Province, some of which also developed medical outlets.

By the mid-1970s, when the State began to take over many of the mission hospitals that had developed from these early beginnings, Natal and Zululand together had the highest concentration of mission hospitals in South Africa. The Lutheran Medical Foundation (LMF) alone had thirteen hospitals comprising a total bed count in excess of two thousand beds,[5] which in reality meant considerably more in terms of daily numbers of in-patients. Neither of these relate to the vast number of out-patients seen both at the hospitals and at their "out-reach" and mobile clinics. With one exception[6] these were all general hospitals although ranging considerably in size and facilities. It is this breach in the otherwise fairly uniform pattern of rural medical deprivation that this chapter is intending to explore. It will also present a somewhat different scenario from that presented in an earlier chapter by David Hardiman which took a broader view of the development of mission medicine across India, China and parts of central and southern sub-Saharan Africa—as always different contexts respond with particular nuances. For example, in her chapter on Lovedale Mission Hospital, Anne Digby has described how the two-tiered system of training male 'native' Africans as 'medical aides' to assist district surgeons and care for rural Africans, accepted elsewhere in Central Africa, was for a long time opposed by much of the medical profession in South Africa.[7] Simultaneously,

[4] P. J. Knutson, "Partnerships in Mission: Mismeeting in Jesus Name?" (unpublished D. Theol. University of the Western Cape, Department of Theology, Cape Town, 1998), 31, states that Natal was the only province in South Africa where all five Lutheran denominations were found together in close proximity to each other.

[5] Lutheran Medical Foundation correspondence file 1972–1977: LMF leaflet, *LMF. Republic of South Africa,* c.1973, Lutheran Archives, St Pauls, Minnesota.

[6] Thulasizwe was a specialist TB hospital.

[7] See also: Digby, *Diversity and Division in Medicine*, 192–98.

within the country's closely-linked, predominantly female, nursing profession [8] and its (medical) provincial regulating councils, [9] there was considerable resistance to the idea of separate, lower-grade state certification of African nurses for acceptance on the Register [10] specifically for 'practice amongst their own people'. [11]

I therefore begin this chapter with an overview of the history of healthcare provision by missions in KwaZulu Natal, followed by a more detailed description of the historical development of Hlabisa hospital, underpinned by using evidence from similar hospitals in the province. It concludes with a discussion of the role this hospital played in the community during its time as a mission hospital. It draws on a three-year post-doctoral research study looking at the roles of mission hospitals in the rural communities of present-day KwaZulu Natal, [12] as well as building upon earlier work, which focused on medical pluralism in the South African Cape. [13] The former concentrated on four mission hospitals scattered across rural KwaZulu Natal. Hlabisa was the focus of the study and was founded by Norwegian Lutherans and later taken over by the American Lutheran Mission. The other three hospitals which were also stud-

[8] Again, unlike much of the nursing mission field elsewhere, male nurses were very much in the minority, see discussion in Shula Marks, *Divided Sisterhood: Race, Class and Gender in the South African Nursing Profession* (London: Macmillan, 1994), 86–88.

[9] For the first 53 years, until Nursing Act No. 45 (1944), regulation of the nursing profession in South Africa was controlled by the Provincial medical councils, and later by the South African Medical and Dental Council. After 1944 the South African Nursing Council took over this role.

[10] Marks, *Divided Sisterhood*, 91. Marks explains in South Africa that: "the class issues were wrapped up in racial agendas".

[11] Charlotte Searle, *The History of the Development of Nursing in South Africa, 1652–1960: A Socio-Historical Survey* (Pretoria: South African Nursing Association, 1980 [1965]), 270.

[12] "Hospitals in the Developing World: A Study of Two former Colonies—Ceylon and KwaZulu Natal", Wellcome Trust funded project led by Professor Mark Harrison.

[13] "Medical Pluralism in the South African Cape", Wellcome Trust funded project led by Professor Anne Digby. My sincere thanks to Professor Digby for allowing me to draw data from the project.

ied in depth but will only be briefly referred to in this chapter, were Tugela Ferry (Church of Scotland), St Mary's KwaMagwaza (Anglican) and Emmaus (German Lutheran). Together they provide a representative sample of medical missions spread across present-day KwaZulu Natal as a whole. In addition the research looked in lesser detail at several others including Mariannhill (German Catholic), Nongoma (Benedictine) and Ceza (Swedish Lutheran). This chapter will be focussing on a particularly rich blend of material located at Hlabisa Lutheran Mission Hospital, now under State control, drawing upon oral history, photographic evidence and a unique full-run collection of the hospital's quarterly newsletters: *Isibani* (or The Lamp) for a "ground-up" insight to mission hospital life from around 1928 to the present time, supporting this with more traditional official documentary sources.

Medical Missionaries: The South African Historical Context

European missionaries arrived in South Africa in the mid- to late nineteenth century, many coming as Protestant married couples supported by missionary societies. Where this was the case, the husband generally served as evangelist with his wife acting as (unpaid) nurse and teacher often having to nurse the sick in her own family and those of fellow missionaries to the best of their ability. This was frequently extended to include the indigenous population—for example, Hanna Otte wife of the pastor at Hlabisa mission in the 1890s, "alleviated the natives" pains at her back door and in the kraals as well as occasionally helping with difficult midwifery cases. [14] Typically they carried with them a medical chest of simple, often homeopathic and herbal remedies and a layman's medical handbook, but missionary provision of paramedical "help in times of illness" [15] was at first merely seen as an additional and relatively minor secondary service to the main missionary duties.

[14] Solveig Otte, *Isibani*: XIV (1972), 3.

[15] Report from Emmaus Mission Hospital, Port Shepstone, Killie Campbell Museum (henceforth KCM) 98/2/09, KCM and Archives, University of KwaZulu Natal (henceforth UKZN), Durban.

Medical handbooks such as *Cox's Companion to the Family Medicine Chest and Compendium of Domestic Medicine* contained "plain rules for taking medicines", to which was added a basic description of "the treatment of fractures and dislocations, and a concise account of Asiatic or spasmodic cholera". [16] Similarly *The Travellers' Medical and Surgical Guide* [17] published a year later, whilst recommending the use of Burroughs Wellcome 'Alkaloidal Tabloids' also suggested whisky as a stimulant including 'per inj, for heat exhaustion, cholera or typhoid', and patent medicines such as 'Livingstone's rousers', 'Peptonising powders', 'Warburg's tincture', 'Dover's powder' and 'Glauber's salt'. [18] The fact that similar books were produced even earlier [19] than these demonstrates an urgent and ongoing need amongst many missionaries, as well as their contemporary lay explorers, military men, traders etc., for access to basic medical advice and support in an alien and often isolated environment.

Caring for the local population was therefore generally seen as a subsidiary, though laudable role for the missionary's wife, and was concentrated on obstetrics and midwifery and on public health measures such as advising on hygiene and sanitation. Likewise, missionary doctors' and nurses' primary role was initially to look after the mission's staff. From basic out-patient or dispensary beginnings

[16] Popular amongst these were: 'a member of the Royal College of Surgeons', *Cox's Companion to the Family Medicine Chest and Compendium of Domestic Medicine: Particularly Adapted for Heads of Families, Ship-Captains, Missionaries and Colonists, with Plain Rules for Taking Medicines, to which are Added a Plain Description of the Treatment of Fractures and Dislocations, and a Concise Account of Asiatic or Spasmodic Cholera*, 48th ed. (London: Simpkin, Marshall, 1887).

[17] 'a physician', *The Travellers' Medical and Surgical Guide: A Brief Manual for Explorers, Missionaries, Colonists and Ship-Captains*, 2nd ed. (London: Whiting, 1888)

[18] For a fuller account of this see Anne Digby, "Self-Medication and the Trade in Medicine Within a Multi-Ethnic Context: A Case Study of South Africa from the Mid-Nineteenth to Mid-Twentieth centuries", *Social History of Medicine* 18, no. 3. 2005, 439–57.

[19] For example, published thirty years earlier, Jabez Hogg, *The Domestic Medical and Surgical Guide, for the Nursery, the Cottage, and the Bush: Giving the Best Advice, in the Absence of a Physician or Surgeon in Cases of Accident or Sudden Illness. Useful to Families, Emigrants, Travellers, Missionaries, Village Clergymen, and Sea Captains* (London: Ingram Cooke, 1853).

they often set up small mud-hut 'hospitals' or 'dispensaries' of one or two four-bedded wards. More permanent buildings were built as and when they became better established within the local communities along with the gradual development of outreach clinics where time and resources allowed. In some, though not all cases this work expanded to such an extent that a larger general hospital might eventually be built. Yet this provides a very simplistic and generalised view of the process of hospital development largely ignoring the complex inter-relationships that influenced the success or failure of individual hospitals—for example, between state medical provision and that of missions and their mission hospitals, or at the grass-roots level between district surgeons and mission doctors and nurses, or between medical missionaries and traditional healers.

On this last point Forster claims that, "Missionaries have had to develop a much closer relationship with Africans than most other Europeans in Africa were prepared to contemplate." [20] In his view this applied to where they had to live, the need to learn language and customs of the local inhabitants, and that they usually had an advantage "even over the anthropologist" of a long period of stay in the same area. However, he cautions us that, "examining missionary accounts is the question of the balance between discussion of the activities of mission staff and of the customs of the local population." [21] This was because certain preoccupations—in particular, religious and spiritual beliefs usually referred to as "magic" and "witchcraft" in missionary accounts were generally condemned outright, whilst

> particular condemnation was often reserved by missionaries for traditional medical practice, especially since some mission staff were qualified medical doctors. . . . the traditional practitioner was seen as flouting

[20] P. G. Forster, "Missionaries and Anthropology: The Case of the Scots of Northern Malawi", *Journal of Religion in Africa* 16, 1986, 101–9. This last reference to M. Gelfand's work, for example, *Christian Doctor and Nurse: The History of Medical Missions in South Africa from 1799–1976* (Sandton: Mariannhill Mission Press, 1984), 307.

[21] Forster, "Missionaries and Anthropology".

Christian doctrine by being a magician, and medical theory by being a quack; and additionally he was a competitor for the mission hospital.[22]

In 1961, Keen[23] a general surgeon at the non-European Hospital, Johannesburg, described the surgeon's approach to African patients as different by necessity from that of a physician or obstetrician. His personal experience was drawn particularly from rural medical practice in Swaziland in the 1940s, where many of those who came to the hospital had already received "treatment from their own doctors and come to us as a last resource, in a state of suspicion and doubt strongly tinged by feelings of hope. In these cases we are competing with the herbalist and witchdoctor and must adopt the right tactics and do better than the witchdoctor at his own game."[24]

As an example of this, he described how he would get the orderly to write down the patient's main symptoms so that he could make a preliminary diagnosis at the outset, just as the sangoma might do and similarly if taking blood, he would explain that this was because: "There is poison in your blood, and I must take some to find out the best medicine to give you".[25] He contested that whilst lay doctors did not consult the ancestors in front of their patients this was "a predominant factor of the witchdoctor's armamentarium. Missionaries [therefore] have a decided advantage over government officials in this respect, as a prayer offered up is an indication of consultation with ancestors". A district surgeon in Eshowe even went so far as to claim that: "religion is sold to the Native with a bottle of

[22] Forster, "Missionaries and Anthropology".

[23] P. Keen, "Surgical Problems in Bantu Practice", in *The African Nurse*, ed. T.N.E.D.G. (unpublished seminar series, 1961), 44–47.

[24] P. Keen, "Surgical Problems in Bantu Practice".

[25] Ibid.

medicine"[26]—adding in a subsequent letter that some missionaries actually "retain their hold by medical quackery".[27]

Writing in 1997, Jaques[28] agreed that a spirit of non-cooperation from the missionary side towards the indigenous healers had existed well into the twentieth century. The significance of these facts and the impact this has had can only be fully appreciated if we understand the extent of the role played by missions and mission hospitals in South Africa not only in providing health care but in the field of health education. Interestingly however, at a conference held at Umpumulu in 1967 on the "Healing Ministry of the Church",[29] the findings reflected a gradual change in attitude, at least on the part of some medical missionaries, with growing awareness of some commonalities between traditional healing and missionary medicine in contrast with secular biomedicine. This led to recommendations for a more sympathetic study of traditional healing in this light, particularly with regard to the spiritual and holistic nature of missionary and traditional medicine compared with standard biomedical practice. Perhaps of greatest significance were the following points set out amongst the Report's conclusory findings:

26 E. Holland et al., "National Health Insurance and Medical Services for Rural Areas", *South African Medical Journal* 10, 1936, 249–56. This strongly worded letter was signed by the district surgeons of Stanger, Manda and Ndwedwe, Umfozoli and Hlabisa and as well as condemning the mission hospitals also denounced the idea of training Africans as medical aids or as midwives to work in the rural areas.

27 E. Holland, "State Medical Service for Native Rural Areas", *South African Medical Journal* 10, 1936, 387.

28 P. H. Jaques and Sam Fehrsen, "The Role of Mission Hospitals in Providing Health Care in South Africa", in *Health Sector Reform: Coping Strategies and Professional Identity of Primary Health Care Clinicians* (unpublished, Discussion Paper, c. 1997)

29 Rev. Rector Gunnar Lislerud (Director), *The Report of the Umpumulu Consultation of the Healing Ministry of the Church*, held at the Lutheran Theological College, Mapumulu, Natal, 19–27 September 1967 (unpublished Proceedings, 1967).

a) The traditional African understanding of health and healing should be sympathetically studied since it is an essential part of the background of the Church's work in Africa. In the past it has too often been dismissed as pagan and unworthy of attention by the Church.

b) Much of the traditional African understanding of health and healing is based on a spiritual and even theistic view of the world, and has much to teach by its positive emphasis on the need for healing the whole man, by its sense of community and by its consciousness of the reality of spiritual powers in the world.

c) Whilst there are non-Christian ideas in this understanding which need to be carefully distinguished and set aside, there are also practices which the church could rid of their pagan associations and use in its ministry of healing. [30]

At the same conference Dr Wolfgang Bodenstein described his unusually pluralistic version of general practice, referring to the "tragedy of our cross-cultural situation [due to] ignorance and prejudice regarding each other's cultural roots and patterns." [31] Indeed, he went further, stating that:

> The Missions summarily branded the whole field of African Medicine as "witchcraft," as "heathen heritage," as something to be condemned, ignored and thrown out. We must accept that this was done in good faith, never mind the consequences. In its place, Western Medicine was substituted and enthroned, although it is probably just as heathen, perhaps more so in some aspects. Due to this fateful initial error, and its subsequent perpetuation, the Christian Ministry of Healing so far just could not get off the ground. [32]

He stressed the holistic nature of the traditional healers' approach and their "intelligence and flexibility in their astonishing capacity for adjusting to a changing cultural pattern in a new era". Indeed he had evidence that some were 'succeeding to rope hospitals, clinics and doctors into their business outfit without those "partners" having the faintest ideas about it.' This provides rare insight to the other

[30] Rev. Lislerud, *The Report of the Umpumulu Consultation*.

[31] W. Bodenstein, "Contemporary Approaches of Healing: African Medicine", *The Report of the Umpumulu Consultation*, 1967, 51–64.

[32] Bondestein, "Contemporary Approaches of Healing".

side of the story—i.e., that of the healers' responses to the threat being presented by biomedical healers invading their territory.

Obstacles to Establishing Sustainable Medical Missions

Looking at the histories of thirty mission hospitals,[33] and bearing these points in mind, there are a number of common factors to their development. Perhaps the most noticeable of these is the tenuous nature of their existence, often surviving with minimal resources, poorly financed, little or no medical cover and until considerably later where this did exist it relied largely upon doctors and nurses from Europe, Scandinavia and America, as opposed to trained South Africans. Relationships between medical missions and country doctors were not always particularly genial, especially where the latter found themselves, 'defending their livelihoods against missionaries who used medical practice or dispensing as a way into the hearts and minds of the unconverted.'[34] On the other hand, several mission hospitals only had limited access to visiting doctors even as late as 1977, so that a heavy burden of responsibility fell on the (mostly white) resident senior nursing staff. This is particularly of significance when comparing the previous working experience many of those nurses would have received in the USA, Scandinavia or Europe—in contrast they were suddenly expected to deal with "medical emergencies such as burns, fractures, snake-bites, difficult maternity cases and malnutrition"[35] with minimal or no advanced preparation, to say nothing of the cultural and language barriers. An English nurse, Alice Hillier, running the small St Augustine's mission hospital near Dundee (northern Zululand) wrote in 1934:

[33] Collection of Histories of Thirty Mission Hospitals compiled by Miss Eva Reynolds in 1974, KCM 98/2/1–30 , KCM and Archives, Durban.

[34] Harriet Deacon, "Medical Gentlemen and the Process of Professionalisation Before 1890", in *The Cape Doctor in the Nineteenth Century: A Social History*, ed. Harriet Deacon, Howard Phillips and Elizabeth van Heyningen (Amsterdam/ New York: Rodopi, 2004), 92.

[35] Report from Assisi Mission Hospital, KCM 98/2/02, KCM and Archives, Durban.

> "We take in Midwifery cases and General. The Doctor only comes once a week—sometimes it is a fortnight. I have to dispense medicines, and diagnose cases, extract teeth, do accounts and housekeeping."[36]

Although matron Hillier had three "Native nurses" who she had to "train and give lectures to", nurse training schools producing nurses with a recognised qualification could not be fully established until medical supervision was in place. If for some reason that failed—for example with doctors not being replaced when they felt the need to return home-nurse training was often forced into deferment or totally suspended. In 1942 Miss Alexander (General President, South African Trained Nurses' Association) stated:

> there is a great deal to be done to create an A1 nation in South Africa. Conditions in Native Territories present a very wide field of activity. . . . Native girls [should be given] the knowledge to help their own people to understand and practice the art of keeping well people well and of helping sick people to regain good health through training in good training schools. . . . African nurses are urgently required in the rural areas and Native Territories.[37]

The article listed all South African Nursing Association-approved training hospitals as well as revealing the differential between salaries for 'European' i.e., white and 'non-European' i.e., black or coloured nurses working in South Africa, stating that there were

> at least 955 non-European nurses and midwives in training in the Union. Last year (1941) the names of 63 non-Europeans appeared in the lists as having passed the SAMC's final examination for medical and surgical nurses and 60 who had passed the Council's examination for midwives.[38]

[36] Alice Mary Hillier to Miss Cox-Davies 20 March 1934, Records of the Royal College of Nursing (henceforth RCN) 22/1/4/2, RCN Archives, Edinburgh.

[37] "Nursing as a Profession for Non-European Women", in *The Health Magazine*, February 1942, 1–15.

[38] "Nursing as a Profession for Non-European Women". In KwaZulu Natal the hospitals that prepared students for the examination to become Registered Nurses (henceforth RNs) were: Nongoma (a Benedictine Mission Hospital [henceforth MH]), King Edward VIII Hospital, Durban, McCord

Listed were forty-six training schools in South Africa, twenty-one of which prepared Black or Coloured students for the government examination of Registered Nurse (RN). Of these five were in present-day KwaZulu Natal—this was from a total of thirteen training hospitals in KwaZulu Natal named as providing nurse training—significantly almost all being Mission Hospitals. In fact Natal and Zululand had pioneered widespread training of black nurses with McCords American Zulu Mission Hospital successfully training African nurses from 1910 onwards, [39] and hospitals at KwaMagwaza, Marianhill and Nkonjeni following that example from as early as 1921. [40]

However, the mission hospital histories referred to above indicate clearly that the principals of biomedicine were alien to the local population and the way these appear to have been handled suggests a major cultural gulf. [41] Not only was it difficult to persuade patients to receive biomedical treatment, but in some cases it was difficult to recruit trainee nurses. For example, at Mangusi Hospital in 1951, German missionary doctor, Dr Schwalbe, "had to institute a training school that would attract nurses from elsewhere as local girls wouldn't work". [42] However, despite difficulties in some places, both nurse-recruitment and take-up of out-patient and in-patient treatment did increase substantially throughout the 1930s and 1940s and this acceptance of biomedicine escalated as more purpose-built institutions were established in the 1950s. This coincided with tuberculosis becoming much more successfully treatable and hospital figures reflect this, suggesting an average of 1:4 beds being provided for treatment of tuberculosis by the 1970s. Materni-

---

Zulu (American MH) Durban, St Aidan's (Anglican MH) Durban, and St Mary's Kwamagwaza (Anglican MH).

39 T. G. Mashaba, *Rising to the Challenge of Change: A History of Black Nursing in South Africa* (Cape Town: Juta and Co. Ltd, 1995), 17–20.

40 *Six Decades of Service: St Mary's Mission Hospital, KwaMagwaza, c. 1973*, 5.

41 See Anne Digby and Helen Sweet, "Nurses as Culture Brokers in Twentieth-Century South Africa" in *Plural Medicine, Tradition and Modernity, 1800–2000*, ed. Waltraud Ernst (London and New York: Routledge, 2001).

42 Report for Manguzi Mission Hospital, Ubombo, KCM 98/2/12, KCM and Archives, Durban.

ty cases also formed a significant proportion of the total with some hospitals providing facilities for ante-natal care as "waiting mothers"[43] and taking the opportunity to introduce these young women to biomedically-based principles of health education, child care and nutrition as well as to Christian evangelism.

Whilst it is clearly not the case that the development of all mission hospitals conformed to a clear-cut pattern, it would be helpful at this point to look at one that appears to have gone through many of the stages experienced by its contemporaries.

Hlabisa—Case Study of a Mission Hospital

Hlabisa is set in a picturesque area of rolling hills and valleys, in the north-east of the province, situated between Mtubatuba and Nongoma on the edge of the Hluhluwe-Umfulozi game reserve which was one of the earliest reserves, established in 1895. The population of the largely rural Hlabisa health district in 1995 was estimated at 205,463 from the 1991 census. Most residents speak Zulu as their first language and the majority live in widely scattered kraals, depending on pension remittances, migrant labour and subsistence farming for money and food. A major national road and trading route crosses the district and a large township is spread out along this road.

The site at Hlabisa[44] was given to the Norwegian Missionary Society by King Cetshwayo in 1869. The following year a small mission was started up there by Pastor Ole Stavem but he only stayed three years, claiming: "there are many wild animals and people almost as wild as animals", suggesting he was very poorly prepared for missionary work in such a remote rural area, particularly at a time of

[43] The "waiting mothers" facilities refer to ante-natal hutted accommodation which was vital for first and 'at-risk' pregnancies where the expectant mother was unable to gain quick access to midwifery care for the birth. They would stay for several weeks before giving birth on a self-care basis and would also receive instruction on how to care for their babies, health and hygiene, cooking and nutrition.

[44] 'Hlabisa' means "to slaughter a beast for one's guests" and is thought to refer to Zulu hospitality and values.

escalating instability in this part of the country. [45] However, this was also influenced by internal politics within Norwegian missionary circles as the Hlabisa station was ceded to the Church of Norway (Shreuder) Mission in 1891 in exchange for exclusive rights to the station at Umpumulu. Bishop Nils Astrup from the Shreuder Mission arrived at Hlabisa the following year, in 1892 to re-establish the mission, and his daughter and son-in-law, Heinrich and Anne Otte settled there five years later, in 1897. With the nearest store more than 30 miles on foot and with constantly unpaid debts, a doctor's fees were clearly too expensive—in fact the nearest doctor at that time was probably in, or close to Durban. Anne's father had provided them with some medicines which he had taken with him on his mission expeditions up the Limpopo and it was these that she dispensed from her stoepe. They included jalopin, polophyllin and quinine for malaria, camphor as an antispasmodic or expectorant, tartar emetic and liquorice. [46]

The first 'nurse', Borghild Andresen, joined them in 1916 [47] coming as housemother and nurse for the girls' home within the mission. [48] It would seem that she also continued providing informal nursing care to the local community, together with Mrs Otte,

[45] Whilst the Anglo-Zulu war was fought between January and July 1879, serious distrust and episodes of open aggression existed over a much longer period, increasing dramatically with the succession of Cetshwayo to the Zulu throne in 1873.

[46] My thanks to Professor Frederick Hale for these details from his current work (in progress) towards a full translation of N. Astrup, *En Missionsreise til Limpopo: gjennem Zululand, Swaziland og Tongaland ind i Riget Umgaza (An Account of a Journey from Zululand Through Swaziland into Southern Mozambique* [Kristiania: Steen, 1891]).

[47] Oral history, Miss Inge Kruse, KZN 14. There is unfortunately no record to confirm or refute whether Borghild had received any formal training as a nurse, but it would seem unlikely.

[48] In his "Superintendent's Report of 1943", in *Khumbulani, the Year Book, 1943–44 of the Board of Foreign Missions of the Norwegian Lutheran Church in America*, Dr Johannes Astrup stated, "During the past 40 years several lady workers have been with us, a good many for shorter periods. As for instance, Miss Halvorson from Norway and with exception of Miss Wessel the following six ladies also from Norway: Miss Carlson and Mrs Falck-Moe, 1915–1928, and the Misses Pettersen, Nafstad, Saeter, Andresen, Wessel and Kwaale."

in much the same way. However, her main role was still primarily to care for the missionaries and the children at the mission. Swedish trained nurse, Anna Standberg who arrived at the sister mission, Ceza one year earlier wrote:

> I have been so unhappy, not being able to do more. My wishes for a doctor have been very strong. During my visits to the homes I have often met with witch-doctors and have seen their methods of treating people and have been astonished at the patient's great faith in them. A nurse often feels her great shortcomings at the sight of all the misery.[49]

In fact Ceza was in advance of Hlabisa as the first trained missionary nurse arrived there as early as 1911 doing her district nursing work on horseback. By 1915 she had established three rondavels serving as small wards doubling to six by 1928 plus a small outpatients' department and maternity ward.

At Hlabisa, Borghild Andresen was succeeded in 1928 by a fully trained Norwegian nurse and midwife, thirty-six year old Petrine Solvik, who immediately increased the momentum by starting a dispensary and she had a small (four-bedded) ward built there by 1932. This grew rapidly so that the first 'hospital' of just thirty-two beds was dedicated in 1935. When she was away on furlough the following year (her last for eleven years because of wartime restrictions) a "qualified native nurse and midwife", Miss W. Miya was brought in as relief sister. Between them they saw 717 out-patients and 37 in-patients, plus 30 maternity cases. Nevertheless, Sister Solvik still experienced similar difficulties (due largely to cultural differences) to those expressed by Sister Sandberg, referring in her annual hospital report of 1936 to

> the disparity in the number of in-patients compared with that of outpatients [is] partly due to the Natives' ignorance of the necessity in serious and neglected cases, of entering a hospital ward for regular nursing and medical attention. The Native wants his sickness diagnosed and minutely described in all its symptoms and expects a remedy for each of them. If his curiosity be not met according to his expectations, that is, if

49 M. Adolfsson and Anna Berntsson, *Ceza, a Roundabout Way to the Goal: Three Decades of Medical Missionary Work in South Africa* (Klippan: Ljungbergs Boktr., 1984), 33.

> the diagnosis does not correspond with his own feelings and opinions, a suspicion is engendered in his mind as to the White man's ability to cope with his particular disease. . . . The natives are as yet most susceptible to the persuasions of the ignorant and superstitious. [50]

She further expressed concern over the high infant mortality and the "barbarous and revolting treatment Native women have to endure during confinement".

After 1 January 1927 when the Norwegian Lutheran Church in America (NLCA) took over the work of the Schreuder Mission, Dr J. R. Birkelund, Director of their Board of Foreign Missions, made a two-month visit to South Africa. In his report, made in the same year that Petrine Solvik arrived at Hlabisa, he also stated:

> There is need for a medical man on our field. The infant mortality is extremely high. It ranges from one-third to one-forth [*sic*] of the children born. It might be expected that the adults who grew out of this sifting would be the strongest of mankind, but the mortality among them is possibly three or four times as great as in America. The causes are many: ignorance, insufficient and unsuitable food, bad water, unclean clothing, unsanitary houses, dangerous insects, such as the mosquito carrying the malaria, the tsetse fly carrying the sleeping sickness, and last those contagious and infectious diseases which come with such virulence upon the people whose blood has not been acclimated to resist attack. [51]

He also referred to Dr J. Astrup's [52] report, which had been presented in the church periodical at that time and which expressed an "ardent wish" to have a medical doctor who could start a hospital within the Zululand Mission, especially in the northern parts of the mission field

> where there is much sickness and where there is no hospital within a radius of a couple hundred miles. I sincerely hope that we will see the

[50] *Hospital Annual Report*, 1936, Hlabisa Mission Hospital.

[51] Dr J. R. Birkelund, Director of their Board of Foreign Missions, Report dated May 1928, NLCA.

[52] Dr Astrup was a Doctor of Theology, not of Medicine.

> day when we have a hospital at Hlabisa under an American doctor and a couple of nurses.[53]

In response to this Birkelund noted that he had visited the magistrate at Hlabisa who had expressed great satisfaction with the idea of a hospital there and offered any assistance within his power. Apparently there were even some government buildings that the magistrate thought could be used for this purpose yet this project did not materialise for another twenty years.

However, supported by grants from the Native Affairs Department and the Provincial Department the mission had been able to construct two large underground water tanks[54] and a laundry, plus a "waiting home" for expectant mothers at the small makeshift hospital. Also from 1935/36 it was being referred to as a "hospital" with annual reports being prepared by Sister Solvik as its "Matron" suggesting a rise in perceived status by those who were involved with the mission. By 1939 the Native Affairs Department had requested that a Hospital Board should be formed, consisting of local magistrate, district surgeon and representatives from the mission, Native Affairs Department and Provincial Health Department—interestingly, this did not include the 'matron' as a board member!

I would argue, however, that the most significant development during this period was the establishment of outreach clinics by Sister Solvik which she visited on a fortnightly basis. The first of these was at Emacibini, on the main road to Somkele, and the Annual Report for 1939 notes that, "A good many have made use of the opportunity to seek remedies for minor ailments [at the clinic]."[55] In less than six months Sister Solvik saw 113 patients at the Emacibini clinic and it can be seen from the graph (see Figure. 11.1) that out-patient numbers at the hospital grew rapidly from this point

[53] *Lutheran Herald*, 1 May 1928. I am indebted to Rev. Jim Knutson for this reference.

[54] As with similar mission hospitals, the supply of a large and reliable year-round supply of fresh water was vitally important to any further development at the site.

[55] *Hospital Annual Report* , 1939, Hlabisa Mission Hospital.

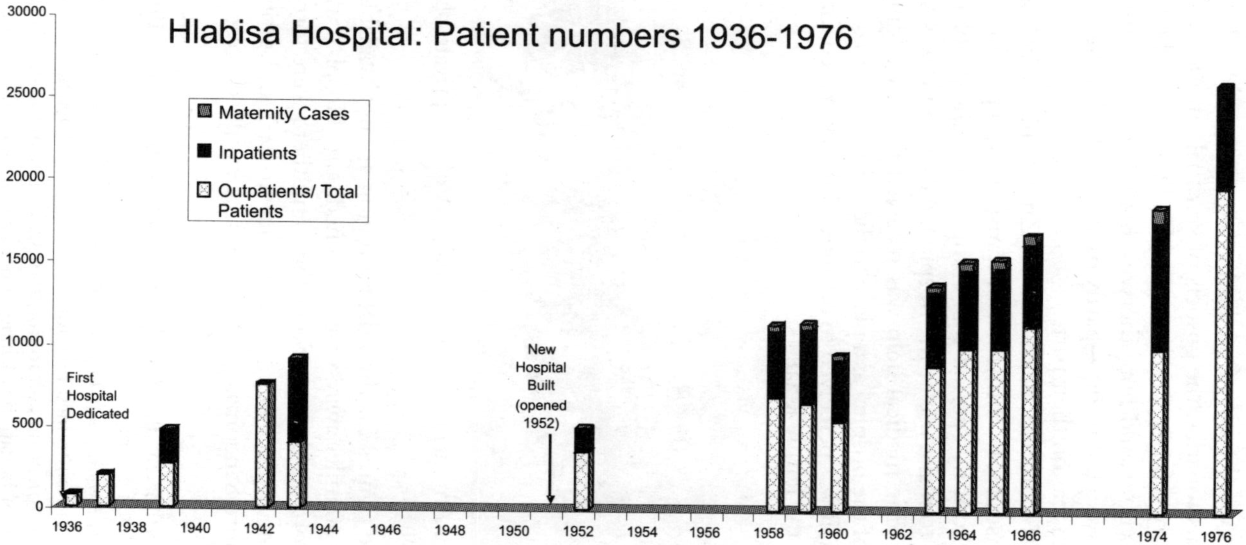

Figure 11.1: Graph showing Hlabisa Hospital's growth in terms of in-patient and out-patient numbers over the forty years between 1936–76 (i.e., the time of the official founding of a mission "hospital" to State take-over as part of the "Comprehensive Health Scheme").

onwards.[56] This was a form of medical evangelism and for Petrine as with many missionaries, the gospels of spiritual salvation and of social and sanitary reform, were inseparable. This also enabled her to see patients who would not otherwise have sought her nursing attention, unless as a last resort—partly because of their remoteness and partly due to fear on their part.

The picture (Figure 11.2 below) of the Zulu "ambulance" taken in the 1950s illustrates the difficulty of transporting a patient to the hospital throughout this period that compounded the problem of getting patients to make use of the hospital. As a result it was often too late by the time medical help was received thereby adding to the reputation of the hospital as a place to die. Also, for a mixture of cultural reasons, it was perceived to be preferable to be cared for and maybe to die at the family kraal.

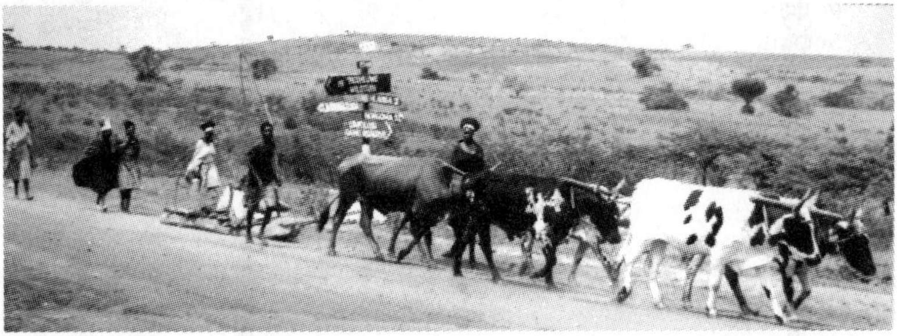

Figure 11.2 Zulu Ambulance, c.1950 (Image: Author's private photographic collection)

Although the figures for the Hlabisa region are not available, in Nongoma, just 30 miles away, where a Benedictine Hospital was in a similar but more rapid stage of development, there were forty-six registered Inyangas practising in the district in 1937 and probably considerably more Sangomas.[57] Oral histories would suggest these

[56] Although unfortunately the reports containing statistics from 1943–58 appear to have been destroyed.

[57] Both are types of traditional healers—the former is generally applied to mean a herbalist often trained by another family member whereas the latter also bases treatment on communication with the 'ancestors' and trains through a period of initiation working under an experienced sangoma.

numbers would have been similar in the Hlabisa district. Certainly they appear to have represented serious competition to Sister Solvik both in terms of biomedical and religious converts. She refers to this again whilst describing the apparently haphazard, organic rather than planned hospital development based mostly on urgent response to immediate difficulties

> Because we needed a place to put our patients, we took a small storeroom in the Zulu School Girls' Home. Very soon this room proved to be too small, because at night when all were asleep on the floor—the sick and those who brought the sick there was no place left to even walk. . . . We needed a larger and better place than this storeroom with its dirt door. . . . Very soon we received the money so that we were able to build the first hospital building, consisting of four rooms. During this time we used a thatched mud and daub building with dirt floor for our hospital. Even though it was a very dark and dreary place, many who came were healed. Dr J. Astrup . . . saw that we needed to enlarge our hospital so he built another small two-room building. . . . When he left Hlabisa, his son, Rev. Hjalmar Astrup, and family came. During his term here he built the laundry, a kitchen, a house for expectant mothers, with kitchen, and a home for white nurses. Up until this time I had lived in the Zulu School Girls' Home. We were very pleased to get these additions to our hospital as it aided us so much in the work. When Rev. Astrup left for his furlough overseas, Rev. Farup returned. It was during this time that we had a very bad epidemic of dysentery and we again found our hospital over-crowded so that all floor space was taken. Again Rev. Farup wrote for help. Again we received help and were able to build a second hospital building of four rooms.

She then added:

> We hope now that the Zulu people will learn to bring their sick people to this place God has given them so that they may be healed—under His blessing and not go to the witch doctor who deceives them and keeps them under his evil control. [58]

This hostile attitude towards indigeneous medicine remained relatively unchanged although perhaps less visible to those working

[58] P. Solvik, "History of Hlabisa Hospital", in *The Missionary*, n.d.

at the hospital—as one nurse who was at Hlabisa in the 1960s and 1970s stated:

> We had the idea that our western medicine was pretty much accepted in the area while also being aware that witch doctors and sangomas and herbalists were being utilized. But Diti and Marlene [two Catholic missionary district nurses] set us straight on our "universal acceptance" theory! They reported that at some of the outlying clinics they served, there were people who would have gladly died at home before they would agree to come near our hospital! [59]

Mostert claimed that throughout this period, "The missionaries and the diviners were fixed enemies", [60] whilst the Rev. J. Knutson remembered that, "In the 1950s some Lutheran mission doctors would even cut off patients' bracelets or amulets before preceding with their treatment". [61] Yet there is no hard evidence to suggest that this represented a two-way antagonistic situation—for example, traditional healers do not appear to have actively prevented their patients from attending clinics or hospital, sometimes accompanying them there rather than relinquishing their care.

Interestingly, however, this uneasy relationship between biomedics and traditional healers would seem to have been changing relatively recently according to the present Matron and Hospital Manager who commented in 2003: "Our clients' first call is at a sangoma before they come to us, so now it was high time that we and the sangomas and traditional healers, would form alliances, because we were looking after the same clients." [62] She attributed much of this change to Ministry of Health directives in the face of the HIV AIDS epidemic.

Despite growing political emphasis on the need for doctors to support the work being pioneered by nurses such as Petrine, and to take it forward to provide a more comprehensive rural health care service, the nearest doctor to Hlabisa throughout the 1930s and 1940s

[59] Oral History, Anne Rabie nee Brownlow, KZN 17.

[60] N. Mostert, *Frontiers—The Epic of South Africa's Creation and the Tragedy of the Xhosa People* (London: Jonathan Cape, 1992), 956.

[61] Knutson, *Partnerships in Mission*, 180.

[62] Oral History, Matron Dawn Zungu, KZN 08.

was the district surgeon, Dr Abel, whose practice was 20 miles away at Mtubatuba, and who made regular but infrequent visits to the mission.

For many reasons, including the depression in the USA and the Second World War, it wasn't until 1948 that Dr Erling Hestenes, the first resident doctor at Hlabisa, arrived from the USA to oversee the building of a much larger, purpose-designed hospital, which opened officially in 1952, when a second resident doctor, Dr Hall also arrived.

This was fundamentally a quite different stage of hospital development from its rudimentary make-shift predecessors, being equipped from the outset with the modern requirements of a general hospital, including in-patient wards and maternity department, an operating theatre, small X-Ray and pathology department, and a dispensary. An administration block, doctors houses and a school of nursing were also included. Existing facilities were either modernised and incorporated into the new building or replaced, and this process of modernisation of buildings and equipment became a feature of the ensuing two decades. Hospital growth had already quite clearly begun in the fifteen years preceding the arrival of the doctors and the larger hospital, and the records point to this being taken up predominantly by female African patients. From its opening in 1952 the hospital grew rapidly to 150 beds and this continued over the next two decades to 276 beds by 1966.[63] Endemic diseases prevalent at that time included tuberculosis, bilharzia, typhoid, amoebiasis, venereal diseases and gastro-enteritis as well as widespread malnutrition including pellagra and kwashiorkor. There are also recorded occasional outbreaks of cholera, malaria, polio, measles and chickenpox which temporarily swamped the hospital's resources. Trauma cases were a regular feature of medical and nursing reports—in particular burns and scalds; lacerations, fractures and head injuries

[63] E. J. Holman, *A Report on the Medical Program of the Evangelical Lutheran Church in Southern Africa South Eastern Region, Natal Province, Republic of South Africa* (Dundee, South Africa: R. A. Burns and Co., 1967), 27–35 gives this as 130 general and 86 tuberculosis beds plus approximately 60 additional 'un-registered' beds. As such it was described as 'one of the key institutions of the Lutheran medical programme in Natal'.

from axe, knobkerrie and stick fights; and bites and other injuries caused by snakes and various wild animals. Figures relating to the latter were substantially higher than other mission hospitals studied due to its proximity to the game reserve, although there was a good relationship between the two.

Preventative medicine or a modified version of "social medicine" formed a prominent part of the hospital's work and a comprehensive vaccination programme within the community was run from the hospital through the mobile clinics from the mid-1950s onwards. With the new hospital in the 1950s came electricity and a more sophisticated water supply and sanitation system with the doctors having to design and oversee the building and installation of these essential services. Most of the doctors interviewed commented on the need to learn non-medical skills such as water and sewerage engineering, electrical engineering, car-mechanics and ambulance driving and a range of building skills in addition to their day-to-day medical responsibilities. At first they also had to be able to take and develop their own X'Rays and carry out basic pathological techniques, until staff could be trained to take over these responsibilities.

In 1967 there was no outward sign of an imminent take-over of the province's mission hospitals by the government—indeed the official line taken by the LMF was that they should come under the wing of the Evangelical Lutheran Church in Southern Africa South East Region (ELCSA-SER).[64] Knutson suggests this was possibly "understood but too painful a subject to declare openly" but that it was also being made clear that "in the 1960s the newly formed indigenous churches could not at that time, nor in the foreseeable future, assume full management or financial responsibility for the church related medical programs".[65] Even as late as 1971, Knutson notes that Hlabisa's Lutheran Pastor, Rev. Rindahl reported on a visit to the Bantu Affairs and State Health Department by representatives of the LMF, "to try and get a better picture of future prospects for our medical work. . . . They [the Health Department]

[64] Holman, *A Report on the Medical Program* , 214–15.

[65] Knutson, *Partnerships in Mission*, 177.

stated emphatically, "We cannot get along without the missions".... We had asked if and when they might want to buy out and take over fully.... Guesses of up to 50 years were made." Rindahl concluded tentatively that "from this interview it would seem the future of our mission hospitals is not quite so dark as we had feared."[66]

Whilst, it had always been a primary aim of the missionaries to train African personnel to the point where they could take over their roles and responsibilities—that is effectively to work themselves out of their jobs gradually—the speed with which this was forced through had clearly not been anticipated.[67] The last mission nurse sponsored by the American Lutheran Church left in 1978 and the last doctor in 1981 so that by 1980 all Lutheran hospitals had been handed over to the South African government. During the missionary period, it is worth noting that several of the doctors and nurses stayed for many years—several nurses such as Olga Guttormson and Petrine Solvik exceeded thirty years each, and many were there for approximately twenty years, whilst Doctors Hestenes, Hall and Rabie were there for twenty-eight, sixteen and nineteen years respectively. Therefore, where others came only for shorter lengths of stay the longer-term doctors and nurses were able to orient them and oversee their early settlement period, thus increasing their level of effectiveness. Dr Rabie pointed out that: "it is difficult to be efficient in deep rural medicine when you have had your training in a more resource-rich environment, not to mention the different [cultural, environmental and epidemiological] challenges."[68] Dr Waalewijn who came from Holland with less post-graduate experience echoed this, explaining:

> And they [the senior doctors] said, "Well . . . with the Caesarean Sections, you . . . you assist the first one, and you do the next one". So I said, "Well, maybe the third one!" Well, I assisted with the first one, and then the second one . . . they said, "You do this, and do that", but then

[66] Ibid., 178.

[67] This subject will be considered in greater depth elsewhere, Helen Sweet, *Medicine with a Mission: The Role and Development of Missionary Nursing and Medicine in KwaZulu Natal, c. 1920–1980?* (monograph in preparation).

[68] Personal Communication, Dr Seig Rabie, 18 May 2003.

> . . . it's not such a difficult operation, so and that's the way it went. They just coached me, and I did it quite well. I must say the work, like in Outpatients Department, was overwhelming in the beginning, so many patients and [presenting at] a stage of illness you'd never see in Holland.[69]

As with the nurses, many of the doctors like Dr Waalewijn, found a need to rapidly learn new medical and surgical skills as they encountered problems beyond their Western expertise. Indeed by the 1970s it was felt that doctors in particular, were beginning to come for shorter-term periods of stay, primarily to gain experience and to offer something positive *before* settling down to their "real lives" elsewhere. This was in marked contrast to their predecessors—both missionary nurses and doctors—who often became a part of the community within which they lived and worked, learning language and customs, and in some cases settling on a permanent (life-long) basis.[70]

A Mission Hospital's Contribution Beyond 'Care and Cure'

One of the main questions my research has aimed to answer is: "what were the contributions of these rural mission hospitals to the larger community beyond the obvious one of providing access to biomedical health care?" The LMF's stated purpose for their hospitals was both the practice of public health and preventative medicine and the educational aim of training nurses and ancillary staff and supporting the training of doctors and other personnel.

Perhaps the most obvious contribution, therefore, is that of providing employment and training. Group photographs and those of individuals which regularly feature in *Isibani* suggest the very considerable extent of this. Several interviewees expressed their appreciation for training or apprenticeship received. These ranged from cooks, carpenters, electricians and mechanics to ambulance drivers, pathologists, and X'Ray technicians. It was further pointed out that

[69] Oral history, Dr Nico Waalewijn 30 May 2003, KZN 03.

[70] Helen Sweet, "'Wanted: 16 Nurses of the Better Educated Type'—Provision of Nurses to South Africa in the Late Nineteenth and Early Twentieth Centuries", *Nursing Inquiry Special Issue* 11, no. 3, 2004, 176–84.

these were valued transferable skills—for the women, for example the training they received as housekeepers, seamstresses or cooks often provided greater marriageable status as well as a valuable income for those living effectively as single mothers whilst under the apartheid regime their husbands were sent away for long periods of time to work in Johannesburg or Durban. Also, looking beyond the immediate hospital employment, there were (and still are) many local services and suppliers who depended to some greater or lesser extent on the hospital and on the hospital staff for their livelihoods.

Possibly the greatest commitment was to nurse-training which began even before the hospital building was completed in 1952. Initially this was for the South African Nursing Council Certificate (equivalent to the Enrolled nurse in the UK but comprising three years' training emerging as 'staff nurses') and a few years later a one-year Midwifery Certificate was added to the School of Nursing's core curriculum until tighter national regulation were introduced in 1962 making this untenable at Hlabisa. Also, a two-tiered training was established to allow nurse-assistants to train first as auxiliary nurses and then to progress to staff nurses. A few nurses went on to up-grade their qualification to become Registered General Nurses, providing themselves with opportunities for promotion into the higher ranks and into the state hospital sector. *Isibani* provides numerous examples of the cultural divide the young probationer nurses had to cross. Many of them were recruited from other parts of South Africa, so had to learn the Zulu language and become proficient in English as well as coping with the ordeals of hospital experience, including living away from home, working in an operating theatre, nursing male patients, and encountering birth and death. Despite this, by the mid-1970s the first black (Zulu) matron, Hermina Nxumalo, was in place, making the nursing staff entirely African. She was a dynamic personality and very popular matron, maintaining both the high nursing standards of the hospital's missionary past and the religious ambience and outlook, as did her equally well-respected successor, Duduzile Biyela.

Medical students from South Africa and from Europe, army doctors, and doctors avoiding military conscription on grounds of religion, also found Hlabisa provided them with a wealth of experience in medicine and surgery—the articles in *Isibani* regularly attest to this, and to their appreciation of the relaxed "family" atmosphere generated at the mission hospital. In addition, the mission established a women's voluntary welfare group that drew from the local community, teaching women skills such as cooking, sewing, reading and basic nursing skills. With some direction from the hospital community staff they then visited the sick and elderly and new mothers helping out as needed in the homesteads.

The cultural support provided by the mission working under the restrictions of apartheid legislation, is particularly interesting. For example, basket making, weaving, clay-pot making, beadwork, shoe repairing and wood carving were all done by Hlabisa's long-stay TB patients, under the label of "occupational therapy". However, it was taught and developed to a very high standard thereby providing an important source of income to patients and their families whilst also maintaining and protecting an important part of cultural heritage. In some cases these crafts were taken back into the wider community creating viable local businesses as popularity and export demand was established. For example, in the 1970s the Vukani Association began marketing locally-made basketry and woodsculpture of exceptionally high quality both in South Africa and overseas, with many of the early pieces being made in Hlabisa's TB wards. This venture was managed by Rev. LöFroth a Swedish missionary working with Baba Elliot Dludla and others providing support and overseeing standards of quality. This is one example of a project intended initially to alleviate poverty but that became instrumental in the renaissance of basket weaving and taken up in the mid-1970s by the Inkatha National Cultural Liberation Movement. [71] A comment in the Killie Campbell Museum relating to the Rorke's Drift Mission art collection recognises the significance of the missions' and mission hospitals' contribution to the preservation of Zulu arts and crafts stating: "Persons of African descent who

[71] At that time Inkatha had a very strong leaning towards Zulu nationalism, and among its founding philosophies were the preservation of traditional culture and customs.

desired an art training in South Africa had little choice but to attend mission art schools."

Finally the lasting religious legacy of the missionaries has to be acknowledged. Thirty years after transfer to state control, mornings on the wards at Hlabisa as with many other ex-mission hospitals still start routinely with prayers, as do most hospital meetings. The chapel is in use every week for services and various gatherings, however, spreading the gospel became increasingly the province of the locally recruited "hospital evangelist" and "bible women" rather than that of the hospital's doctors and nurses. Several doctors who worked there in the 1970s and 1980s commented that, whilst they considered themselves to be Christians, they were not "missionaries" or "evangelists", and left the spiritual care of their patients to others.

Conclusion

The pattern of hospital development outlined here, suggests four quite separate phases which can be recognised in most of the other mission hospitals I have looked at, although these are not always such clearly defined watersheds. Firstly, the informal stage in which health care was provided to members of the local community on an ad hoc basis often by untrained or semi-trained missionaries or their wives. Secondly, one or more nurses joined the mission working largely as district nurses and evangelists with minimal medical support. During this time the mission might have found itself providing a small number of beds for the more seriously ill cases. Medical care during this time was generally provided by a visiting district surgeon, but on a day-to-day basis the nurse or nurses would work independently. Where a hospital emerged, this was (initially, at least) purely responsive to wants and needs as the community developed a trust in biomedicine and the individual nurses and doctors providing it. Thirdly, a more formal stage in which the missionary society committed itself to building a more substantial "hospital" with associated facilities and a support framework of service, maintenance and administrative staff. It was in this phase that the need for nursing staff demanded that the hospital must provide training facilities and accommodation for student nurses.

The final stage covers the transfer from mission control to state management although in reality there was often considerable overlap with the State being asked for increasing amounts of money to support the hospital as it developed, coming in grant form from several sources, some of which might also include local businesses and voluntary bodies—in the example of Hlabisa these included the Native Affairs Department, supplemented by the sugarcane farmers and lumber businesses and a women's charitable group in nearby Mtubatuba. This also required that the (largely African) staff were able to take over responsibilities from foreign missionaries.

During the first two phases of Hlabisa's development, the relationships discussed earlier in the chapter, between local community and the emerging medical aspect of missionary work, were at their most fragile state. Outreach in the form of clinic and district nursing provided the vital link in this stage for establishing trust and understanding, but the barriers created by language and cultural differences cannot be over-stated. Once the third stage was reached and a purpose-built hospital created, biomedicine appears to have become more easily accepted although traditional medicine remained relatively unscathed and probably still is the first option for many. Training nurses and ancillary staff was a high priority and throughout this period, practical problems such as finance, water supply, sanitation, building and servicing feature heavily in the *Isibani* newsletters. By the fourth stage, as State takeover loomed large, the focus shifted towards the fears of the unknown and transfer of managerial responsibility to African nursing and administrative hands in line with apartheid policy.

Today, Hlabisa hospital is a 450-bed district hospital additionally providing full maternity, child-health and general medical care through the seven village clinics and two mobile clinic teams. The life expectancy is sixty-three years, however the HIV epidemic in rural KwaZulu Natal has been rapidly escalating throughout the last decade, posing a major challenge, in terms of both prevention and care, for healthcare provision, with an estimated 35 per cent of the population being HIV positive. In 2001 the province of KwaZulu Natal had an estimated eighty thousand HIV/ AIDS-related deaths.[72] The combination of understaffing and 1/3 more in-patients than the official number of beds, is probably the most serious test the hospital has had to face—high levels of HIV/AIDS and of unemployment, exacerbate this, and the role of preventative medicine tends to be sacrificed to the curative one.

An important recent development has been the evolution from a small research area set within the hospital and run on a part-time basis by its medical staff, to a purpose-built research centre, "The Africa Centre for Health and Population Studies" based at nearby Somkele. This was officially opened in 2002 and is supported by the Wellcome Trust and South African Medical Research Council and a number of other charitable trusts. It continues to work closely both with the local community and its leaders and with Hlabisa hospital, with further continuity provided by its liaison officer, ex-matron, Mama Dudu Byela. Local, national and international community all benefit from the work carried out there with at times a new kind of (secular) missionary zeal echoing its earlier origins. Following a Presidential visit in 2004, Hlabisa Hospital was identified by a Presidential Task Team to serve as a pilot project or prototype for similar developments currently being planned at a national level for improving rural primary health care provision. Major re-building work has now replaced much of the original mission hospital with modern, purpose-built facilities including new male and female wards, a modern Central Sterile Supply Department, new laboratories and accommodation blocks and recreation facilities for doctors and nurses—the latter in a bid to encourage health professionals to work in a rural hospital.

[72] Report of speech by KwaZulu Natal Premier Lionel Mtshali http://www.afrol.com/News2002/sa004_mtshali_aids.htm (accessed 26 February 2002).

12

Lost in the Labyrinth: Patients in a Bangladeshi Hospital Ward

Shahaduz Zaman

Introduction

This chapter is based on a larger ethnographic research project in an orthopaedic ward of a government teaching hospital in Bangladesh. In seeking reference points to contextualise such a study, one is struck by the lack of literature on the social, cultural and historical dimensions of biomedicine and modern hospitals outside Europe and America. This is true of some classic sociological studies of hospitals such as those of Eliot Friedson and Bryan S. Turner, who ignored hospitals beyond the West.[1] The same goes for the renowned studies on biomedicine of Margaret Lock and Deborah Gordon, and Hahn and Gaines, who were quite explicit about the narrow focus of their work: "the study of biomedicine will contribute to the ethnography of U.S. and Western society", they stated.[2] The lack of such studies has been noted by, among others, Finkler, who discussed at length how the biomedical practice has not been generally the subject of anthropological inquiry outside the Western setting.[3] When biomedicine is discussed in non-Western contexts,

[1] Eliot Friedson, ed., *The Hospital in Modern Society* (London: The Free Press, 1963); Bryan S. Turner, *Medical Power and Social Knowledge* (London: Sage, 1987).

[2] Margaret Lock and Deborah R. Gordon, eds., *Biomedicine Examined* (Dordrecht: Kluwer, 1988); Robert A. Hahn and Atwood D. Gaines, eds., *Physicians of Western Medicine: Anthropological Approaches to Theory and Practice* (Dordrecht: Reidel, 1985), 9.

[3] K. Finkler, "Diffusion Reconsidered: Variation and Transformation in Biomedical Practice; A Case Study from Mexico", *Medical Anthropology* 19, no. 1, 2000, 1–39.

it is generally discussed in the light of medical pluralism and is juxtaposed with traditional systems of healing and medical choice.[4] These studies assume that biomedicine is a monolithic enterprise that follows the core universal characteristics of biomedical practice, irrespective of the cultural setting. M.J. Del Vecchio Good,[5] however, rightly argued that although biomedicine or 'cosmopolitan medicine' (the term popularised by Charles Leslie in 1976)[6] is fostered through international medical scientists and educators, it is taught, practised, organised and consumed in local contexts.

The lack of representation of the culture of biomedical settings in non-Western countries inspired me to do an ethnographic study of a Bangladeshi hospital. The goal of my ethnographic study was, first, to give a thick description of the life in a ward of one of the main Bangladeshi government hospitals. This enabled me to show how the actors involved in the setting give a local character to the hospital, which was otherwise a cosmopolitan institute. The second problem with existing hospital ethnographies is that they followed the conventions of traditional anthropological research that focused only on the micro-level phenomena of a small-scale society. For example, decades back, Baziak and Denton wrote:

[4] L. Crandon-Malmud, *From the Fat of Our Souls* (Berkeley: University of California Press, 1991); J. M. Janzen, "Therapy Management: Concept, Reality, Process", *Medical Anthropology Quarterly* 1, no. 1, 1987, 68–84; M. Last, "Professionalization of Indigenous Healers", in *Medical Anthropology: A Hand Book of Theory and Method*, ed. T. M. Johnson and C. F. Sargent (New York: Greenwood Press, 1990), 349–66; R. P. L. Lee, "Comparative Studies of Health Care Systems", *Social Science & Medicine* 16, 1981, 629–42; M. Nichter and C. Nordstrom, "A Question of Medicine Answering: Health Commodification and the Social Relations of Healing Sri Lanka", *Culture, Medicine, and Psychiatry* 13, 1989, 367–90; L. Sachs and G. Tomson, "Medicine and Culture: A Double Perspective on Drug Utilization in a Developing Country", *Social Science & Medicine* 34, 1992, 307–15; D. Weisberg, "Physician's Private Clinic in a Northern Thai Town: Patient Healer Collaboration and the Shape of Biomedical Practice", *Culture, Medicine and Psychiatry* 8, 1984, 165–86; Lock and Gordon, *Biomedicine Examined*.

[5] M. J. Del Vecchio Good, "Cultural Studies of Biomedicine: An Agenda for Research", *Social Science & Medicine* 41, 1993, 461–73.

[6] Charles Leslie, ed., *Asian Medical Systems: A Comparative Study* (Berkeley: University of California Press, 1976).

"From an anthropologist's point of view, a hospital is an isolated subculture".[7] Similarly, Coser termed the hospital as a 'tight little island'.[8] These studies ignored the link between local level events and the forces operating in society-at-large. Some relatively recent hospital ethnographies done in America and Europe have also focused mainly on the biomedical culture and medical discourse within the hospital, and do not pay attention to the link between the hospital life and the locality in which the hospital is situated.[9] My argument is that the hospital is not an isolated subculture or an 'island'; rather it is a microcosm of the larger society. A hospital ward, therefore, is a mirror that reflects and reveals the core values and norms of the broader society. Thus, the second goal of my study is to discuss how various features of the broader Bangladeshi society became expressed in hospital life.

Although, in my larger study, I explored the experiences of different actors in the Bangladeshi hospital including patients, doctors, relatives of the patients, nurses, ward boys, and cleaners, this chapter deals only with the experiences of the patients.

The Hospital

The hospital where I did my fieldwork is one of the thirteen government medical college hospitals of Bangladesh. The hospital that started as a 'Medical School' in 1927, during the British colonial period originally had a capacity of 500 beds, gradually increased to its present capacity of 1,000 beds. It is the only tertiary level hospital in the south-eastern part of the country and caters to the medical needs of over three million people living in an area of about 50,000 square kilometres. Although, officially, the hospital has a capacity of

[7] A. T. Baziak and R. K. Denton, "The Language of the Hospital and Its Effects on the Patient", *Social Interaction and Patient Care*, ed. J. K. Skipper and R. C. Leonard (Philadelphia: J. B. Lippincott, 1965), 272.

[8] Rose Laub Coser, *Life in the Ward* (East Lansing: Michigan State University Press, 1962).

[9] Paul Atkinson, *Medical Talk and Medical Work: The Liturgy of the Clinic* (London: Sage, 1995); C. P. Germain, *The Cancer Unit: An Ethnography* (Wakefield: Nursing Resource, 1979); Lorna A. Rhodes, *Emptying Beds: The Work of an Emergency Psychiatric Unit* (Berkeley: University of California Press, 1995).

1,000 beds, 400 to 500 additional patients are usually admitted and placed on the floor. The hospital has nearly all the major departments of modern medical practice. Except for a nominal admission fee, services at the hospital are virtually free; however, there are serious constraints on medical and surgical resources, equipment, instruments and manpower. There is always a shortage of medical and surgical resources, including insufficient amounts of medicine, instruments, linen, gauze, bandages, laboratory chemicals, furniture and oxygen. The administrative office stated that the hospital can supply only about 20 per cent of the medicines required every day in the hospital. There is also a shortage of manpower in the hospital. Though the hospital has been upgraded from a 500 bed to a 1,000-bed hospital, the staffing has not been increased commensurately. The chronic scarcity of resources is clearly related to the budget constraints of the hospital; each year the hospital receives only about half of the proposed budget from the government.

I did the ethnography in the orthopedic ward of the above mentioned teaching hospital. The ward has 100 beds, but additional patients can be admitted and placed on the floor. It is worth mentioning at this point that I, myself, am a medical doctor but later on took the career of a medical anthropologist. The data was collected solely by me in a period of about five months in the year 2000. The anthropologist Rob Van Ginkel once remarked that the problem faced by anthropologists doing research at home is how to get *out* of their culture, while their colleagues working in foreign cultures struggle to get *in*.[10] The intellectual and emotional challenges that I experienced whilst a 'native among the natives' are beyond the scope of this paper, however. During the study, my role in the hospital was that of a researcher and I collected data mainly through participant observation.

Patients: Broken Limbs, Broken Lives

Following are some demographics of the admitted patients, at one point of time during my fieldwork.

[10] Rob Van Ginkel, "Writing Culture from Within: Reflections on Endogenous Ethnography", *Etnofoor* 7, no. 1, 1994, 12.

About 80 per cent of the patients in the orthopaedic ward were adult males, while only 18 per cent were adult females and 2 per cent were children below twelve years. The small number of female patients in the ward is remarkable and can probably be attributed to the restricted mobility of Bangladeshi women in the outside world. Though Islamic rules of *purdah* (female seclusion) are not strictly followed in everyday life, women are generally discouraged from working outside their homes. And, as the mobility of women outside the home is limited, they are not much exposed to the dangers that typically cause orthopaedic casualties.

The majority of the patients are between fifteen and forty years of age. This can be explained by the fact that this is the most mobile and active age group, who are most exposed to road traffic accidents and work related casualties, which cause orthopaedic problems. The majority of the patients are bus, truck and taxi drivers and their helpers, day labourers, and low salaried workers. Most of the patients are illiterate or have low levels of education. It is obvious that the patients are mostly from low-income groups, which is to be expected, as government hospitals are generally the cheapest option for Bangladeshi people and this medical college hospital is the only such hospital in a vast area.

Traffic accidents are the most frequent cause of admission, followed by occupation-related accidents, criminal violence-related cases and accidents due to falls. In 2002, a Bangladeshi national daily newspaper (*Daily Janakantha*) reported that countrywide, there is an average of seventy deaths daily due to road traffic accidents.[11] However, this definitely does not tell us the full story of the casualties, for it is not known *how* the casualty actually occurred, which would give the context in which the hospital is situated. The following are a few brief accounts the patients shared about their casualties.

The Stories Behind the Casualties

Gafur is a day labourer. Every day he travels from his village to the city, to find work, by commuter train. As he is poor, he usually does

[11] *Daily Janakantha*, 8 January 2002.

not buy a ticket for the train. To avoid the ticket-checker he climbs up to the roof of the train while it is moving, where other ticketless passengers ride. He has done this for years. On the day of his accident, he tried to jump from the roof of one compartment to another while the train was moving, which he had done many times before. But on that day he fell in the gap between the two compartments and his legs were crushed.

Jasimuddin drives a lorry, although he does not have an official driving licence. He travels all over the country transporting goods. On his last trip, he was carrying a heavy machine in the truck, which he was supposed to deliver to another corner of the country. The trip had already taken three days; he was supposed to have reached his destination by the second day, but his journey was delayed due to several traffic jams. Though he had not slept during his second night on the road, he did not take a break because he was already late. He felt sleepy, but continued driving. Past midnight, on the third day of his trip, he smashed into a roadside tree. He was trapped in the truck; his hands and legs were broken. People from the nearest village came to rescue him and brought him to the hospital.

In addition to traffic accidents, the hospital contains many victims of accidents at work. For example, Riajuddin is a mason. He was working on the construction of a high-rise building but used no supports or braces while he was working on the roof, nine storeys above the ground. He fell and fractured both the legs. Another patient—Sobhan—works in the ship-demolishing industry; an industry where old, out-of-order ships are broken down into pieces and then sold as raw material. While Sobhan was cutting off a part of the ship with an electric saw, a big piece of iron fell on his leg, which was broken.

The third main category of patient injury is physical assault, as evinced by the following cases. One patient—Kabir—had a bad quarrel with his parental cousin over a piece of land. The cousin maintained that he bought the land from Kabir's father, so it belonged to him. However, Kabir knew that the cousin made some false papers regarding the ownership of the land. His cousin told him to surrender the land to him; otherwise he would not treat him properly. Kabir challenged him and told him that he will never give him the land, no matter whichever way he wants to treat him. The following night the cousin hired some professional criminals who kidnapped Kabir, took him to a nearby jungle and cut his hand off. They told him that, from now on, he should no longer claim the land that his cousin was asking for.

Another patient—Abdur Rob—is a school teacher. A young boy from a neighbouring locality wanted to marry his daughter, a college student. But Abdur Rob rejected his proposal as the boy was disreputable and not educated enough. The boy persisted with his proposal, so Adbur Rab threatened to inform the police. One day when Abdur Rab was walking on a deserted road, the boy approached and beat him with a stick. His right hand was broken.

Our last example is Rashida Khatun. Her family had been feuding with a neighbouring family over various issues. One morning, while she was feeding her cow, the neighbour came to her house. He complained that the vines of her bean tree had climbed the branches of his mango tree. He then kicked her in her hip. Rashida's hipbone was broken.

Uncertainties of the Patients

As mentioned above, most of the patients are poor, illiterate, predominantly male, young adults fifteen to forty years of age. They are mostly victims of traffic accidents, criminal violence and occupational hazards. In relation to other illnesses, these musculo-skeletal injuries have a tremendous impact on the patient, their family and society in general. Such injuries result in great physical and psychological pain, disruption in daily activities, loss of independence and reduced quality of life, as well as direct and indirect economic loss. This study thus found that the physical misery was multiplied in various ways for the orthopaedic patients of this Bangladeshi hospital.

The first uncertainty experienced by patients arises from confusion about how the ward functions. It is a great hurdle for the poor, illiterate, patients to familiarise themselves with the different departments, rules, and procedures of the hospital administration. For many patients this was their first visit to a big city and many have never before entered such a big building. It takes quite some time for the patients to understand how the ward operates and to differentiate between the roles and attitudes of the many new people, especially the staff members s/he suddenly faces. Patients struggle to learn the difference between the ward boy and the cleaner, the male nurse and between the different kinds of doctors. Patients eventually find their own system for identifying them in the course of time. One patient told me about his strategy:

> You can see who is cleaning the floor, who is carrying the trolley. Though the person cleaning the floor sometimes carries the trolley, the trolley man never cleans the floor. You know the nurses, both male and female, because they dress in white. I had some problems recognising the doctors, because they don't wear white coats. But you can say who is a doctor from their manner of behaviour. They are the bosses of the ward.

It also takes some time for patients to understand the ward routine and the behavioural expectations that are made of them during each of the shifts. For example, during the morning shift patients are more alert in their movements and activities because this is the time for the professor's round and all sorts of doctors and students are present. Patients are under the scrutiny of many eyes. In the evening they are relatively relaxed; that is when they are surrounded by many visitors. At night, they again come under the close supervision of the staff members. Patients find it difficult to shift their mood according to the change of the ward shift, which causes continuous friction between the staff members and the patients.

After the initial matters of admission are settled, patients enter into a long, monotonous process of treatment in which most of them must remain immobile and confined to bed. During this stage, patients' experience various kinds of uncertainties, anxieties and feelings of loss. Most of the patients are also unsure about their treatment plan and prognosis. The staff of the ward barely explain either of these to the patients and patients are unsure what the doctors and staff members of the ward are doing for their broken hands or legs, for nothing about their condition is clearly communicated with them. To make matters worse, during the professor's round, the patients are asked to remain passive. Medical discussion goes on over the patient's bed and s/he is not allowed to speak except to answer the questions directed at him or her. If someone dares to ask a question, he or she is immediately scolded by the doctor for hampering the round, and asked to keep his/her mouth shut. Sometimes the patients direct their questions to the nurse after the round, who usually ignores their questions or tells them to ask the doctor. Usually, one of the intern doctors or the CA later tells them about their condition, though in a vague manner. Doctors say, "You are improving", "It will take time" and so on. It is generally very difficult for patients to resolve any confusion they may have regarding their condition.

Ramjan Ali is a bus helper (an assistant to a bus driver) who hurt his legs in an accident. Since his admission he has been sceptical about the treatment procedure in the ward. He has X-rays of both of his legs, which show the fractured sites, but Ramjan thinks that one of the X-rays is not of his legs and was put into his file by mistake. He tried in vain to convey his suspicion to the staff members. First he told a ward boy who chided him for such thoughts: "Don't you dare say it to the doctor; he will just beat you up". Ramjan still tried to persuade the nurse. The nurse also became very angry and said: "Don't try to be too smart. Doctor will see whether the X-rays are correct or not. If you don't like the treatment here, just leave." One day when he was trying to see the X-ray plate against the light, a duty doctor was passing by and told him: "You! What are you doing with the X-ray? Want to be a doctor? Keep those in the file and don't mix up with other papers." Ramjan did not dare to tell him about his suspicion.

The financial consequences of hospitalisation worry patients the most, for their economic losses are manifold. First, there are the costs that come from being in the hospital. Though the government hospital is officially virtually free of charge, there are many expenses involved in the hospitalisation process. The patient must buy almost all of the medicines and other materials for daily use in the hospital as the hospital has very few supplies. For example, the relatives of Jasimuddin who was admitted after having a head injury in a road traffic accident, had to buy all the medicines, injections, saline sets, cotton, gauze, X- ray film and even the blood that was transfused to him including a piece of brick. Bricks are a curious, but essential, part of the orthopaedic ward. All around the ward, red bricks hang by plastic ropes from the arms and legs of the patients. These bricks are used to give traction to fractured lower limbs. Ideally, metallic weights with specific measurements are used for this purpose, but they are expensive and beyond the means of poor patients. However, traction is one of the most important practices in an orthopaedic ward and must be done. The use of local material as weights, namely different sizes of bricks, makes this possible. Though they are not precise, the general purpose is served. Ward boys keep a pile of building bricks in one corner of the storeroom to sell them to the patients' families.

There are other sorts of informal payments in the ward. Informal payment begins upon entry to the hospital. The liftman demands money for taking the patients to their respective wards, the ward boy demands money for bringing the patients from the outdoor patient's consultation room to the ward, the gate keeper asks for money for allowing the relatives to enter the ward a little earlier then the official visiting time or to stay past the official visiting time, the X-ray technician wants money for taking the X-ray to the patient and cleaners demand money in exchange for helping the patient to go to the toilet in the absence of his or her relatives. All these informal payments are known as *bakshees* (tips).

The second type of economic loss is the loss of personal income. The patients' profiles indicate that most of them are day labourers, employees with low salaries and small businessman. In most cases their inactivity means a complete loss of income, which is a huge economic burden for most of the patients. They try to find various ways to cope with the economic loss. In most cases the poor patients do not have any savings, so they take loans from relatives or sometimes from the people for whom once they worked. When such loans are not possible, they sell their property. It is worth mentioning that there is no health insurance system in Bangladesh. Many patients told me that they are economically ruined by their accident and subsequent hospitalisation. They have lost their jobs, businesses and property, and do not know how they will recover from the loss.

For instance, Izzat Mia, who drives a baby taxi, was admitted to hospital after breaking a leg in an accident. He said:

> My *malik* [owner of the taxi] didn't give me money. I looked for loan. But who wants to give a loan to a poor man? Then I told my wife to sell the cow that she was raising. I am managing to buy the medicines and take care of other expenditures in the hospital with that money. But now doctors are saying that I need an operation. That will require 7000 or 8000 more *Taka* [Bangladeshi currency]; I don't know how I will arrange that money. Maybe I will have to sell my piece of cultivable land in the village.

Considering the resource constraints of the hospital and the poor economic condition of the patients, doctors try to find innovative and cheaper ways to deal with orthopaedic problems, falling some way short of the biomedical ideal. One day I saw in the operation theatre a doctor using a razor blade to do skin grafting. The doctor told me:

> For small-scale skin grafting we often use this. Ideally you should use Hambi's knife for skin grafting, but where can I get that knife? Moreover it will cost about 300 taka [6 USD] while I can buy a shaving blade for 2 Taka [0.04 USD]. It works quite well. You only need to have practice.

For the immobilisation of lower limbs the doctors usually use only a half-leg plaster, even when a full-leg plaster is indicated, because of the scarcity of plaster materials. Likewise, whenever possible, the doctors use local anaesthesia for correcting orthopaedic problem, though it is advised to use general anaesthesia by the academic books. Doctors also find ways to minimise the drug and material shortage of the hospital. The CA once told me: "We use the suction method". "What is that?" I asked. He replied:

> You see, every now and then we find one or two patients in the ward who are relatively financially better off. We immediately seize the opportunity. When we write the list of the drugs and materials required for the patient and hand it over to the relative to buy those from outside, we always increase the number of the items. If the patient needs twenty antibiotic tablets, we write thirty, if he needs two gloves we write four. Sometimes we tell the patient about it, but sometimes we do not. We

'suck' some of their money to buy extra medicines and materials, which we can use later for the poorer patients who cannot afford to buy them.

Another issue creating anxiety for patients is the lack of privacy. J. D. Thomson and G. Golding have shown that the issue of privacy in hospitals has been the centre of many debates in America, and that is has influenced hospital architecture. [12] The demand for privacy in Bangladesh is definitely less than in the West and it is almost impossible for a poor Bangladeshi to afford that level of privacy in his or her personal life. However, in a hospital, amongst strangers, the lack of privacy can be felt acutely. The orthopaedic ward is an open hall with more than 100 beds placed in rows, the gaps between which are generally four or five feet at most. Sometimes a mattress is placed in this gap for extra patients when the beds are full. Everyone's privacy is therefore compromised in some way or other; particularly in their use of toilet facilities. Most of the patients in the orthopaedic ward are non-ambulatory as their traction or plasters confine them to bed. These patients have to use bedpans for their toilet needs and, despite this, no curtain is available to shield them. I observed that when patients defecate into a bedpan, with the assistance of their relatives, they usually keep their eyes closed, probably to avoid embarrassment. One patient told me: "See, what punishment Allah has given me, now I have to defecate in front of so many people."

To avoid such a state, most patients try to delay defecation as long as possible. A number of patients defecate only once in two or three days. I found that a strategy patients use to avoid needing the toilet is to avoid food completely, or just to eat very little. A school teacher whose hand was broken during an assault said: "I was afraid to eat, because then I would have to go to the toilet."

The physical examinations performed by doctors, medical students, and staff members, during the clinical and teaching rounds are also humiliating. When the professor talks about a certain case, ten to fifteen people gather around the patient's bed. They expose the injured part of the patient as the professor demonstrates medi-

[12] J. D. Thomson and G. Golding, *The Hospital: A Social and Architectural History* (New Haven: Yale University Press, 1975), 225.

cal facts, examines the damage, and talks about clinical features and treatment plans. The other doctors and students also examine the patient. They generally do not look at the patients face, but rather concentrate on the injury site. For the duration of their examination, patients remained passive and indifferent. Some just keep their eyes closed while some stare at the roof. If someone hesitates to cooperate with the doctor during the examination, s/he receives a vigorous scolding.

Tajul Isam, a 35-year-old man, was lying on his bed while eight fourth-year medical students surrounded him. The assistant professor was giving a clinical lecture and asked the students to examine Tajul Islam's fractured patella. The students felt Tajul Islam's knee, one by one. Tajul remained silent and kept a vacant look throughout the duration of the examination. None of the student talked with him as they examined him; they only discussed his X-ray.

The whole day prior to his operation, different doctors and students came to examine Tajul. He kept his leg exposed to the thigh for the most part of the day, so that he would not need to continuously uncover and then re-cover it each time a doctor visited him. He told me later:

> That's my fate. What to do? Now I am trapped and people are pulling and pushing my body from all sides. I am particularly scared about the big doctor. When he examines me, he catches the very point where I have the most pain and presses it. I feel that my heart will stop, and want to scream aloud. But I cannot because I know he will be very angry and give me *boka* (scolding) me. I keep my eyes closed and bear it.

Boka is a form of humiliation that patients receive from all the staff members, from cleaners to professors, regardless of their rank. Indeed, scolding the patients and their relatives is an integral part of the ward scene. They are scolded for a multitude of reasons, but especially when they do not act according to the expectations of the staff. The scolding starts right from their admission, when patients are reprimanded for delaying their visit to the hospital and for visiting local bonesetters instead. The nurses also scold them for not following the medication and other instructions properly or for attempting to elicit any information regarding the treatment. Patients are also scolded by ward boys for not cooperating properly with the ward boys' jobs, such as changing the patients' beds, taking the patient to the X-ray department or changing a dressing. Cleaners also continually scold the patients and their relatives for making the ward dirty. Physical humiliation is also a possibility; on a few occasions I saw doctors slap patients for non-cooperation.

Relatives: Crucial Players in Patient Care

In Bangladesh, the relatives of patients are crucial and almost inseparable actors in the whole process of hospital care. As the hospital is severely under-resourced and understaffed, it is not feasible for a Bangladeshi public hospital to provide all the necessary support to the admitted patients. As a result, the relatives of a Bangladeshi patient do not rely completely on the hospital facilities and take up various responsibilities of patient care themselves. Usually, closely related kin members of the patients like the wife, father, mother, brother, or sister stay with the patient. Less often, this role is performed by a more distant relative: an uncle, brother-in-law, sister-in-law, father-in-law or even a fellow worker also acts as an attendant.

The attendants perform a number of functions that are crucial to the care of the patients and the running of the ward. Orthopaedic patients are generally bed-ridden, so they are very much dependent on their attendants to meet their bodily needs like going to the toilet, feeding and washing themselves. Most patients are unable to move to the toilet alone or even at all. In these cases, relatives help them with the bedpan. Attendants also feed the patients. Patients with plasters on their hands cannot eat by themselves. Attendants also help the patient with washing. It is almost impossible for patients to take a complete bath due to their plasters and traction. The attendants therefore regularly wash the patient's body by sponging them off with a wet cloth as they sit or lie in bed.

As previously discussed, the government hospital has a limited and irregular supply of drugs. As a result, patients have to buy nearly all of the crucial drugs from medicine shops. The physically disabled patients depend completely upon their attending relatives to purchase medicines for them. The doctors on duty usually give the attending relative a small slip of paper on which the names of the required drugs are written. After the relative buys the drugs from a nearby shop, he or she hands them over to the doctor, nurse or ward boy. This is a crucial task; the treatment does not start until the attendant brings the medicine. Many a time, relatives also share the cost of the medicine. Likewise, it is imperative for a relative to remain present just outside the operating theatre during surgery, because they are responsible for fetching additional medicine or surgical supplies should they be necessary during operation. Relatives also help to administer medication to the patients. The nurse usually instructs the relatives about the appropriate dose and asks them to follow up the schedule of medication. Illiterate relatives remember the doses according to the colour and size of the tablets and capsules. It was also interesting to notice that the relatives sometimes dress the patient's wounds. As the limited number of staff cannot manage to give all the necessary dressings indicated for the day, nurses and intern doctors train the attending relatives on how to wash the wound with antiseptic or how to apply a new bandage.

By bribing the lower staff, it is possible to get preferential treatment in the ward and these negotiations are mostly carried out by the relatives. Through bribes and negotiations with the ward boy, relatives can insure that the patients sleeping on the floor will be shifted to a proper bed. Even if the doctor prescribes an X-ray examination, it will not be done unless the ward boy takes the patients to the X-ray department or calls the X-ray machine man to come with the portable machine. These and countless other tasks like bringing the bed pan to a patient in time or being allotted a bed near the window will be accomplished much more quickly if the patient, or the patient's caretaker, greases the palm of the ward boy or the cleaner.

Relatives are also the medium through which the patient communicates with the outside world. On behalf of the patient, the relatives settle matters with the business, work place and/or academic institution with which the patient is involved. If the patient wants to leave the hospital to receive treatment from a bonesetter or in a private clinic, the relatives must also negotiate the matter with the relevant people.

Most importantly, relatives provide emotional support to the patient. Hospital staff never speak with the patients about anything other than that which is medically relevant, and often not even about that. Instead, patients receive only harsh comments from them for any number of reasons. It is the relatives who console them in their agony. One patient said:

> It would have been hell if my brother would not be here with me. There is no one to listen to me, no one to say a few soft words. It is my brother who puts his hand on my head and says to me: "Don't worry every thing will be all right". My frustrations go away.

The Hospital: A Mirror of Society

As mentioned earlier, the hypothesis of my larger ethnographic study was that a hospital is not an isolated institution; that it mirrors various features of the life of the country of which it is a part. In the original study, I described the experiences of different actors of the government teaching hospital of Bangladesh including patients, doctors, nurses, relatives, ward boys, cleaners. Although this chapter is based on the experiences of patients only, it is still possible to identify certain features of Bangladeshi society in hospital life.

Most obviously, the hospital reflects the general impoverishment of the country. One can see, feel and smell the poverty in every aspect of hospital life. The cycle begins when the hospital receives only half of its required budget. This limited budget, in turn, generates an environment of chronic scarcity of materials. Poor patients need to buy nearly all required drugs and even some instruments for their treatment. These expenditures ruin the patients financially and impinge on their families who take over all the nursing responsibilities, as there are not enough nurses in the ward. The low-paid lower-level staff exploit their indispensable position by demanding tips from the patients. Poverty thus broadly dictates the reality of life on the ward.

Poverty is a recurrent theme in any discussion concerning Bangladesh and there are a range of explanations for it. At a general analytical level, applicable to most of the developing countries, it has been argued that poverty arose from the way these countries were incorporated into an international economic and political system dominated by the industrially-developed capitalist countries that were also colonial powers. In addition, natural disasters and lack of natural resources have contributed to poverty in Bangladesh. Thus, the current situation is the result of a mixture of external and internal factors. In spite of some progress since independence, high rates of population density, population growth, illiteracy, morbidity and mortality, as well as low industrialisation and inequitable distribution of income and social opportunities, continually challenge the alleviation of poverty in Bangladesh. [13]

Bangladeshi government hospitals suffer disproportionately from the nation's poverty, in part because the health sector receives a smaller slice of the already small national budget than other ministries. Maniruzzaman, for example, has shown that the legacy of direct and indirect army influence in Bangladesh politics has directed a large amount of the country's expenditure to the defence forces. [14] And, of the small amount allocated for health, less then one-fifth of sector expenditure is on hospital services. [15]

The hospital also reflects the social hierarchy of Bangladeshi society. A marked social hierarchy exists in Bangladesh, just as in many other South Asian countries, and a number of observers have noted the remarkable preoccupation of Bangladeshis with social status and rank:

> Every individual [in Bangladesh] knows and is quick to estimate who is above and who is below him. Indication of rank is displayed in casual conversations and official inquiries, whereby persons are specified by references to skin colour, size of salary, academic degree and birth order within the family. [16]

[13] *Bangladesh Human Development Report*, BIDS (Dhaka: Bangladesh Institute of Development Studies, 2000).

[14] T. Muniruzzaman, *Politics and Security in Bangladesh* (Dhaka: University Press, 1994).

[15] Henry B. Perry, *Health for All in Bangladesh: Lessons in Primary Health Care for the Twenty-First Century* (Dhaka: University Press, 2000), 29.

[16] Jitka Kotalova, *Belonging to Others: Cultural Construction of Womanhood in a Village in Bangladesh* (Dhaka: University Press, 1996), 148.

Life within the hospital ward that I have observed, clearly demonstrates the social importance of hierarchy. Interactions within the ward show a robust concern on the part of the staff with the definition of boundaries and the maintenance of institutionalised inequalities between the doctors and the patients and their attendants, and between the different grades of staff. The language, gestures, and overall demeanour of the staff members indicate who is 'big' and who is 'little' in the ward. The patients are incorporated into the ward at a level lower than any hospital staff. Thus the poor and physically- and mentally-crushed patients remain the most vulnerable within the hospital hierarchy.

From a Marxist perspective, hierarchical behaviour is a feature of a class-divided society. Hierarchical behaviour is more likely in countries like Bangladesh, where there is extreme inequality of power, influence and opportunity. However, various traditional values also generate hierarchical behaviour in Bangladesh. A number of authors have commented that the wider social customs of hierarchy have shaped the bureaucratic and training institutions of Bangladesh.[17] Clarence Maloney, for example, has argued that the principle of hierarchy in interpersonal relations in Bangladeshi—*samaj*—is inculcated from childhood, when people first experience themselves in subordinate-superior relationships.[18] As in the orthopaedic ward, where there is a concentration of people of different social status, it becomes a platform where the practice of social hierarchy takes on an intense form.

[17] Emajuddin Ahmed, *Bureaucratic Elites in Segmented Economic Growth: Pakistan and Bangladesh* (Dhaka: University Press, 1980); A. S. Huque, *Paradoxes in Public Administration: Dimensions of Development* (Dhaka: Dhaka University Press, 1990); I. Jamil, "Administrative Culture in Bangladesh: Tensions Between Tradition and Modernity", *International Review of Sociology* 12, no. 1, 2002, 93–125; Monique Selim, *The Experience of a Multinational Company in Bangladesh* (Dhaka: International Centre for Business Studies, 1995).

[18] Clarence Maloney, *Behaviour and Poverty in Bangladesh* (Dhaka: University Press, 1986).

The Value of Family

We have observed that family members play a crucial role in the life of the patients of the orthopaedic ward. One family member usually accompanies the patient in the ward throughout the period of hospitalisation and provides all kinds of nursing care for the patient. The lives of the patients in the ward reflect the crucial role that families play in an individual's life in Bangladeshi context. A Bangladeshi patient is never an individual actor or decision maker; the family provides all sorts of economic, social, emotional and psychological support. Medical care involves expenditure of time and energy by the patient's relatives, and money for the treatment also comes from family funds. Although family involvement in a kin member's sickness is common in almost every culture, [19] the degree and level of involvement varies greatly. For example, the role of family members in a Western hospital contrasts sharply with what has been described here. Family members have limited access to Western hospitals, and they have a limited role to play once the patient has been admitted. When writing about the Mount Hermon hospital in the USA, Coser observes: "Family and friends belong to past or future, and wear an air of unreality". [20]

In contrast, in Bangladesh, relatives are almost inseparable actors in the whole process of hospital care. The obvious presence of relatives in the ward has both structural and cultural dimensions. As the hospital is severely under-resourced and understaffed, it is not feasible for a Bangladeshi public hospital to provide all the necessary support to the admitted patients. As a result, the relatives of a Bangladeshi patient do not rely completely on the hospital facilities and take up various responsibilities of patient care themselves.

There are also deep-rooted cultural reasons behind this family involvement. Like in many other non-Western countries, social sys-

[19] P. Frank, T. I. Campbell and C. G. Sheilds, "Social Relationship and Health: The Relative Roles of Family Functioning and Social Support", *Social Science & Medicine* 34, 7, 1991, 779–88; J. T. Litman, "The Family as a Basic Unit in Health and Medical Care: A Social Behavioral Overview", *Social Science & Medicine* 8, 1973, 495–519.

[20] Coser, *Life in the Ward*, 4.

tems in Bangladesh are mostly based on primary relationships and family is a crucial unit in the society. In most cases, family influences the important decisions of an individual's life concerning issues like selecting a marriage partner, choosing a career, buying property and so on. In contrast to the individualism in the Western societies, 'familism' (the subordination of individual goals and decisions to those of the family) plays a very important role in the day-to-day decisions that people make about present and future plans.[21] As a result, whenever an individual becomes ill, the family members become involved in selecting and organising the therapy.

This appears to be true not only of Bangladesh but of many 'non-Western' societies. Janzen, for example, has shown that the management of illness and therapy by close kin is a central aspect of the medical scene in central Africa and developed the concept of 'therapy management group' to describe it; that is, the set of individuals who take charge of therapy management with or on behalf of the sufferer.[22] In some respects, therefore, hospitalisation may be seen as a culturally alien experience, as indicated in Joanna Kirpatrick's study of patients in India. She observed the unwillingness of families to permit a member to be separated from kin control, care and observation, quoting Gluckman,[23] whose comments are equally applicable to Bangladeshi society:

> People in societies organized mainly through kinship (primary relations) cannot easily segregate the activities of everyday life and the persons associated with these activities from each other to the extent possible in structurally more complex societies. A dire event befalling an individual in the traditional society has wider implications for a greater number of 'significant others' and for strain within the role system than is the case in societies like that of U.S. or those of industrialized Europe. In the

[21] M. E. Abasiekong, "Feminism and Hospital Admission in Rural Nigeria: A Case Study", *Social Science & Medicine* 15(B), 1981, 45–50.

[22] Janzen, "Therapy Management".

[23] Max Gluckman, ed., *Essays on the Ritual of Social Relations* (Manchester: Manchester University Press, 1962).

latter social roles are more segregated and the range of significant others tend to be restricted.[24]

The stories behind the criminal assault cases in the orthopaedic ward tell us about the level of violence and intolerance in the society outside of the ward: one cuts off his relative's hands to acquire a piece of land, one political group cuts the limbs off of the members of rival political group in order to take revenge, one attempts to murder his employer for dismissing him from the job, one kicks his neighbour simply because the vines of her bean tree have climbed over his mango tree. Violence, aggression, murder and blood are, indeed, persistent themes in Bangladeshi social life. A UN Report states that Bangladesh has seen a nearly 40 per cent increase in the incidents of crime in the period of 1991–1996. The crimes include assaults on individuals, destruction of property, shootings and homicides.[25]

Violence generally erupts from conflicts over the exercise of the right to control or acquire resources, especially in a hierarchical situation where such power and/or resources are unequally distributed.[26] Frequent eruption of conflict and violence is therefore a common feature in a hierarchical society like Bangladesh, where the inequality of power and resources between individuals and groups is intense. Violence is also a consequence of bad governance by the government of Bangladesh.[27] As a result Bangladesh, once a peaceful land of the Buddha, has become a violent country in recent years.

[24] Gluckman, quoted in Joanna Kirkpatrick, *The Sociology of an Indian Hospital* (Calcutta: Firma KLM Private, 1979), 4.

[25] United Nations, *The Common Country Assessment: Bangladesh* (Dhaka: University Press, 2000).

[26] Roushan Jahan, *Hidden Danger: Women and Family Violence in Bangladesh* (Dhaka: Women for Women, 1994).

[27] J. Berenstein, *Overcoming Fuzzy Governance in Bangladesh: Policy Implication in Least Developed Countries* (Dhaka: University Press, 1994); Akbar Ali Khan, *Discovery of Bangladesh: Exploration into Dynamics of a Hidden Nation* (Dhaka: University Press, 1996); Kamal Siddiqui, *Towards Good Governance in Bangladesh: Fifty Unpleasant Essays* (Dhaka: University Press, 1996).

The orthopaedic ward also reflects the stark gender divisions of Bangladeshi society. The 'maleness' of the orthopaedic ward is prominent. Most of the patients are young males, as they are the main work force in Bangladesh and have greater likelihood of becoming victims of orthopaedic injuries. The majority of the attending relatives are also male, which is in contrast to the stereotype that women are caregivers, but is indicative of the fact that women have restricted mobility in public places. The majority of the staff members are also male. There are fewer female doctors in Bangladesh than male doctors, by contrast to some Western countries.

This relative invisibility of women in the public sphere is a characteristic feature of Bangladeshi society. To a great extent this is related to the Islamic notion of purdah, the system of isolation of Muslim women from outsiders and the imposition of high standards of female modesty.[28] Although the practice of putting women in purdah is changing, it is still socially valued in Bangladesh, where it serves to sanction and legitimate the separate and unequal worlds of women and inhibits them from directly participating in activities carried out in public sphere. Katalova has observed that:

> The most striking characteristic of the agnatic emphasis in Bengali Muslim culture is that half of its population [46% of Bangladeshi population are women] those who retain an eminent role as life sustainers are defined by their absence. Unless thoroughly concealed, women are not to be seen at public events, in the street or on public transport.[29]

Although remarkable change has also taken place in the life of Bangladeshi women in recent years, the invisibility of women in the public sphere is still the characteristic feature of Bangladeshi society.

The orthopaedic ward also shows the characteristically inventive ways in which Bangladeshi people cope with the difficulties of everyday life. In response to limited resources, the patients and doctors invented cheap, locally available options to manage ortho-

[28] Najmir Nur Begum, *Pay or Purdah: Women and Income Earning in Rural Bangladesh* (Dhaka: Winrock International Institute for Agricultural Development, 1987), 11.

[29] Kotalova, *Discovery of Bangladesh*, 16.

paedic cases. Patients use bricks instead of metallic weights, doctors use shaving razors instead of surgical knife. They have also developed various alternative measures to solve administrative problems, like extracting money from rich clients and pharmaceutical companies. In the context of manpower shortages, the relatives of the patients have made themselves informal partners in the hospital organisation.

When Bangladesh achieved independence from Pakistan in 1971 and was recognised by the whole world as a sovereign state, the first question asked was: "Could it survive?" Bangladesh was referred as a 'test case of development'.[30] That basic question has now been answered: Bangladesh has survived its first three decades, thanks in part to Bangladeshis' many coping skills. Despite repeated disasters, political instability and poverty, the people of Bangladesh have found their own survival techniques and also made considerable progress in many sectors, meanwhile disproving conventional assumptions of development scholars. As James Jeremiah Novak wrote:

> They [first time visitors to Bangladesh] were expecting poverty, degradation, and hopelessness, as most television news shows and aid agency advertisements focus on the poor, who generally are portrayed as passive victims of floods or worse. But Bangladeshis are anything but passive sufferers. They are doers.[31]

Through the experiences of the patients of the orthopaedic ward in a Bangladeshi teaching hospital, I have presented the social and cultural dynamics of life within a non-Western hospital, which is generally missing in the literature on hospital ethnography. I have also argued that the hospital ward is not an isolated subculture, as assumed in number of hospital ethnographies done in Western hospitals, but rather a mirror that reflects the core values and norms of the broader Bangladeshi society. Through the orthopaedic ward, I have seen a Bangladeshi society that is poor, hierarchical, family-oriented, male-dominated, and violent, and, at the same time, which is adaptive and endlessly inventive.

[30] Just Faaland and John Richard Parkinson, *Bangladesh: The Test Case of Development* (Dhaka: University Press, 1975).

[31] J. Novak, *Bangladesh: Reflections on the Water* (Dhaka: University Press, 1994), 18.

13

Tale of Two Halves: The Contradictions of Apartheid Medicine; A Case Study of Baragwanath Hospital in the 1980s

Simonne Horwitz

Introduction

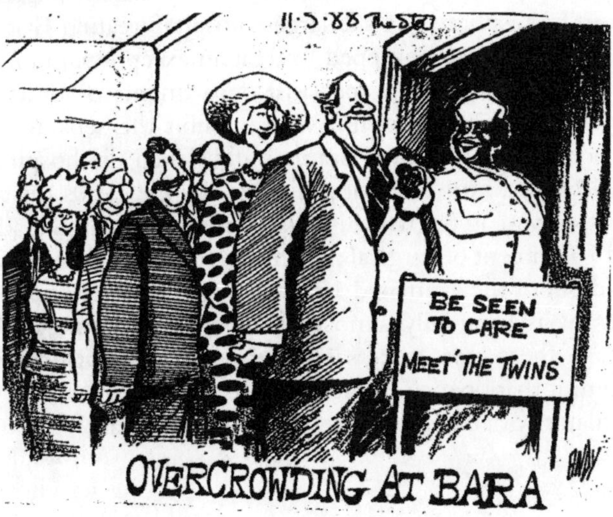

Figure 13.1 Cartoon: "Overcrowding at Bara" [1]

I wish to thank Dwight Newman, Peter Delius, Bob Stock, Helen Sweet, Anne Digby, Haroon Saloogee and especially William Beinart and Megan Vaughan for their comments on earlier drafts of this paper. Thanks also to the Rhodes Trust, Skye Foundation and Wits Foundation for the funding which made this research possible.

1 'Andy', "Overcrowding at Bara" *The Star,* 11 May 1988. My thanks to 'Andy' and Independent Newspapers for permission to publish this cartoon.

The above cartoon appeared in *The Star* newspaper on 11 May 1988, just a few days after the high-profile, successful separation of conjoined twins Mpho and Mphonyana Mathibela at Baragwanath Hospital in Soweto.[2] The separation of the twins—a medical first for South Africa—attracted the attention of the media and the medical community, both locally and internationally. The cartoon also cleverly points to another critical issue shaping the hospital. While the twins were fighting for their lives, there was another struggle being fought at Baragwanath, a struggle by doctors, nurses and patients against massive overcrowding.

The juxtaposition of reports on these two issues—the advanced medical care available at the hospital and chronic overcrowding—highlight the central contradiction of Baragwanath's services during the 1980s. By this time Baragwanath, the largest specialist hospital in the southern hemisphere and the largest hospital treating Black South African patients, was equipped to treat an exceptional range of diseases within its seventeen specialist departments or units.[3] The Department of Surgery, within whose ambit the separation of the twins occurred, had grown dramatically. When the hospital opened in 1948 it had nine operating theatres, by the 1980s thirty operating theatres were in use to deal with the massive surgical load. About 60 and 70 per cent of surgical patients were admitted because of trauma, and out of the estimated 15,000 patients admitted to the general surgery wards annually, almost 4000 were head injuries.[4] A small number of these cases were seen in the highly sophisticated neurosurgical unit that opened in the 1950s, yet a lack of resources meant that a majority of cases never received specialist care.[5]

[2] "Conjoined" is the term now preferred to "Siamese" to describe these twins.

[3] W. Sakalo, "Letter from . . . Soweto, Baragwanath Hospital", *British Medical Journal* 1, no. 6165, 17 March 1979, 740.

[4] H. H. Lawson, Preface to *Modern Surgery in Africa: The Baragwanath Experience*, ed. Desmond Pantanowitz (Johannesburg: Southern Book Publishers, 1988).

[5] B. Rabinowitz and D. Demetriades, "Resuscitation", in Pantanowitz, *Modern Surgery in Africa*, 3.

Neverthless, the existence of such specialist care and the image of the hospital as technically advanced was important for the Baragwanath staff, provincial administration—under whose immediate control the hospital fell—and for the state. For the doctors it was a justification for their association with the hospital, and the provision of high-quality care corresponded with their role as healers. In the context of apartheid South Africa, the government stressed the high-quality, highly technical care available at Baragwanath, which was considered their "showpiece", to illustrate the kind of services they were providing for the Black population. This was particularly important during the 1980s when the apartheid state was coming under increasing internal and external pressure. Economic sanctions were becoming more intense as pressure from the United States and the United Kingdom increased towards the end of the decade. Internally, the rise of the United Democratic Front and the increasing action of Trade Unions led to a period of intense boycotts, strikes and violence that rendered the townships "ungovernable".[6] As the townships burned during the mid-1980s, Prime Minister P. W. Botha imposed a state of emergency that lasted for the rest of the decade and brought with it increasingly violent state-sponsored oppression. Simultaneously, the limited reforms which were introduced during this period did see an increase in state funding of Black hospitals. However, this had almost no effect on relieving the major inequalities in South Africa's health service. In this context the image of Baragwanath as a hospital that provided high-quality care to the urban African population became increasingly important to the state.

While areas of high-quality care did exist at Baragwanath, by the 1980s it was running at a bed occupancy rate of well over 100 per cent. The structure of apartheid health services meant that for tertiary level hospital care, the large majority of Soweto's growing population of well over a million people, as well as innumerable Black patients who were referred from smaller centres, had to rely

6 William Beinart, *Twentieth Century South Africa* (Oxford: Oxford University Press, 2001), 243–53; and B. Bozzoli, "Why Were the 1980s 'Millenarian'? Style, Repertoire, Space and Authority in South Africa's Black Cities", *Journal of Historical Sociology* 12, 2000, 78–110.

on the twenty-seven hundred beds at Baragwanath Hospital.[7] A few smaller private clinics were in operation during this period but these catered to a limited number of diseases and patients. There was also limited access to doctors in private practice.[8]

The average intake per ward in Baragwanath's Department of Medicine was between 10 and 15 patients per day in the mid-1950s. These numbers increased to an average intake of approximately 100–130 patients per day during the 1980s.[9] At the same time the bed occupancy rate was between 155 per cent and 265 per cent,[10] with the estimated shortfall in beds for Black patients at hospitals in the Southern Transvaal region at almost 2000 in 1988.[11]

By comparison, during the same period, Pretoria's H. F. Verwoerd Hospital for White patients seldom saw an occupancy rate of above 60 per cent and the Johannesburg General Hospital, also serving White patients, was rarely more than 70 per cent full.[12] White patients in Johannesburg had not only a choice of state hospitals but also a far greater choice of private hospitals and clinics.[13] For the country more generally, it has been estimated that during the mid-1980s there was one state hospital bed for every 337 Black per-

[7] Cedric de Beer, *The South African Disease: Apartheid Health and Health Services* (Johannesburg: Southern African Research Service, 1984), 37.

[8] P. Morris, "Soweto: A Brief History", *The Black Sash* 24, no. 2, 1981, 13; and N. Anderson and S. Marks, "Apartheid Health in the 1980's", *Social Science & Medicine* 27, 1988, 677.

[9] Copy of Petition by seventy Baragwanath Doctors to the Registrar of the South African Medical and Dental Council, 12 June 1980, Baragwanth Hospital and Archives Department of Medicine Files (henceforth DMF), Soweto, South Africa.

[10] J. Smith, "Baragwanath: The Squalor of Segregation", *British Medical Journal* 298, March 1989, 773–74; and A. Dubb, Acting Head of Department of Medicine to G. Louw, Deputy Superintendent Baragwanath Hospital, 7 July 1987, DMF, Soweto.

[11] Cedric de Beer, "How Many Beds Does Baragwanath Hospital Need?", Occasional paper no. 10, Centre for the Study of Health Policy, Department of Community Health, Johannesburg, unpublished, 1988, 4.

[12] "Apartheid Health—A Disease", *New Nation*, 12 August 1986, 9.

[13] J. Trescott, "South Africa's American Dreams—Divided, a Continent Away", *The Washington Post*, 7 August 1977.

sons and one state hospital bed for every sixty-one White persons.[14] Funding for Black and White hospitals also remained vastly uneven during this period. In the early 1980s White hospitals received a budget from the provincial authorities that translated to between R75.76 and R107.47 per patient per day, while hospitals serving black, Indian and coloured patients received between R20.54 and R40.56 per patient per day.[15]

During the 1980s the hospital also experienced a massive, almost crippling strike. This was the manifestation of simmering labour tensions and broader political upheavals in the country.[16] Successive states of emergency in 1985 and 1986 saw far greater powers being placed in the hands of the security forces. The combination of constant overcrowding, a chronic lack of staff, serious underfunding and the pressures of the apartheid state made conditions at the hospital almost unbearable for patients and staff alike.

This chapter seeks to explore the tensions outlined above. It highlights the contradictions in the way that the hospital functioned and the image it communicated and presented to local and international audiences. More broadly the chapter argues that the dichotomy between the existence of areas of clinical excellence within a setting where basic health care was often lacking and general facilities were horribly overstretched, is essential to understanding the history of Baragwanath Hospital and indeed apartheid medicine more generally.

I begin by analysing the separation of the conjoined twins. It is argued that their separation became an icon of the sophisticated care available at Baragwanath and changed the way the hospital was viewed both locally and internationally. At the same time the simmering issue of overcrowding at the hospital was thrust into the public domain by a letter of protest, signed by 101 Baragwanath doctors, deriding the deplorable conditions at the hospital. The let-

14 Anderson and Mark, "Apartheid Health", 678.

15 Ibid.

16 B. Bonner and L. Segal, *Soweto: A History* (Cape Town: Maskew Miller Longman, 1998), 104–5; and Tom Lodge and Bill Nasson, *All Here and Now: Black Politics in South Africa in the 1980s* (London: Hurst & Co., 1992).

ter, printed in the *South African Medical Journal* (*SAMJ*) in September 1987, and the subsequent fallout will be used to highlight the other side of Baragwanath Hospital. An analysis of responses to the letter by various groups reveals a great deal about attitudes to medical care in apartheid South Africa.

The Mathibela Twins: A Tale of Two Children and a World of Attention

Conjoined twins are rare—conjoined twins born alive with a viable possibility of separation, are even more so. By 1964 it was estimated that only twenty-six surgical separations had been attempted worldwide. That number had grown to about two hundred by the mid-1990s.[17] By the early 1980s only four successful separations had been recorded in South Africa.[18]

The conjoined twins destined to become arguably South Africa's most famous twins were born on 7 December 1986. They were Mpho and Mphonyana Mathibela, a pair of craniopagus conjoined twins born at the small regional Tshepong Hospital in Klerksdorp.[19] Shortly after their birth the twins and their mother, Sophie Mathibela, were moved to Baragwanath. They soon became household names in South Africa and abroad.

The initial discussions and investigations concerning the separation were not in the public domain. The medical team determined that the babies had separate brains but shared some brain tissue and

[17] A. D. Dreger, "The Limits of Individuality: Ritual and Sacrifice in the Lives and Medical Treatment of Conjoined Twins", *Studies in the History and Philosophy of Biology and Biomedical Science* 29, 1988, 5.

[18] For a description of these operations, see S. Cywes and C. E. Bloch, "Conjoined Twins: A Review with a Report of Case", *South African Medical Journal* 38, 1964, 817; S. Cywes and J. H. Louw, "The Siyepo Conjoined (Siamese) Twins", *South African Medical Journal* 41, 1967, 1050; J. Wolfowitz et al., "Separation of Craniopagus Twins", *South African Medical Journal* 42, 1968, 412–24. The fourth operation, the first to take place at Baragwanath, took place in 1980, when Nicholette and Nicholine Nthene, joined at the upper abdomen, were separated. The weaker of the two, Nicholine, who also suffered from spina bifida, died, but Nicholette survived.

[19] Craniopagus twins are fused at the head.

importantly had a common superior sagittal sinus, one of the major veins draining blood from the brain. From the outset, some doctors were sceptical about the outcome and were concerned that the amount of money allocated for the operation and the twins' care, which cost the state approximately R1.5 million, could be better used elsewhere.[20] One paediatrician recalled:

> There were lots of other needs for children in the institution, for example spinal defects or meningoceles.[21] There were many babies who have these defects who require treatment and the earlier you do any procedure the better the outcome. . . . During the time of the Mathibela twins we kept raising the issue of babies not with brains that were joined but spines that needed fixing. There was certainly very little enthusiasm for neurosurgeons to do anything serious about the problem. . . . That is the game we play all the time at Baragwanath, it is a resource-poor setting. So therefore to me the twins' operation was a case of the bad use of resources but glamorous.[22]

By contrast, for the superintendent at the time, and a hospital Public Relation Officer, the calculation was rather different.

Chris van den Heever: If the patients are here they are here. Lipschitz got his salary whether he was operating on the twins or not. Bernice Peltz (one of the anaesthetists) got her salary whether she was doping the twins or not, it was part of the job. The only thing that we got extra were a few seals, and those were lent to us.

Hester van den Heever: We bought those clamps that they had to fly in—that was the most expensive thing that we had to get.

Chris van den Heever: But we used those clamps afterwards for other neurosurgical procedures.

20 The estimated cost is based on comparable costs in the private sector, see Legislature Documents, Replies to Written Questions, Pretoria-Witwatersrand-Vereeniging Provincial Legislature, no. 70, 1994: First Session, First Legislature, 5 December 1994, 203, section 1 (b), http://www.gautengleg.gov.za/Publish/LegislatureDocuments/House-Documents (accesed 2 December 2005).

21 Meningocele refers to a form of spina bifida where the vertebrae fail to fuse.

22 Interview with Haroon Saloojee, 31 August 2004.

Hester van den Heever: If you look at the cost on that it was minimal because as Chris explained everybody was still doing their jobs and getting their salaries. . . . They kept throwing at me questions like "how can you allow this type of surgery to take place if you have waiting lists for other types of surgery?" You know, it is not the question. As long as we can do this surgery we can extend our teaching facilities to include training more people to do that type of operation that is important at a teaching hospital. [23]

These recollections point to disagreements and tensions around resource allocation and priorities that existed at the hospital at the time. However, despite such concerns, Baragwanath's Chief Neurosurgeon Robert Lipschitz was keen to undertake the operation.

The ultimate decision about separation was, however, left to the twins' mother, who reportedly stated, "you must operate Prof. God will help you, you will see". [24]

Once the decision was made, the issue of making the story public was considered. Historically, conjoined twins have often been the centre of public attention, whether in the fairs and freak shows of the early nineteenth century, the circuses and the "scientific" exhibitions of later periods or under the media spotlight when display became unacceptable. [25] The Mathibela twins received a large amount of media coverage, some of which was specifically facilitated by the hospital.

In March 1987, while discussions around a media strategy were in progress, *Bona* reporter Ike Motsapi, who had heard about "monstrous children at Bara", approached the hospital about writing a story on the twins. The media-astute superintendent felt that Bona,

[23] Interview with Chris and Hester van den Heever, 6 October 2004.

[24] Chris van den Heever, "Ons Tweeling", unpublished paper, July 1988, van den Heever Papers (henceforth vdH Papers), Johannesburg, South Africa; and *Barameter*, July 1988, 4, Baragwanath Public Relations Department Archives (henceforth Bara PR Archives), Soweto, South Africa.

[25] Cf., K. Loughlin, "Spectacle and Secrecy: Press Coverage of Conjoined Twins in 1950s Britain", *Medical History* 49, no. 2, 2005, 197–212; and Jose Van Dijck, "Medical Documentary: Conjoined Twins as a Medical Spectacle", *Media, Culture and Society* 24, no. 4, 2002, 537–56.

a widely read Black general-interest pictorial monthly magazine, would be an appropriate vehicle for the story.[26] With the consent of Sophie Mathibela the story was printed in June 1987 with the mother and children on the front cover.[27]

The story had the effect of making the twins the centre of concern for the magazine's Black readers. Floods of letters began arriving at the hospital wishing the twins well, offering prayers and support.[28] Framed pictures of the twins appeared alongside those of the Madonna and Child and revered African leaders at market stalls around the country.[29]

Things had begun to change not only for the twins but also for the hospital. It was known that a set of similarly-joined twins, the Binder twins, had recently been separated in a fairly successful twenty-two-hour operation at Johns Hopkins Hospital in the United States.[30] Sceptics wondered if the same could be done in South Africa and at a hospital such as Baragwanath. Lipschitz is recorded as saying:

> [m]ost likely Baragwanath Hospital is one of the only hospitals in Africa that is capable to do such an operation and can hold its own against any other in the world. It would be unnecessary to send the twins overseas while we have the skills and a very good team of doctors here at Baragwanath, who could do the operation.[31]

[26] Interview with Chris and Hester van den Heever, 6 October 2004.

[27] I. Motsapi, "These Babies Are a Gift from God, says Mother", *Bona*, June 1987, 59–61.

[28] *Barameter*, July 1988, 4, Bara PR Archives, Soweto.

[29] My thanks to Professor David Coplan for alerting me to these pictures.

[30] G. Drummond, P. Scott, D. Mackay and R. Lipschitz, "Separation of the Baragwanath Craniopagus Twins", *British Journal of Plastic Surgery* 44, no. 1, 1991, 49.

[31] Chris van den Heever, "New Hope for Siamese Twins", *Transhosp Nuus/News* 4, no. 1, 1987, 1. Lipschitz's quote appeared in an article written by the hospital's superintendent, who had a vested interest in proving that Baragwanath was unique in its ability to perform this operation. In his own writing Lipschitz's makes no mention of the relationship between the hospital and the operation.

The hospital administration and its Public Relations Department took up the challenge of proving that Baragwanath was a world-class hospital where such an operation could take place. At this point the media strategy began to focus on "introducing the media to the medical and nursing staff who were going to be the technical side".[32] Lipschitz and other members of the team addressed the media at press conferences explaining the technique they would use. The stress was on the fact that South Africa, and more specifically Baragwanath, had the expertise and the skills to carry out such an operation. Propelled by the prospect of the unusual separation the story spread far beyond the Bona readership and the twins became world news.[33]

The hospital administration felt, or at least publicly expressed, that this effort was a success. When the last pre-operation press conference was held, the superintendent pointed out that it was "now clear that the media were looking at us with new eyes, no sign of doubt or cynicism".[34] When asked about this during an interview he expanded on the point:

> I think that what was important, was the perception, true or false that this was an overcrowded hospital with insufficient everything, and what . . . the separation of the twins did was to show that there was another component to Bara. It marked a turning point. Up till then it was always a question of trying to defend the indefensible—after that it was a question of this is what we did with limited resources.[35]

Unlike the single-operation separation of the Binder twins, the Baragwanath team had developed a unique multi-step process.[36]

[32] Interview with Hester van den Heever, 6 October 2004.

[33] The twins' progress was followed closely by the Sowetan and City Press which had a predominantly Black readership and by the English newspapers *The Star* and *Citizen* as well as the Afrikaans language paper *Beeld*. Among the international newspapers that reported on the twins were *The Washington Post*, *New York Times*, *Toronto Star*, *The Times* (London) and *The Herald*.

[34] Chris van den Heever, "Ons Tweeling", vdH Papers, Johannesburg.

[35] Interview with Chris van den Heever, 6 October 2004.

[36] *The Medical Record of the Separation of the Mathibela Siamese Twins*, Wits Central Television Network, video recording, 1988, Wits Health Science Library (henceforth WHSL), Johannesburg, South Africa.

The first operation took place on Monday, 20 October 1987 and was followed by a second a week later. Six months later, having spent their first birthday at Baragwanath, the date of the twins' final separation dawned. A week before the operation a full dress rehearsal was held.[37] Wits Central Television Services were on hand to take photographs and to video the procedure.[38] The emphasis was on the fact that the operation was a medical breakthrough, and would be watched by generations of medical students to come.

On the day of the Mathibela twins' final operation, 3 May 1988, the hospital's council chamber was converted into a press office and dozens of media people waited for tidings from the theatre to feed through to the world. By mid day over 230 reporters had either visited or called the hospital.[39] In the hospital's chapel, a group of women from Soweto, nurses and patients prayed with the mother.

The intricate operation was completed in just over ten hours. The news then reached those waiting at the hospital; it was over—they were alive. The superintendent commented: "suddenly we realised, we had planned everything except for a bottle of Champagne to celebrate!"[40]

The operation was hailed as a breakthrough. Both twins survived. The stronger of the two, Mpho, whose name translates as Gift, was able to leave hospital in November 1988—although not unscathed. She suffered some brain damage and partial paralysis on one side of her body. Mphonyana, the smaller of the twins whose name means Little Gift, spent months in hospital. In July 1989, she had improved enough for doctors to agree to transfer her back to Tshepong Hospital so that she could be nearer her mother and sister. She died in 1991.

In essence, the separation of the twins focused a spotlight on Baragwanath and on the technically advanced medical expertise

[37] A detailed discussion of the plans of the operation can be found in P. Makhetha, "The Matibela Siamese Twins", *Nursing RSA* 4, no. 7, 1989, 10–13.

[38] *The Medical Record of the Separation of the Mathibela Siamese Twins*, WHSL, Johannesburg. See also, "Bara's Twins", Baragwanath Hospital Yearbook 1992/93 vol. 3, 1993, 80–83.

[39] *Media Book—April–June 1988*, Bara PR Archives.

[40] Van den Heever, "Ons Tweeling".

available at the hospital. The operation was portrayed not only as a success but one that made medical history. In an anniversary review fifty years after Baragwanath's opening, it was said that "the birth of the Mathibela Siamese twins in 1986 and their subsequent successful separation, will go down in Baragwanath's history as one of its greatest triumphs".[41] Similarly, a congratulatory message from the Link Chain of Pharmacies paid "tribute to Professor Robert Lipschitz and his medical team on their history-making achievement which has once again placed South Africa at the forefront of world medical attention".[42] For some of the staff, too, this was a historic event. One nurse pointed out, "I remember that very well, I nursed them. It was one of Baragwanath's limelights, something that put us on the map more than anything before".[43]

In the wake of the final operation a stream of high-profile people visited the hospital. Mrs Elize Botha, wife of the State President, was photographed delivering personalised Northern Sotho Bibles as gifts for the babies.[44] The Administrator of the Transvaal, Willem Cruywagen and his wife Snow Cruywagen, Vice-Chancellor of the University of the Witwatersrand (Wits), for which Baragwanath was a key teaching hospital, Robert Charlton, Member of the Executive Council (of the government) for Health Daan Kirstein, and Executive Director of Hospital Services Dr Hennie van Wyk were all reported to have visited the twins.[45] It was not only South African or high-profile visitors who were drawn to the hospital. As Hester van den Heever stated in regards to the years immediately following the separation of the twins:

[41] Van den Heever, "Ons Tweeling" 80.

[42] *Barameter*, July 1988, 3, Bara PR Archives, Soweto.

[43] Interview with Harriet Gwebu (name changed on request) 16 August 2003.

[44] Cf., "Elize Botha Visits Twins", *Sowetan*, 11 May 1988.

[45] *Barameter*, July 1988, 2, Bara PR Archives, Soweto; Foto 19862, "Mr W. A. Cruywagen, Administrator of Transvaal, and Mrs S. Cruywagen during their visit to the Siamese twins born in the Baragwanath Hospital", South African National Archives (henceforth SANA).

> all of a sudden we found that we had between 2000 and 3000 outside visitors coming here per year to know what we are doing and to see what the hospital looked like. We also found that busloads of tourists would come in here and demand to see the hospital. We found out that overseas the touring companies put advertisements into the magazines and newspapers and they advertised Baragwanath Hospital as part of the itinerary.[46]

Among the celebrities who came to the hospital were 1980s Swedish movie star Britt Ekland, and Ursula Andress, the "Bond Girl" from the 1962 James Bond movie *Dr. No*. Having heard about the Mathibela twins, the actresses raised R24,000 for the hospital and the Sithole conjoined twins who were transferred to Baragwanath a few years after the Mathibela twins.[47] This is particularly interesting given that it was a time when few people visited South Africa due to apartheid. Those who came to the hospital in highly publicised visits found themselves linked to the humanitarian and technical success of the operation.

The creation and maintenance of this image of the hospital was clearly important not only to the hospital itself but also to the state. The letter of congratulations from the National Minister of Health, Dr Willie van Niekerk, highlights this point. He wrote:

> Congratulations to the medical [and] nursing members of Baragwanath Hospital staff on their success with unique operation on Siamese Twins. You have demonstrated to the world that your hospital has the capability which compares with the best.[48]

The operation and the positive stories it created linked well to the government propaganda around their provision of medical services to Black South Africans.

The question remains: why was there such a strong outpouring of support for the twins? Initial interest might have been sparked by the macabre sight of the "monstrous children" and a voyeuristic in-

[46] Interview with Hester van den Heever, 6 October 2004.

[47] Minutes of the 251st Hospital Board Meeting, 25 January 1989, 3, Baragwanath Hospital Board Records; and "Bond Girls Raise R24 000 for Bara", *Barameter*, June 1989, 4, Bara PR Archives, Soweto.

[48] *Media Book—April–June 1988*, Bara PR Archives, Soweto.

terest in the process of their separation, yet the intensive media coverage humanised the twins, who were, after all, innocent children. This humanisation of Black patients was unusual at a time when it was more common for Black patients to be dehumanised and to be blamed for their diseases. The twins captured the hearts and minds not only of the Baragwanath staff but of South Africans across racial, gender and generational divides. South Africans felt that they knew the twins and were in some way responsible for their future. Paediatrician Lucy Wagstaff remembers, "I was at Bara and there was all this hype—about consultations with America and enormous expense and the people talking about the separation—and ordinary people from Soweto said to me 'you know those twins have been here about a year have they been immunised?' I remember calling neurosurgery and they were not!"[49] The concern for the twins can also be gauged from the number of high-profile public companies that pledged donations of clothing and groceries.

Support from the Black community was clear. For many there was a sense of pride in the technical advances that had led to the operation taking place at their hospital: "to me it was good that something good was done in this so-called Black hospital and I don't know why it should not be known the whole world over!"[50] It is also possible that there was pride in the active participation of Black health care professionals in the operation. All the nurses, including the head of the nursing team, were Black and there was at least one Black neurosurgeon in the team, Professor Sam Mokgokong.[51] These members of the medical team could have been seen as playing an important role in healing the twins in a modern urban way.

There was a strong outpouring of support for the twins from the government. As has already been mentioned, part of the reason for this was linked to the way the story chimed with government propaganda. The operation highlighted the quality of medical care avail-

[49] Interview with Lucy Wagstaff, 14 September 2004.

[50] Interview with Harriet Gwebu, 16 August 2003.

[51] Makhetha, "The Matibela Siamese Twins", 10–13. Mokgokong is currently Professor and Chief Neurosurgeon at Ga-Rankuwa Hospital and Medunsa. He headed the teams that separated the Makwaeba conjoined twins in 1994 and the Banda twins in 1997.

able to Black patients at a time when hospital services were coming under extreme pressure and scrutiny, as will be shown below. The success of the operation also seems to have created feelings of pride in South Africa across the racial spectrum, a rare uniting event.

Finally, the question must be asked: to what extent the separation of the twins can be seen as a success? This is especially relevant at a time when there was a generally accepted medical belief that separation was the desired state for conjoined twins.[52] There were some doctors who argued that the operation was not a surgical triumph at all. One surgeon commented, "I personally don't think it was a big surgery triumph to separate the twins, it was just a long tedious operation".[53] A paediatrician brings out the complexities of the argument around the operation's success within the Baragwanath context:

> Then there was the whole issue of the success of the operation. I was not at Baragwanath at the time—I was at Coronation. I think while we all prayed for the babies and were hopeful for a positive outcome, certainly in my view, in terms of a medical operation the operation was a disaster. You had one baby who died and a second baby who has ended up with cerebral palsy and the consequences of that for the rest of her life. Now there were problems at the time of the operations that were not predictable, there was blood loss, but to go on and assume that this was a great success for Baragwanath is, I think, misconstruing the facts. I understand the reputation of Bara is intimately linked, certainly in the 1980s, with the success of the twins operation, but I think at a more micro level I would argue that the whole reasoning behind the operation and its outcome were in fact far from glorious for the hospital.[54]

At the same time the operation was vital to the image of the hospital as one in which highly specialised care was available. This was important for the institution and the staff who worked there. Doctors and nurses who were often criticised for the services at Baragwanath, and who were looked down upon by their colleagues at White hospitals, found opportunities such as this reassuring. This

52 Loughlin, "Spectacle and Secrecy", 197–98.

53 Interview with Desmond Pantanowitz, 15 July 2004.

54 Interview with Haroon Saloojee, 31 August 2004.

emphasised their professionalism, technical excellence and capability to perform operations that were on a par with those around the world. Max Price noted that "very sophisticated neurosurgery was done at Bara and it helped raise the status and image of the hospital . . . the twins operation was an example of that".[55]

While there were arguments about the success of the operation, the twins were certainly celebrities in the hospital. They were cared for in a separate part of Ward 7:

> let me tell you the majority of patients did not stay like this. . . . They were also physically separated from the rest of the hospital; they had a very different level of care. We, as residents (who often ended up seeing the majority of cases in the hospital), were not allowed in the area in case we would say something or do something which might upset the public relations apple cart.[56]

The twins had two registered nursing staff on duty for each child at all times. Before the procedures, the operating theatre was cleaned and specially painted.[57] All this occurred amidst the "normal" chaos, overcrowding, underfunding and understaffing of Baragwanath Hospital in the 1980s. It is to an exploration of these conditions that I now turn.

A Tale of "Disgusting and Despicable" Conditions

The wards at Baragwanath Hospital were overcrowded almost from the time the hospital opened in 1948 with four hundred beds. By 1957 Vernon Wilson, the head of the Department of Medicine, was warning that increasing admissions in the medical wards were leading to overcrowding.[58] Although the hospital had grown to just over two thousand beds by the early 1960s, these were insufficient to serve an estimated million-plus people living in the Soweto environs. It was the medical wards, which admitted the chronically ill,

55 Interview with Max Price, 30 August 2004.

56 Interview with David Seftel, 7 July 2004.

57 Makhetha, "The Matibela Siamese Twins", 13.

58 V. H. Wilson, "Ten Years' Medical Experience at Baragwanath Non-European Hospital", *Medical Proceedings* 4, no. 10, 1958, 251.

that bore brunt of overcrowding. This overcrowding hit the newspaper headlines in the early 1960s and never really left them.[59]

During the early 1970s, Leo Schamroth, Professor of Medicine at Wits and Chief Physician at Baragwanath for fifteen years, repeatedly warned about overcrowded wards, lack of staff, and unhygienic conditions. Conditions were made worse when the upheavals in Soweto during the 1970s brought a further increase of patients to the hospital. During this same period the number of doctors began to decline as they left Soweto fearing for their safety.

During the early 1980s, the population seeking healthcare continued to expand. While the number of doctors increased slightly, the number of nurses remained static due to the policy that allocated nurses according to bed numbers and not according to patient activity.[60] The policy was changed in the mid-1980s but new posts were frozen.[61] Thus during this period the ratio of nurses to patients was 0.75 at Baragwanath, 1.66 at Pretoria's H. F. Verwoerd Hospital, and 1.75 at the Johannesburg General Hospital.[62] In 1983 it was estimated that the Department of Medicine needed forty-two junior doctors to function adequately, yet the provincial administration allocated only twenty-eight junior doctors to the department.[63]

The conditions in the wards were unacceptable. One patient wrote, in 1980, that she would "prefer to be discharged from hos-

[59] "Hospital Crowding Difficult to Avoid—Director", *Rand Daily Mail*, 28 November 1962; B. Pogrund, "Who's to Blame for Hospital Where a Person Dies Because a Doctor is too Exhausted", *Rand Daily Mail*, 15 March 1965; and "Baragwanath Battles to Keep up with the Pace: Swamped on Saturdays", *The Star*, 26 May 1969.

[60] Schamroth to van den Heever, 19 August 1985, DMF, Soweto; Medical Advisory Committee, Extra Ordinary meeting, 10 May 1985, 1–2, DMF, Soweto.

[61] "Full Report of the Du Plessis Commission", 9 August 1988, Annexure 12.1, 14–19, Adler Museum, Johannesburg.

[62] Medical Advisory Committee, Extra Ordinary meeting 10 May 1985, 1–2, DMF, Soweto.

[63] L. Schamroth to C. van den Heever, 10 January 1983, DMF, Soweto. See also L. Schamroth to H. Stein, Chairman Medical Advisory Committee, Baragwanath Hospital, 14 July 1983, DMF, Soweto; and L. Schamroth to H. Grove, 27 July 1983, DMF, Soweto.

pital due to the fact that I am obligated to sleep on the floor with no possibility of obtaining a bed. I fully realise that I am not yet well but would prefer to be discharged".[64] Another glimpse into patient conditions can be obtained from an evocative account written by Thandeka Gqubule, a journalist who found herself admitted to Baragwanath during the 1980s. While this is an individual case expressing the story of one night's stay at the hospital, it is representative of a number of statements and comments made by doctors, nurses and patients. Having arrived by ambulance, Gqubule was examined relatively quickly but thoroughly. The examination was watched by three nurses, other patients and anyone else in the wards. This led her to comment that "privacy was not a priority here".[65] She was eventually admitted and taken, "by a drunk middle aged man—who had brought me a grubby hospital gown—to another ward—he wore a brown suit and I could not work out what his job was".[66] Gqubule described the wards she was taken to as comprising three floors: a top floor that consisted of closely packed rows of beds, a ground floor with two rows of mattresses beneath the beds, and then the basement which consisted of thin rubber mats on the floor between mattresses. It was not only the sleeping arrangements that were inadequate. Gqubule noted that in her ward sixty patients had to share four toilets and because there were no baths the patients had to wash in six basins. These conditions led her to comment that "not even during my 4 month detention at Diepkloof prison had I felt so uncomfortable".[67]

Throughout this period the provincial administration publicly expressed some scepticism about Baragwanath's actual patient numbers. Where they did acknowledge overcrowding they blamed this on the medical staff's lack of work ethic. The administration repeatedly hinted that doctors were unnecessarily admitting patients

64 Alina Mtshweni to Dr Mendelson, 24 March 1980, DMF, Soweto.

65 Thandeka Gqubule, "My Night under the Bed at Bara", *Weekly Mail*, 9 December 1988.

66 T. Gqubule, "My Night under the Bed at Bara".

67 Ibid.

and keeping them in hospital longer than necessary.[68] To counter this scepticism Leo Schamroth, who was by then an internationally renowned cardiologist, wrote regular letters to the hospital and provincial authorities recording intake numbers and the "desperate situation" in the medical wards. He also showed that contrary to the belief of the administration, doctors were using increasingly strict criteria to admit patients and were often forced to discharge them early in order to make room for others.[69]

Schamroth's famous "voluminous correspondence" with the hospital authorities and provincial administration is perhaps the fullest account of conditions at the hospital during this period.[70] He was determined to demonstrate that the inaction of the administration—rather than inadequate commitment and service by the medical staff—was responsible for the hospital's problems. While many of Schamroth's letters did not result in direct action they were a thorn in the side of the provincial and hospital administration and a constant reminder of what was going on in the wards. Schamroth's letters cut at the very heart of the image that the administrators were trying to portray.

Schamroth was not the only doctor who called on the administration to address conditions at the hospital. In the early 1980s, doctors launched a number of campaigns to goad the administration into action. These included a delegation of registrars visiting the Director of Hospital Services in Pretoria to call for a solution to the suffering of patients. A delegation led by Schamroth also met the Vice-Chancellor of Wits in an attempt to gain the University's support.[71]

68 "The Problem: A Racial Imbalance in Services", *Sunday Express*, 14 August 1983.

69 Cf., L. Schamroth to C. van den Heever, 10 November 1982, DMF, Soweto; and L. Schamroth to C. van den Heever, 8 November 1983, DMF, Soweto.

70 These letters now form part of the DMF and thanks are due to Professor Ken Huddle for alerting me to and providing me with access to these files.

71 K. Huddle, D. Blumsohn and B. Traub, "A Proud Record of Protest", Draft Submission by the Department of Medicine, Baragwanath Hospital to the Truth and Reconciliation Commission, 1, DMF, Soweto .

When neither of these efforts bore fruit, the doctors changed tack and attempted to appeal to the South African Medical and Dental Council (SAMDC) which was responsible for registering medical practitioners and maintaining the standards of practice and training. Seventy doctors signed the petition in the hope that the council might react either on ethical grounds or on the basis of the substandard conditions for training.[72]

The SAMDC decided that they were satisfied with the training at Baragwanath and referred the issues of the hospital's service delivery to the Director of Hospital Services and Wits arguing that the issues were in their domain.[73] The lack of further action on the part of the SAMDC is hardly surprising: the majority of the council's members were appointed by the Minister of Health and were reluctant to speak out against the government. The Truth and Reconciliation Commission hearings pointed to a long history of inaction in the face of gross inequality and human rights abuses on the part of SAMDC.[74] Having obtained no satisfactory action by early 1983, the staff in the medical wards threatened to make information about the conditions at the hospital available to the media, medical associations around the world, and to the International Red Cross.[75]

In the mid-1980s, senior Baragwanath physicians Blumsohn, Huddle, Kurt and Marinopolus met to decide on a course of action which might at last bring some relief to the patients and staff at the hospital. It was decided that a letter of protest would be written

[72] To the Registrar, South African Medical and Dental Council, signed by Seventy Members of the Department of Medicine, Baragwanath Hospital, 12 June 1980, DMF, Soweto.

[73] N. M. Prinsloo, "Conditions at Baragwanath Hospital", *South African Medical Journal* 72, 1987, 643.

[74] Laurel Baldwin-Ragaven, Jeanelle de Gruchy and Leslie London, eds., *An Ambulance of the Wrong Colour: Health Professionals, Human Rights and Ethics in South Africa* (Rodebosch: University of Cape Town Press, 1999), 143–48; and *Truth and Reconciliation Commission of South Africa: Final Report* (Cape Town: Juta, 1998), 4: 5 and 156.

[75] L. Schamroth, records of meeting with Dr S. Cronje, TPA, 19 July 1983, DMF, Soweto.

and submitted for publication to the *SAMJ*. [76] 101 doctors, almost the entire Baragwanath Department of Medicine, signed the letter which appeared in the *SAMJ* in September 1987.[77] The letter and responses to it caused an outcry that catapulted the situation at Baragwanath into the public eye and into the courts.

In the letter the doctors repeated criticisms that had been made in the early 1980s. They deplored the "disgusting and despicable" conditions of the medical wards, and further accused the Transvaal Provisional Administration (TPA) of indifference to the problems faced by staff at Baragwanath and their callous disregard for the patients. The letter asserts that "the attitude of the responsible authorities can only be described as deplorable. The state of affairs is inhumane". [78] It goes on to criticise the authorities for their lack of action and to suggest that any promises to improve facilities at Baragwanath, or to build a new hospital in Soweto "have proved to be devoid of truth". [79] The letter outlines the hypocrisy of the provincial administration's stance that there was no money for new medical facilities at Baragwanath when an expensive administration block had been erected at the hospital beginning in 1983 and a second R300 million hospital for Whites was being planned in Pretoria. [80]

The intent of the 101 doctors who signed the letter was clearly stated in its conclusion: that it would evoke enough response from the profession to bring about some action. The letter certainly caused a furore. Letters of support, comments and reproachful letters flowed into the *SAMJ* and a number of those were published in successive editions. The media picked up the story and in the months following the letter's publication a number of reports and exposes appeared in the *Sunday Times, Sowetan, Rand Daily Mail* and *The Star.*

[76] Medical Advisory Committee, Extra Ordinary Meeting, 10 May 1985, 1–2, DMF, Soweto.

[77] "Conditions at Baragwanath Hospital", *South African Medical Journal* 72, 1987, 361.

[78] "Conditions at Baragwanath Hospital"; and J. Smith, "Baragwanath".

[79] "Conditions at Baragwanath Hospital".

[80] Ibid.; and K. Huddle and G. Marinopoulos, to *The Star*, 3 March 1987, DMF, Soweto.

In the immediate aftermath of the letter the TPA swung into action. The accusations, especially those regarding their inaction and callous attitude, were immediately denied by the administration. At the same time doctors were threatened with disciplinary action, dismissal or non-promotion if they did not sign a grovelling apology.[81] In the apology letter, drafted by the TPA and then altered by the doctors, they did not apologise for statements made about the overcrowding itself. Rather the focus was on "incorrect" and "derogatory" statements, ranging from accusations made about the state's focus on white hospital care to comments about the authorities' attitudes towards doctors and patients at Baragwanath. It was signed by forty-nine doctors and was published in the *SAMJ* in April 1988.

The apology letter did not calm the fracas; rather it stimulated a debate around the circumstances in which the doctors made the apology. A number of letters to the *SAMJ* and in the press suggested that the apology might have been extracted under duress, and that doctors were facing "active victimisation and intimidation".[82] For some, especially Black doctors, Baragwanath was one of the few places they were able to work in the public sector. It is therefore possible that they signed the apology out of a commitment to remain in the public sector and continue to serve their patients despite the conditions.

The majority of senior doctors emerged from the affair with little more than an official reprimand.[83] However, a number of junior

[81] Bara. B2, A. Byrne, "Press Statement by the Public Relations Officer of the Transvaal Provincial Administration", 7 January 1988, University of the Witwatersrand Central Registry (henceforth Wits Archives), Johannesburg, South Africa; and Provincial Secretary to Dr K. Huddle, "Publication of a Letter in the South African Medical Journal, 5 September 1987: Baragwanath Hospital", 28 January 1988, DMF, Soweto.

[82] Medical Graduates Association, University of the Witwatersrand, "Conditions at Baragwanath", *South African Medical Journal* 73, 1988, 438; N. C. Lee, "Bara: An Editorial Dilemma", *South African Medical Journal*, 73, 1988, 449; and C. le Grange, "Signatories Are Being Victimised, Say Doctors", *Business Day*, 7 January 1988.

[83] Dr M. H. A. Ismail from H. Van Wyk, "Publication of a Letter in the South African Medical Journal, 5 September 1987—Baragwanath Hospital", 23

doctors faced punitive action. Beverly Traub and Hubert Hon were both refused reappointment as Senior House Officers while Linda Jivhuho, Zolela Ngcwabe, Gideon Grame and Mark Friedman, who were all completing periods of internship, were not appointed as House Officers as per the usual practice.[84] All had signed the original letter—none had signed the apology.[85]

The six doctors then sought to have the administrator's decision reversed through the courts. When the case was first heard in December 1987, Mr Justice Richard Goldstone demanded that the six be given the opportunity for a fair hearing with regard to their applications. At the hearing the applicants were claimed to be "not suitable" for appointment. Feeling they had no other option, five doctors apologised. However, Beverly Traub did not. She had held the position of Senior House Officer for two 6-month terms and had been recommended by her seniors, yet the TPA considered her "not suitable" for re-appointment.[86] One gets the sense that "not suitable" had less to do with her medical qualifications than with the TPA's sense of what constituted loyalty and "correct" behaviour.

Traub again instituted legal action against the Administrator of Transvaal, the Director of Hospital Services, the Superintendent of Baragwanath Hospital and the Director of Personnel of the TPA.[87] In August 1989 the court decided that Traub and the other doctors had been refused appointment or reappointment due to their association with the original *SAMJ* letter and their refusal to sign

April 1988, DMF, Soweto; and "Official Wrist-slaps for Bara Doctors", *Weekly Mail*, 13 May 1988.

84 Dr K. D. Bolton, Acting Head Department of Paediatrics Baragwanath Hospital to C. van den Heever, "Re: S. H. O. Appointments for 1988", 29 October 1987, DMF, Soweto.

85 "Bara Dossier of Shame", *Sunday Times*, 2 October 1988.

86 C. Rosendoff, Faculty of Medicine, University of the Witwatersrand, "Fact Sheet Relating to the Non-Appointment of Medical Personnel at Baragwanath Hospital", 8 December 1987, DMF, Soweto; and Administrator, Transvaal, and Others vs Traub and Others 1989 (4) SA 731 (A), Founding Affidavit, B. Traub, 1–18, Johannesburg Magistrates Court.

87 Administrator, Transvaal, and Others vs Traub And Others 1989 (4) SA 731 (A) and "A Judgment Reserved in Medic's Plea on Bara Decision", *The Citizen*, 30 September 1988.

the apology. The court upheld the earlier judgment of the Witwatersrand Local Division that the doctors should be given a fair hearing and should be hired because they fulfilled all the stated criteria. Traub had not only questioned a decision taken by four top officials, including the Administrator of the Transvaal, but she had won.

During this time the public stance of the government was that improvements were being made and that more would be done as soon as the money was available. The TPA did spend more than R23 million on Baragwanath during the 1980s. Among the projects undertaken was the building of the new administration block, the construction of a new R8 million nurses' home and training centre, the building of new gateposts, the installation of new boilers and a telephone exchange. None of these projects eased the overcrowding nor addressed the central concerns of the staff and patients.

This period also saw the growth of a number of medical specialties at the hospital, some of these funded in part by the TPA. This expenditure ensured that the hospital offered the possibility of highly specialised training for the students who passed through it and that it maintained the appearance of a modern academic hospital. This type of expenditure also reflected a broader focus on advanced, technical hospital medicine rather than primary health care. At Baragwanath the lack of basic funding and infrastructure, coupled with its huge patient load, militated against provision of basic health care on a large scale.

The 101 doctors' letter also brought Wits into the debate in an active way. In direct response the university set up a commission of inquiry into conditions at the hospital under the leadership of Professor D. J. du Plessis, former Wits Vice-Chancellor and former head of the Department of Surgery at Baragwanath. The commission had a rather limited remit—it was to investigate the effect of conditions in the medical wards on teaching and research, and to propose solutions. The commission's report, issued late in 1988, confirmed many of the claims made in the original letter about inadequate facilities at the hospital. It stated that

> the degree of congestion and human activity was considerable . . . the toilets could be smelled from some distance away . . . the noise level was unacceptably high. . . . Preparations were being made to accommodate

patients for whom there were no beds by placing mattresses under the beds. [88]

The commission found that although many doctors and nurses tried to provide optimum care amidst appalling conditions, these conditions negatively affected staff morale. The report concluded that the heavy workload and congestion on the wards made teaching and research almost impossible. It also disputed the TPA's claim that patients were admitted unnecessarily. Rather, it found that most patients admitted were seriously ill and needed a high level of care and that they were kept in hospital no longer than necessary.

The report also made a number of suggestions including increasing medical staff numbers at the hospital as well as the urgent provision of more beds and facilities for patients. It suggested that this could be done through reopening closed wards, constructing temporary wards, and the use of empty beds at White hospitals in Johannesburg. The latter was a suggestion that had often been mooted by clinical staff and just as regularly refused by the TPA administrators. [89] In the longer term, the report recommended building another hospital to serve the people of Soweto.

The Wits Medical Faculty accepted most of the findings and recommendations of the commission, thereby endorsing most of the doctors' original criticisms, albeit more moderately. Wits's engagement also brought some material benefits in the wake of the unproductive response by the authorities to the commission. The university raised R3.9 million from private sources to provide an extra 325 beds at Baragwanath and to erect prefabricated structures to accommodate the overflow. [90] While the TPA had not undertaken any such initiatives themselves they seemed happy to support those

[88] Bara. B2, "Abridged Report of the Du Plessis Commission", 24 November 1988, 5, Wits Archives, Johannesburg.

[89] Bara. B2, "Full Report of the Du Plessis Commission", 9 August 1988, 14–19, Wits Archive, Johhannesburg.

[90] Bara. B2.4/7, C. Rosendorff, Dean, Wits Faculty of Medicine, "Press Statement", 18 January 1989, Wits Archives, Johannesburg. See also media reports, such as T. Younghusband, "We're Going to Help Bara, Says Wits", *The Star*, 26 January 1989; and P. Devereaux, "Shot in Arm for Crowded Bara", *Saturday Star*, 4 March 1989.

of the university and to take advantage of the opportunities this created not only to ease the overcrowding in the wards but to provide some positive publicity.[91]

Conclusion

In the byline that accompanied the cartoon with which this chapter began, the question is posed: "Where were these powerful people when Baragwanath really needed them?" While the good intentions of the well-publicised flow of important visitors expressing their concern for the Mathibela twins were not necessarily being challenged, the question posed by the cartoon is an important one. As the case of the twins shows, the hospital was a place capable of specialised medical services. Yet it was a hospital in which the daily functioning of medical services was grossly hampered by chronic overcrowding and a serious shortage of facilities. Government officials and provincial administrators showed concern for the twins, yet they were quick to spring into action against doctors who spoke out about the conditions at the hospital.

The responses to both issues, although seemingly very different, were rooted in the image of the hospital that different interest groups were attempting to present. In both cases it was the image of a modern technologically advanced academic hospital that was the "show-piece" of the TPA that played an important role in driving the response.

The story of the twins was important for the image of the hospital. It brought fame and renown to Baragwanath, partly as a result of the superb way in which the media (including the Black press) were brought into the case and the way the image of the hospital was managed. It is very clear that the babies got the finest treatment; neither they nor their mother were placed into overcrowded wards. This had an effect on the quality of their care and the way conditions at the hospital were viewed. At the same time, the technical detail that became a focus of many of the media reports about the twins

[91] Cf., T. Younghusband, "Bara's Patients get Beds", *The Star*, 29 September 1989, which contains a photograph of Transvaal MEC for Hospital Services, Mr Daan Kirstein, standing smiling next to a patient in a new ward.

served to reinforce the technical capabilities of the hospital staff. It is thus clear that the hospital was managing its image, presenting itself as a hospital where good quality, highly technical medical care was provided to the African population. At the same time there seems to have been a very real feeling of fondness that developed between the hospital staff and the twins who were affectionately called "Ons Tweeling" (our twins).

The case of the Mathibela twins was also used by the state and provincial administration to tell a story about medical progress, technical excellence and South African ability. At the same time, the provincial authorities were asked to demonstrate concern and interest, albeit in a very paternalistic way, for Black health and medical care. The interest in the case shown by government officials and the coverage of it in government publications also suggests that the case was being used to highlight the kinds of high-quality medical services provided for Black patients. Baragwanath as a state-run hospital was a key institution in the apartheid machinery and events like this could be used to highlight the "separate but equal" strategy of the government. This was particularly important at a time when issues around the overcrowding had reached their zenith.

It was, to some extent, what officialdom saw as an attack on their image and the image of the hospital that precipitated their response to the letter 101 doctors signed. The attempt to protect their image through threats and punitive action backfired. Once this became public it fuelled criticism of the authorities. The letter was significant in that it brought to light not only the horrific conditions that the ordinary patients in the wards at Baragwanath faced, but also the power structures and attitudes that were preventing improvements.

In discussions around the 101 doctors' letter, the hospital administration seemed rather quiet—sandwiched between their bosses and their staff, who were at loggerheads. This was a time when the hospital management was moving far beyond the provincial authorities' understanding in response to the rapidly changing political tides in the country. Unlike the provincial administration, the hospital administration was in the hands of people who, although of varying political persuasions, were in Soweto on a daily basis and had far greater contact with the community they served.

These two cases also highlight the irony of care at the embattled institution. The case of the twins is but one example of the provision of sophisticated technological care in some areas when basic care was very often lacking in others. David Seftel angrily elaborated on this contradiction:

> I found it morally and ethically objectionable that you could have an environment where the majority of patients were denied basic medical care and then you had these kinds of pillars of excellence which were developed exclusively to facilitate personal professional research orientations on behalf of the individual surgeon or medical doctor who was building a reputation on the backs of unsuspecting patients. [92]

This contradiction, one of the central themes in the history of Baragwanath and at the heart of apartheid medicine more generally, is made vivid by comparing the case of the twins and the 101 doctors' letter. The two cases are two sides of the same coin—the very real material benefits of Western biomedicine and the difficulties that a majority of the population had in accessing these benefits. Put another way, "[d]octors say that the technology and life saving functions at Baragwanath are superb, but overcrowding severely compromises follow-up care".

[92] Interview with David Seftel, 7 July 2004.

14

Franco-African Familiarities: A History of the Pasteur Institute of Cameroon, 1945–2000

Guillaume Lachenal

The overseas Pasteur Institutes have been central elements of the French colonial medical system, especially in French Africa. [1] These laboratories, formally linked to the Pasteur Institute in Paris and paired with the main hospital of colonial capitals, served both as technological "tools of Empire", providing vaccines and microbiological expertise, and as sites of scientific "raw material" extraction. Moreover, they were the privileged centres of elaboration of a colonial hygienism, ambitiously covering urban planning, mass medical campaigns, and the regulation of individual conduct. As central institutions of the colonial bio-government of populations, they stood at the symbolic and material heart of the colonial state.

Pasteur Institutes, however, outlived the fall of colonial rule and even in independence found a unique moment to strengthen their presence in Africa. Remarkably, the era of African decolonisation saw Pasteur Institutes maintained in Dakar, Brazzaville, and Tananarivo and actually *created* in Yaoundé, Bangui and later in Abid-

[1] The tie between Pasteurians, Pasteur Institutes and French colonial expansion in Africa has been discussed in Jean-Pierre Dozon, "Pasteurisme, médecine militaire et colonisation," in *L'Institut Pasteur: Contributions à son histoire*, ed. Michel Morange (Paris: La Découverte, 1991), 269–78. The role of the Pasteur Institute of Dakar in designing and applying colonial health policies in Senegal has been analysed by Myron J. Echenberg, *Black Death, White Medicine: Bubonic Plague and the Politics of Public Health in Colonial Senegal, 1914–1945* (Oxford: James Currey, 2002), especially 193–97.

jan and Kinshasa.[2] Such post-colonial vitality is an intriguing but largely unexplored phenomenon, of which this article presents a case study.

"Pasteurians", who defined themselves as the heirs of the French bacteriologist Louis Pasteur, have been partly responsible for that dynamism, through the cohesion and opportunism of their professional body. Almost exclusively issued from the French colonial army, "overseas Pasteurians"[3] were indeed an elite corps of doctors and pharmacists, galvanised by a common training in tropical medicine, which usually culminated in study at the Pasteur Institute in Paris. Once appearing as a "battalion of microbiologists", Pasteurians also formed a "family" or more precisely a "scientific brotherhood". Embodying Republican mythologies, Pasteurians were the first to describe themselves as "disciples", and frequently celebrated their "founding fathers".[4] As such, they have displayed ambivalent ties with colonial administration, oscillating between sincere commitment to its civilizing mission, impatient demand for consequent funding and sometimes, distance. Questioning this ambivalence and the concomitant success of Pasteurians in non-colonial settings,

[2] A factual overview is available in J. P. Dedet, *Les Instituts Pasteur d'Outre-Mer: Centvingt ans de microbiologie francaise dans le monde* (Paris: L'Harmattan, 2000). Note that the Institute created in Kinshasa by French Pasteurians in 1986 never took the appellation of "Pasteur Institute". The Pasteur Institutes of Northern Africa (Morocco, Algeria, Tunisia) would deserve an analysis of their own post-colonial history, for an insight see Anne Marie Moulin, "Les Instituts Pasteur de la méditerranée arabe: une religion scientifique en pays d'Islam", in *Santé, médecine et société dans le monde arabe*, ed. Elisabeth Longuenesse (Paris: L'Harmattan, 1995), 129–64.

[3] As we will see, the term "Pasteurian" has been the subject of never-ending debates over its exact definition. In the more restrictive sense, a Pasteurian designates someone who has succeeded in the *Cours Pasteur*, a practical and theoretical course at the Institut Pasteur in Paris. In an extended meaning, Pasteurians are the employees of Pasteur Institutes throughout the world. "Overseas Pasteurians" more particularly refers to the structured body of colonial doctors working in Pasteur Institutes of (former) French colonies.

[4] The analyses of Kim Pelis on the articulation of Catholic, Republican and Pasteurian ideologies are particularly relevant here. Kim Pelis, "Prophet for Profit in French North Africa: Charles Nicolle and the Pasteur Institute of Tunis, 1903–1936," *Bulletin of the History of Medicine* 71, 1997, 583–622.

Anne Marie Moulin[5] has emphasised the flexibility, through time and space, of the Pasteurian identity. Combining French chauvinism and an internationalist credo, the Pasteurian enterprise was essentially "transformist", skilfully reformulating its history, its missions as well as its distinctive scientific ethos according to political circumstances and local cultures. This beguiling ability for redefinition and the solidity of kinship may thus explain how "this scientific imperialism survived without the Empire".[6]

In addition to that, the surprising expansion of Pasteur Institutes in former African colonies by 1960 can be read as a reflection of the spectacular tightening of Franco-African links following the independences. The system of "La Coopération" was inaugurated at that time, and incarnated by unprecedented numbers of French expatriates working as technical experts in African countries. Their massive presence was not the post-colonial vestige of a vanished French Empire: it rather re-asserted the strategic and economic importance of French deployment in Africa.[7] A geographic and symbolic extension of France's domestic space, known as the African "*pré carré*" was consolidated after 1960. Vigorously secured by mighty and secretive figures,[8] it constituted the very condition of French *grandeur* on the international scene. It is thus widely acknowledged that independence revealed and ratified the existence of a stable—and singular—historical formation: the "Franco-African realm". Close and deeply

[5] Anne Marie Moulin, "The Pasteur Institutes Between the Two World Wars: The Transformation of International Sanitary Order," in *International Health Organisations and Movements, 1918–1939*, ed. Paul Weindling (Cambridge: Cambridge University Press, 1995); Anne Marie Moulin, "Patriarchal Science: The Network of the Overseas Pasteur Institutes," in *Science and Empires*, ed. Patrick Petitjean et al. (Dordrecht, Boston: Kluwer Academic Publishers, 1992), 307–22.

[6] Moulin, "The Pasteur Institutes", 318.

[7] Jean-Pierre Dozon, *Frères et sujets: La France et l'Afrique en perspective* (Paris: Flammarion, 2003); Jean-Pierre Dozon, "L'Etat franco-africain," *Les Temps Modernes*, nos. 620–21, 2002, 261–88.

[8] I refer here notably to Jacques Foccart, President De Gaulle's advisor for Africa. He is commonly described as the secret organiser of French-African independences, and held responsible for the planning of several "Coup d'Etats" in post-colonial Africa.

ambivalent relations—of "brotherhood and subjection"[9]—shaped it over two centuries, and informed its post-colonial aspects. A vast set of political, institutional and social nexuses, partly constructed during the late-colonial experience, was thus redefined and reinforced at the time of independence: techno-scientific cooperation lay at "the core of this interweavement".[10] Instead of merely "surviving *without* the Empire", the Pasteur Institutes would have drawn on the reshaping of imperial relations, after and despite the end of colonial government.

While recent works have described the policies and politics that frame these reconfigurations,[11] the micro-mechanics of their negotiation at the level of collaborative institutions remains largely untouched.[12] To address this issue, this study is conceived as a micro-history[13] of the *Institut Pasteur du Cameroun* (IPC), a Cameroonian branch of the Pasteur Institute, which involved French expatriates up to the present. It attempts to delineate the story of this medical laboratory and research centre, from its emergence after World War II as a colonial project, to its confrontation, as a public Cameroonian institution, with the drastic economic and social crisis of the late 1980s and 1990s. For much of its history, the IPC was closely integrated within a hospital/ health complex, for which it provided

[9] Dozon's inspiring title, "Brothers and Subjects", is borrowed from Hannah Arendt, *L'Impérialisme, Les Origines du totalitarisme* (Paris: Fayard, 1982).

[10] "La science . . . au coeur de l'entremêlement", Dozon, *Frères et sujets*, 215, translation is mine. Several non-academic (and often hagiographic) accounts of Franco-African history are celebrating the role of military doctors and particularly of Pasteurians, e.g., Jean De La Guérivière, *Les fous d'Afrique: Histoire d'une passion française* (Paris: Le Seuil, 2001), 297–310.

[11] Tony Chafer, *The End of Empire in French West Africa: France's Successful Decolonization?* (Oxford: Berg, 2002); Frederick Cooper, *Decolonization and African Society: The Labour Question in French and British Africa* (Cambridge: Cambridge University Press, 1996).

[12] The recent work of Gabrielle Hecht is one of the first attempts. Gabrielle Hecht, "Rupture-Talk in the Nuclear Age: Conjugating Colonial Power in Africa," *Social Studies of Science* 32, nos. 5–6, 2002, 691–727.

[13] For a discussion on the relevance of micro-historical methods for the contemporary history of Africa, see Stephen Ellis, "Writing Histories of Contemporary Africa," *Journal of African History* 43, no. 1, 2002, 1–26.

laboratory services, although latterly it attained greater independence as a research centre in its own right.

The following account makes use of the polysemic notion of "familiarity"—as a tie and a style, referring to acquaintance as well as license—for it has been a systematic depiction of Franco-African relations. [14] Familiarity, as we will see, characterises not only the nature of personal and political relations structuring the universe of Pasteurian cooperation, but also the ambiguous expression of its management rules and its deconstruction.

This article first considers the apparent paradox of the Institute's foundation by French colonial doctors as late as 1959, in the eve of Cameroon's independence (1960). While the creation of the medical laboratory materialised a long-standing presence of Pasteurians in the French colony, the "pasteurisation" of the Cameroonian health system eventually coincided with its formal decolonisation. Pasteurians, once sincere French patriots, had to re-invent themselves, in times of political uncertainty, as mediators of Cameroonian national modernity. Analysing this moment sheds light on the continuity of post-war modernisation policies, beyond rigid "pre-/post- independence" framings. [15] It evidences that the negotiations over the creation of the IPC were embedded in a system of *intimate* relations between Pasteurians figures and emerging local elites. A Pasteurian connection between the French state and the Cameroonian elite neatly appeared, at the turn of independence, as a set of *familiar* relations [16]. Crystallised then, the Pasteurian contribution to

[14] "Familiarity" and "intimacy" are systematically used to qualify Franco-Africain relations, for the denunciation of their "pathological" aspects or for their celebration. Jean-François Bayart, *L'état en Afrique: la politique du ventre* (Paris: Fayard, 1989), 246–47.

[15] For discussions on the question of pre- and post-independence framings, see the introduction by Frederick Cooper, *Africa since 1940: The Past of the Present* (Cambridge: Cambridge University Press, 2003); and Ellis, "Writing Histories".

[16] The focus on the proximity of the personages is not an artefact of our micro-historical lens; on the contrary it is the very modality of insertion of our case-study in the "Great History" of decolonisation. In addition, envisaging the originality of the Franco-African microcosm may help us to avoid, in the case of the IPC creation, simplistic oppositions between resistance

Franco-African familiarity was reproduced and flaunted throughout the decades of "La Coopération".

The second part of the paper embraces the post-colonial history of the Pasteurian institution (which has taken several successive names), by focusing on the harsh negotiations concerning the political status of the institution and its inner workings. Oscillating for forty years between French and Cameroonian control, the institution eventually concretised an original form of post-colonial compromise, after a time of severe friction. Inside the institution, while the staff was commonly described as an appeased Franco-Cameroonian "family", the socio-technical hierarchies [17] ruling the laboratories were contested permanently. Far from being fixed or unequivocally defined, pedigrees such as "Pasteurians" or "laboratory technicians" were informed by racial categories, and constantly disputed too. Moments of conflicts often coincided with major institutional crises. More originally, these conflicts, for example about the integration of Cameroonians as managers, were dramatised on an *intimate* scene—that is, not only in the confined space of laboratories, but precisely on the ground of body conducts. As recent works in the historical anthropology of colonialism have shown, the delimitation and exhibition of racial categories were "matters of intimacy" [18]—just as they were matters of government. Affective, sexual, or domestic behaviours were the "social and cultural space where racial classifications were defined and defied, where relations between coloniser and colonised could powerfully confound or confirm . . . the categories of rule" [19]. We will discuss how the

---

and collaboration and great narratives of nationalism or neo-colonialism. See the introductory remarks of Achille Mbembe. Achille Mbembe, *La naissance du maquis dans le Sud Cameroun, 1920–1960* (Paris: Karthala, 1996).

17 On this notion, the work of Gabrielle Hecht on the management of uranium miners by French expatriates in Gabon and Malagasy has been particularly inspiring. Hecht, "Rupture-Talk in the Nuclear Age", 691–727.

18 Ann Laura Stoler, "Matters of Intimacy as Matters of State: A Response," *Journal of American History* 88, no. 3, 2001, 893–97.

19 Stoler, "Matters of Intimacy". This article presents an extensive discussion on the notion of the "imperial politics of intimacy" in cultural studies of colonialism.

hierarchies of the era of "La Coopération" reproduced, in a similar manner, intimate frontiers. In addition, the Cameroonian example will stress that, with corporal privacy at its core, the enunciation of rule as well as its "ludicrous deconstruction"[20] became expressions of familiarity. Pasteurian ethos and emblems went "cameroonised", and the Pasteurian house eventually embodied Franco-African familiarity, in its conflicting, convivial, and obscene dimension.

Pasteurisation and Decolonisation

The Institut Pasteur du Cameroun was inaugurated on 1 January 1959, one year exactly before Cameroon's declaration of independence. This foundation actually consisted in a "pasteurisation" (taken here in the sense of the official labelling as a "Pasteur Institute") of a laboratory constructed in 1956, which had already been renamed several times. A hundred metres long, the three-floor building represented a concrete outcome of massive public investments in health infrastructure during the post-war decade. Its latest label was clear evidence of the deep influence of Pasteurian experts on post-war politics in Cameroon: at the very moment when Cameroon was experiencing self-government, an allegiance to the French scientific empire was simultaneously surfacing. The paradox is only apparent. I want to suggest here that it reflects what constitutes the core of French decolonisation process: to reaffirm intimate ties.

In 1944, the Conference of Brazzaville defined a "new French colonialism".[21] In many ways, it also celebrated, in the heart of the Empire, the re-birth of the French State, and presumed its post-war developmentalist ambition. The grandiose "reconstruction" policy that France launched in the immediate after-war period, in its colonies as well as in the metropolis, reflected the ambition of the Brazzaville agenda. It even went beyond the past expectations of the official *mise en valeur* programme. In 1946, the FIDES (Fonds d'Investissement Economique et Social) became the funding agen-

[20] Achille Mbembe, *On the Postcolony* (Berkeley: University of California Press, 2001).

[21] See for an analysis of the ambiguities of the "reformist imperialism" of Brazzaville, see Cooper, *Decolonization and African Society*, 177–83.

cy of an unprecedented state intervention in overseas territories, while technocrats, experts and planners became its guiding lights. In that imperial experimentation, science not only took the crucial role of rationalising interventions "from above", it was also considered as a means for local modernisation.[22] Also in line with the Brazzaville recommendations, health infrastructures received particular attention throughout African colonies. Conceived as a medical research centre, the Pasteur Institute of Yaoundé was one of the by-products of this reformist and modernising zeal, like most hospitals in Cameroon. Their common architecture—imposing and modernist shapes—still testifies today to the concrete importance of the "FIDES years" in Cameroon.

With FIDES investments equalling those of the entire colonial federation of French Equatorial Africa, Cameroon was one of the most favoured French territories in terms of metropolitan backing. Cameroon was indeed a "trusteeship territory" (a "mandated territory"[23] before World War II) since the conquest of German Kamerun during the First World War, under French and British administration. The effectiveness of French sanitary action was evaluated annually by the League of Nations and, after 1945, by the United Nations. Consequently metropolitan investments for health in Cameroon, compared to the bordering territories, had been considerable since 1925,[24] and not only because of the dramatic epidemiological situation. Fuelled by intense Franco-German rivalry in the scientific field and under the pretext of the Germans' covetousness for their ex-colony, French patriotism literally obsessed medical officials in Cameroon. It had enabled them to obtain the political and financial support of the metropolitan funds and galvanise public opinions. The famous Pasteurian Albert Calmette,

[22] Christophe Bonneuil, "Development as Experiment," *Osiris* 14, 2001, 258–81.

[23] The territory was under French control for the main part of the actual Republic of Cameroon, except a western band bordering Nigeria, under British administration.

[24] Rita Headrick and Daniel Headrick, eds., *Colonialism, Health and Illness in French Equatorial Africa, 1885–1935* (Atlanta: African Studies Association Press, 1994), 404–5.

as early as 1923, had underlined the patriotic implications of public health in Cameroon:

> Cameroon, which is almost entirely French since the war, used to be an admirable ground of colonial experiments for the Germans . . . , where they exerted their undeniable talent for organization . . . and their utilitarian concern for the safeguard of native labour, by means of an effective protection of public health. . . . It would be a disaster, for our national self-esteem and for the prestige of "the great civilizing nation", if the prosperity of this rich domain does not increase in our hands. [25]

More than any other territory, Cameroon had therefore been considered as a living laboratory where the French had to prove—and could objectivise—their civilising abilities. After 1945, France was willing to demonstrate, with Cameroon and under the scrutiny of international experts, its capacity to enter the era of modernisation. In that context, the creation of a prestigious medical laboratory was a mobilising plan.

Actually, behind the determined and rational guidelines of French experts, tensions over the significance of such a costly research tool appeared in the years before the construction. While Pasteurian experts, from the *Ministère de la France d'Outre Mer* [26] or the Pasteur Institute, were advising the creation of a "modern research centre in Cameroon", [27] officials of the colonial administration in Cameroon, supposedly in charge of the future functioning expenses, were defending a less ambitious project: "a simple laboratory for visiting missions". [28] Continuous debates over the plan and the exact aims of the institution delayed the project: whereas a building designed as a "Laboratory of Hygiene and Microbiology" was attributed a credit in the first "quadriennal plan" for Cameroon (1948–1952),

25 Gustave Martin, *L'Existence au Cameroun* (Paris: Emile Larose, 1921), vii. All translations by author.

26 The new name, after the launch of the Union Française in 1946, of the *Ministère des Colonies*.

27 Health Service Documents, May 1949, 1 AC 7358, Archives Nationales du Cameroun, Yaoundé, Cameroun (henceforth ANY).

28 Letter of *Secrétaire Général* Soucadaux (*Haut Commissariat*, Yaoundé) to the director of the Health Service, 21 April 1952, 1 AC 7358, ANY.

its construction was not decided though.[29] The construction of "the new Institute" was included in the second FIDES plan and effectively began in 1953. Significantly, by 1954, the first *Zeiss* microscopes were ordered and in 1956, Jean Languillon, a Pasteurian military doctor coming from Indochina, was appointed director of the Institute. It was at the time named IRMCAM[30]. Although it had been contested, the creation of this impressive medical facility was nonetheless giving a new dimension to the privileged ties existing between Cameroon and French colonial medicine.

The site chosen for the new institute was the administrative and European district of Yaoundé, on top of the north-east side of the Messa Hill—also known as the Health Hill. Around the *Hôpital Central*—a vast concession of spaced pavilions built in the mid-twenties surrounded by modern "FIDES" blocks—the few square kilometres of the hill were occupied by the Pasteur Institute, the direction of the Colonial Health Service (which became Ministry of Health after independence), the base of the SHMP,[31] a field-oriented and mobile medical service, and their attending villas. The Health Hill was therefore organised as a functional space, which defined the future *Institut Pasteur* as the medical laboratory of the hospital (a footbridge was built to connect them efficiently) and as the vaccination centre and biomedical research laboratory of the territory.

As an operatively specialised space, and as a healthy site—elevated and windy—the hill was also exemplifying the medical rationalisation of urban planning. The latter mainly consisted in rejecting natives, in the name of hygiene, in lower and/or outlying areas—a policy still

[29] Delays seem to have been a regular feature of the first FIDES plan: a commission evaluating the realisation of the first plan regretted that "most of the major infrastructures remained projects". "La Santé Publique dans le 2eme Plan d'Equipement et de Modernisation des Territoires d'Outre Mer," *Medecine Tropicale* 14, no. 3, 1954, 204–32.

[30] Institut de Recherches Médicales du Cameroun, Jean Languillon, retired French director, Letter to the author, April 2003.

[31] Service d'Hygiène Mobile et de Prophylaxie.

remembered in Yaoundé as the *déguerpissements*.[32] Coincidentally a *symptom* of this "sanitation syndrome",[33] and its *cause* as a decision centre, the Health Hill was eventually representing the connection between medical science and colonial power in the heart of the administrative capital.

For the past thirty years, the Health Hill had been one of the organising centres[34] of a medical government of populations, which functioned under the form of centralised, collective and coercive sanitary action.[35] What the new laboratory brought on the Hill was somewhat different. In addition to the central administration of some public health services,[36] the institution offered charged medical exams, and voluntary and individual vaccinations. The new

32 *Déguerpissements* can be literally translated by the "chasing-away-s". For an overview of their history in Yaoundé, see Athanase Bopda, *Yaoundé et le défi camerounais de l'intégration*, *Espaces & Milieux* (Paris: CNRS Editions, 2003), 265–71.

33 I am using here the expression of Maynard Swanson. Maynard Swanson, "The Sanitation Syndrome: Bubonic Plague and Urban Native Policy in the Cape Colony, 1900–1919," *Journal of African History* 18, 1977, 387–410.

34 The decision centres as regard health were also located in Ayos (*region du Haut Nyong*), where a school of Health auxiliaries had been created for sleeping sickness fight, and in Douala, the economic capital.

35 For an example, from the urban, area programmes of expropriation—the *déguerpissements*—were inspired by Germans projects of racial segregation for malaria control and started in Douala, under the auspices of French Pasteurians experts, as early as 1920; they were replicated in Yaoundé since 1923 and until the late colonial and post-colonial period. The rural areas of southern Cameroon were also the theatre, from 1925 to 1960, of the most intense campaigns of compulsory vaccination and prophylaxis in the French Empire, and their Pasteurian organisers are still celebrated today, in hagiographic accounts, as the inventors of the "French methods" to fight endemic diseases. See Jean-Pierre Dozon, "Quand les pastoriens traquaient la maladie du sommeil," *Sciences sociales et santé* III, no. 3–4, 1985, 27–56; Wolfgang U. Eckart, "Malaria and Colonialism in the German Colonies New Guinea and the Cameroons: Research, Control, Thoughts of Eradication," *Parassitologia* 40, no. 1, 1998, 83–90.

36 Mainly, the pilot programme of the WHO for the eradication of malaria. See pp. 151–54 in Matthieu Fintz, "Moustiques et gouvernement du paludisme en Afrique". Thèse de doctorat en science politique (Université Robert Schuman, Strasbourg III, 2004), 504.

laboratory—and maybe the newly enlarged hospital—significantly embodied an innovative mode of government, targeting individual bodies and inviting them to *modern* care, which contrasted with the population-scaled actions of public health previously prevailing in Cameroon.

The Health Hill was not only the material centre of medical power, it was also sheltering its *incarnations*: great Pasteurian figures. By the late 1950s, the entire Hill was indeed stamped by the presence of Pasteur's disciples, which had been there for a long time. The statue of Eugéne Jamot, a doctor who was consecrated "hero" of the fight against sleeping sickness fight during the 1920s, silently kept the entrance of the Hill, in front of the Health Service building; Pasteur himself was celebrated on the first "pavillon" of the Central Hospital; Jamot, again, exposed himself on another memorial in the hospital yard. The great men were ritually celebrated, on almost every official visit since 1939. In a very Republican way,[37] they explicitly commemorated and exhibited colonial power "at its most reformist, its most interventionist, (and) its most arrogantly assertive",[38] and if possible, its most desirable manner. Given the "oppressive" presence of Pasteurians on top of the Hill, the name Institut Pasteur in place of the IRMCAM erected in 1956, fits well in a linear narrative: a body of experts was progressively affirming its hegemony, by obtaining the funding of a laboratory and by naming it after their "founding father". Nevertheless, such a narrative brushes aside not only several obvious paradoxes, but also series of negotiations between Pasteurians and the emerging Cameroonian political class.

The late fifties were indeed times of uncertainty for the French medical experts: the WHO, for example, was beginning to question the Pasteurian monopoly in the field of public health. Notably, it launched in Yaoundé its international Program for Malaria

[37] The tie between Pasteur, colonial policies and republican ideologies is spectacular in Dakar, where the Pasteur Institute reroute on its facade the "republican pray" of the Panthéon ("Aux grands hommes, la patrie reconnaissante", "A Pasteur, l'Afrique Noire reconnaissante"). On this point, see Pelis, "Prophet for Profit".

[38] Cooper, *Decolonization and African Society*, 451.

Eradication. Simultaneously, French scientists from Orstom,[39] the agency for colonial research created in 1943, were visibly competing with Pasteur on the ground of research, while the "Loi Cadre" voted in 1956 in Paris had paved the way to Cameroon's independence. In an even more distressing set of facts, French militaries were fighting the nationalist movement in southern Cameroon; the European population of Yaoundé was regularly targeted by what it called "terrorists"; scientists were carrying guns in the field; and the Health Hill even experienced, in 1955, the deadly repression of a protest in front of the Central Hospital.[40] To sum up, the emblems of the long dated Pasteurian presence were hardly hiding signs announcing changes in the Empire.

On 30 December 1958, two days before the inauguration of the Institut Pasteur, the Cameroonian State was officially declared "fully autonomous", and its independence was announced for 1 January 1960. Early in 1959, Prime Minister Ahmadou Ahidjo, and Jacques Trefouel, director of the Institut Pasteur in Paris, signed a convention defining the status of the Cameroonian institute. One of the first official acts of the "autonomous state", the name however clearly re-asserted, through the tie to the Parisian motherhouse, a form of colonial subjection. The convention[41] ambiguously created a *Cameroonian* institution, funded in part by state subventions, but also defined it as a "subsidiary of the Pasteur Institute at the scientific level". Significantly, the convention demanded that the director and the scientific staff should be "proposed" and chosen by the Pasteur Institute in Paris to "the agreement of the government of Cameroon"—*de facto* a very unequal repartition of power. The new

[39] Office de la Recherche Scientifique et Technique Outre Mer, previously Office des Recherches Scientifiques Coloniales. For a history of the creation of the Orstom and its articulation to colonial policies, see Christophe Bonneuil and Patrick Petitjean, "Les chemins de la création de l'Orstom, du Front Populaire à la Libération en passant par Vichy, 1936–1945: recherche scientifique et politique coloniale," in *Les sciences coloniales, figures et institutions*, ed. Patrick Petitjean (Paris: Orstom éditions, 1996), 113–61.

[40] Riots of 27 May 1955, see Mbembe, *La naissance*, 325.

[41] Reproduced in the first Annual Report of the Pasteur Institute of Cameroon. A. Gamet, *Rapport sur le fonctionnement technique de l'Institut Pasteur du Cameroun*, 1959.

status of the IPC thus associated an affirmation of Cameroonian sovereignty and its negation.

When compared, the official narratives of the history of Cameroonian institution underline a similar paradox. Firstly, the *national* signification of the Pasteurian label is frequently stressed, for example by the first director of the Pasteur Institute, André Gamet: "September 1957. Cameroon is on the eve of independence. It is up to the Cameroonian leaders to determine the interest of Pasteur Institute for their country". [42]

Viewed "from below" also, the pasteurisation did mean national pride—at least retrospectively—particularly when considering that the neighbouring Central African Republic and Congo [43] had their own Pasteurian branch. A laboratory technician, whose career began in 1958, remembers:

> Cm2: In 1960, Dr Gamet decided to transform the "National Laboratory of Public Health" [44] into a Pasteur Institute.
>
> GL: Why did it take the name *Pasteur ?*
>
> Cm2: In those days, there was already the Pasteur Institute of Brazzaville. And there was also the Pasteur Institute of Dakar. Not to mention the other "oldies": the Pasteur Institute of Madagascar . . . and the Chinese one . . . in Indochina. . . . *The independent Cameroon had to have its own Pasteur Institute.* Brazzaville has its Pasteur Institute. Even Bangui had its Pasteur Institute! [45]

The national affirmation was no mere rhetoric. For example, the IPC was by status an institution of the Cameroonian Ministry of Public Health, while the other African outposts of the Pasteur Institute were defined as "belonging" to the Pasteur Institute, and were therefore not national institutions. [46] Moreover, the other African

42 Gamet, *Rapport*, 1959, 1.

43 Previously Afrique Equatoriale Française, territory of Ubangui-Chari and Moyen Congo, respectively.

44 One of the many names of the institution between 1954 and 1959.

45 Interview with retired laboratory technician (Cm2), 16 September 2003 Yaoundé. Emphasis added by the author.

46 This difference had financial consequences, "national" Pasteur Institutes being financially independent from Paris.

branches of the Pasteur Institute were named after their city[47] and not after their nation, which explicitly distinguished Cameroon as owner and master of its Pasteur Institute. Yet the health institution, involving several French military doctors, pharmacists, and technicians, still resembled a sort of Trojan horse, with a philanthropic facade beyond suspicion, to reinforce French presence in Cameroon—a territory watched after by France with an extreme and coercive attention.[48]

A tempting, yet unsatisfactory, way of making sense of these two conflicting readings is to melt them into a Great Narrative: "neo-colonialism". The premises of such thinking are well known: fine-sounding words of self-government would hide agendas of colonial control and exploitation, and independence would be nothing but a 'face-lift'. On the Health Hill however, the facade did change during independence, but precisely not in the sense of hiding something: the 'face-lift' was rather celebrating French science. Although they offer a comfortable intellectual posture, the commonplaces of "neo-colonialism" miss in this case the ambiguity of the historical moment: the confrontation between French control and Cameroonian sovereignty was not a "zero-sum game". Pasteur, though a symbol of the former colonial power, also became in Cameroon a label of national modernity.

What is needed to unravel the paradox is an analytical turn towards the ties binding French doctors and Cameroonian elites. The IPC creation then appears as an expression of the "politics of intimacy" which organised the decolonisation process. Conversely, the role that Pasteurians played between 1955 and 1965 in Cameroonian politics also reveals that science lay at the core of Franco-African relations, which were redefined as ambivalent brotherhood ties.

The Pasteurians' renewed presence in Cameroon constituted a central nexus between the emerging Cameroonian elites and the French State. Three main personalities, involved by 1958 in the ne-

[47] The Institut Pasteur de l'AOF was renamed Institut Pasteur de Dakar after independence, the Institut Pasteur de l'AEF was renamed Institut Pasteur de Brazzaville, and in Central African Republic was created the Institut Pasteur de Bangui.

[48] Mbembe, *La naissance*.

gotiations about the IPC creation, are telling examples: Pasteurian Marcel Vaucel,[49] head of the Office for Overseas Pasteur Institutes in Paris, the military doctor Journiac,[50] head of the Colonial Health Service in Yaoundé, and Dr Louis Paul Aujoulat,[51] a former Deputy for Cameroon in the French parliament and a former Minister in Paris. All three shared brilliant politico-administrative careers in France, which largely benefited from their respective experiences in Cameroon—a manifestation of the continuity of colonial and metropolitan spaces. These Franco-African figures had an impressive political influence in Paris and Yaoundé, reflecting a more general medicalisation of Cameroonian politics.

[49] A military Pasteurian, Marcel Vaucel served in Equatorial Africa and was director of the Health Service of Cameroon in 1939, when he officially proposed the construction of a Pasteur Institute in Cameroon. While his project had to be adjourned, Dr Vaucel quickly rallied, with many military officials from Cameroon and French Equatorial Africa, including A. Sicé, the director of the Institut Pasteur of Brazzaville, the "Free France Epic". This rallying gave a decisive turn to his medico-political carreer: given quickly a prominent place in the Gaullist political apparatus, he was named director of the Health Service for "Free French Africa" in 1942, and put in charge of the health section in the Conference of Brazzaville in 1944. After a spell at the Ministère de la France d'Outre Mer, his career culminated in 1952 when he was appointed head of the office for the "Overseas Pasteur Institutes" at the Pasteur Institute in Paris, from where he carefully followed the creation and the functioning of the Pasteur Institute of Cameroon, until his retirement in 1972.

[50] "Journiac", as he was called by his fellow army doctors, has been the last director of the Colonial Health Service of Cameroon. He became the director of the Health division of the Ministry of Cooperation in the 1960s where he stayed until his retirement. It is worth mentioning that he was the brother of René Journiac, who, after a career as a magistrate in Cameroon, became a prominent figure of Franco-African politics and secret services, an assistant of Jacques Foccart, and the official advisor to Pdt Giscard d'Estaing for African affairs.

[51] A Catholic missionary, eulogist of Jamot and thurifer of French colonial medicine, Dr Aujoulat was continuously elected from 1946 to 1956 into the Cameroon Assembly and the French parliament. This notable of the French *colonat* in Cameroon was eventually appointed, by several government of the Fourth Republic, *Secretaire d'Etat à la France d'Outre Mer* (1949–1952) and *Ministre du Travail et de la Protection Sociale* in 1954.

The medical profession—doctors and auxiliaries—had a major influence during the experimentation of electoral politics in Cameroon, beginning in 1946 by the creation of a local assembly with European and African deputies. This influence was not only due to Dr Aujoulat, who was the "patron and promoter"[52] of numerous local politicians—of diverse regional and ideological affiliations—including Ahmadou Ahidjo (President between 1959 and 1982), André Marie Mbida (Prime Minister, 1957–58), Kamden-Ninyim (Minister of Health, 1960–61), and Dr Marcel Bebey Eyidi,[53] a major figure of the Cameroonian opposition in the 1960s. The Pasteurian body, holding on the colonial Health service, played a similar role: Dr Bebey Eyidi, who became the first biographer of Eugène Jamot in his MD thesis, was a former medical auxiliary of the great man, like Charles Assalé, the first Prime Minister of independent Cameroon (1960–65). Dr Simon Pierre Tchoungui, who became Minister of Health (1961) and Prime Minister (1965–72), was also a former auxiliary of the colonial Health Service. To cap it all, the son-in-law of Jamot (who had left in Cameroon a *metis* daughter), Dr Plantier, was himself a colonial doctor and a deputy at the local assembly. The impressive filiation reflected that indigenous elites had capitalised, materially and symbolically, on their medico-administrative positions.[54] More significantly, the affiliation set a norm for political exchanges: cordial—and willingly dramatised—personal relations. As they shared the same master, relations between Cameroonian ministers and French experts (who became "technical advisors") were literally *fraternal*. The head of the entomological service of the Institute between 1957 and 1960 recalls his relationships with the local government:

52 Jean-François Bayart, *L'Etat au Cameroun* (Paris: Presses de la Fondation nationale des sciences politiques, 1979), 38.

53 For biographical sketch of these personages, see Mark W. DeLancey and Mbella H. Mokeba, *Historical Dictonnary of the Republic of Cameroon* (Metuchen: Scarecrow Press, 1990).

54 Cooper points out that in the absence of a developed associative life, for example, as in Senegal, the logics of cultural capital (notably the positions within the colonial bureaucracy) initially structured the electoral field in Cameroon, more visibly than elsewhere. Cooper, *Africa since 1940*, 75.

> The first Minister of Health that we had . . . was Arouna [NB: Arouna Njoya]. He was a delightful man. He was quite disappointed that I did not marry his niece. Ah, he was not perturbed by the fact that I already had a wife! Then the second was Tchoungui, who then became Prime Minister. He was a doctor. I was on the best of terms with him. This is when I left, because I did not accept his offer . . . to work in Cameroon as his assistant at the Ministry of Health. [55]

Such intimacy predated the strength of the post-colonial Pasteurian presence, and blurred the usual re-partition of roles between (de-)colonisers and (de-)colonised. Familial relations were not, of course, without tension. Notably, some seeds of French colonial doctors joined the Union des Populations du Cameroun, the leftist and nationalist party, which was violently repressed by French and Cameroonian authorities. Two of them were killed. [56]

The creation of the IPC, far from being a peripheral and paradoxical *peripétie*, thus intersects with the Great Histories of Gaullist decolonisation and of Cameroonian independence. This intersection shows that metropolitan and colonial spaces criss-crossed in a confined, convivial and central arena. An expanded brotherhood was formed at the top of French, Cameroonian and Pasteurian States, by the common affiliation of French and Cameroonian to the symbols of Pasteurian science. The Franco-African familiarities

[55] Interview with former French expatriate (Coop 5), 12 April, 2004, Paris. "Même les premiers ministres de la santé que l'on a eu, Arouna, . . . c'était un homme délicieux. Il a était un peu décu que je n'épouse pas sa nièce. Ah le fait que j'ai déjà une femme ça ne le perturbait pas. Et puis ensuite le deuxième c'était Tchoungi, qui est devenu ensuite premier ministre, qui était médecin et avec qui j'étais au mieux. C'est là ou je suis un peu parti parce que j'ai pas voulu accepter l'offre de venir travailler au Cameroun comme adjoint du ministre de la santé."

[56] Dr Felix Roland Moumié, a former medical auxiliary of the colonial Health Service, became a leader of the nationalist leftist party, the UPC, which was violently fought by French army between 1955 and 1961. A French secret agent poisoned him in 1963—a well remembered episode of Franco-African manoeuvres. Pierre Kamden-Ninyim, a protégé of Aujoulat, was appointed Minister of Health in 1960–61. Linked to the UPC, and long suspected of contacts with rebellion, he was convinced guilty of a crime and eventually shot by a firing squad in 1963.

here described in their Pasteurian dimension[57] have thus something singular. When seen at the level of microscopes, French experts were, far from assuming "the more possible task of sitting in judgement",[58] standing on the front line of Cameroonian development. In telling words, Fernand Merle, a French military doctor who was on the Health Hill on 1 January 1960, reminds us the taste of the independence:

> In a good-natured atmosphere, the independence of Cameroon is being celebrated. . . . The behaviour of Cameroonians has not really changed, at least for those who are next to us. May be more sloppiness in the Health service, but no animosity toward us.
>
> The ceremony of colours is imbued with dignity. We feel a twinge of sadness when seeing our flag coming down, but the smile of Eugène Jamot, from the top of his stela, is still caring for the Health of Cameroon.
>
> A big parade takes place. The new little Cameroonian army, flanked by French officers, is brilliantly marching. . . . After a series of delegations, here comes the housewives, singing an unexpected chorus:
>
> *Indépendance*, tcha tcha tcha
>
> *Indépendance*, tcha tcha tcha.[59]

[57] Other brotherhoods have been structuring the Franco-African microcosm, as Dozon has pointed, notably the Freemasonry and the Communist Party. Dozon, *Frères et sujets*, 297–336.

[58] Cooper, *Decolonization and African Society*, 472.

[59] Fernand Merle, *Un voyage au long cours: les aventures d'un médecin outre-mer* (Paris: Albin Michel, 1984), 163–64. "Dans une ambiance bon enfant, on célèbre l'indépendance du Cameroun. . . . Le comportement des Camerounais n'a guère changé, du moins ceux que nous cotoyons tous les jours. Un peu plus de laisser-aller peut être dans le service, mais aucune animosité à notre égard.

La cérémonie des couleurs est empreinte de dignité. Avec un petit pincement au cœur, nous voyons descendre notre drapeau, mais le bon sourire d'Eugène Jamot au haut de sa stèle veille toujours sur la santé du Cameroun. Un grand défilé est organise. La petite armée camerounaise naissante . . . encadrée par des officiers français, défile superbement. . . . Après les delegations de ceci, de cela, voici les ménagères, chantant sur un rythme à la mode, un refrain imprévu: Indépendance, tcha tcha tcha, Indépendance, tcha tcha tcha".

The Intimate Rules of Pasteurian Brotherhood

Since its creation in 1959, the Pasteurian laboratory has known three main institutional configurations, identified by its different names. In 1975, the Institut Pasteur du Cameroun was renamed Centre Pasteur. In 1980, it was renamed Centre Pasteur du Cameroun, with a new status conserved up to the present.[60] My interest in this section lies in linking the turbulence of the institute's history with moments of definition and contestation of the hierarchical categories ruling its inner workings.

As it took a Franco-African dimension, the Pasteurian brotherhood has reproduced, by softening or sharpening it, the essential tension of French colonialism: the hesitation between the ideals of "assimilation"—the republican idea of creating "black Frenchmen" through civilisation and modernisation—and the pragmatics of "association"—using and consolidating local hierarchies in the name of "cultural specificities". For instance, French doctors in Cameroon have continuously claimed their will to train locals as "genuine Pasteurians" and to "Cameroonise" the management of the institute, while holding not less continuously onto the scientific and administrative direction of the Institute. Subtle labour division and distribution of responsibilities were established; their legitimation (or contestation) implied the definition (or denial) of socio-technical hierarchies.[61] "To be—or not to be—*Pasteurian*" has thus been a subject, during forty years, of desire and conflicts. Conversely, the issue of the "Cameroonisation" of the Pasteur Institute—i.e., its effective direction by Cameroonian scientists—has been a recurrent wish expressed in official guidelines for cooperation, and has inspired political struggles from 1959 to 2002.

[60] The post-colonial history of the Pasteur Institute of Cameroon has been extensively documented in my Master thesis. Guillaume Lachenal, "Le Centre Pasteur du Cameroun: trajectoire historique, stratégies et pratiques de la recherche biomédicale en coopération, 1959–2002" (Mémoire de D. E. A d'Epistémologie, Histoire des Sciences et des Techniques: Université Paris 7 Denis Diderot, 2002), 173.

[61] Gabrielle Hecht aptly discussed the notion of socio-technical hierarchies, its link to racial dichotomies, and its partial destabilisation in the post-colonial context. Hecht, "Rupture-Talk in the Nuclear Age", 691–727.

Such "socio-technical" and "national" pedigrees have not only been defined by allegedly objective qualifications like academic curricula or citizenship: they were implicitly framed in overlapping dichotomies, whether racial or "cultural", like "Europeans/Blacks" and "expatriates/Cameroonians". Ultimately, the corresponding boundaries were *intimate frontiers*: their conflicting definitions were not only dramatised on a confined scene, but, above all, literally centred on body privacy, and on sexual and affective conduct and misconduct. They were, as such, permeable.

From 1959 to 1975, four military doctors succeeded each other as IPC directors, in an apparent continuity. In the meantime, approximately five to ten French expatriates permanently headed the scientific and administrative services, while the Institute rapidly came to employ more than a hundred Cameroonians. "La Coopération"[62] was the new name of Franco-Cameroonian relations. It turned out to be a rather efficient tool of management: the activity of the Institute regularly grew, according to all indicators.[63] Medical analysis and vaccine delivery flourished, increasingly orientated to individual clients after the link with the neighbouring Hospital was progressively dropped. Massive research projects were initiated, with field activities involving numerous unskilled workers. The Cameroonian staff consisted also of many nurses and, interestingly, a couple of "laboratory technicians", who had benefited from training in the "school" established at the IPC since 1960. Training thus specifically concerned skilled but *subaltern* technicians, as had been a regular feature in Pasteur Institutes overseas, and particularly in Africa, where the late colonial policy in medical training maintained hierarchic distinctions between Africans and French people.[64]

Nevertheless, the integration of Cameroonian doctors in the staff rapidly came on the agenda. The question was not merely a reformulation of assimilation, or an anticipation of "capacity build-

[62] The Ministry of Overseas France was renamed Ministry of Cooperation in the run-up of African independences.

[63] The number of analyses was 100 per cent during the period 1960–75.

[64] The famous example being the category of "Medecins Africains", naming the Africans doctors trained as "auxilliary doctors" in the Ecole de Medecine de Dakar. Echenberg, *Black Death, White Medicine*, 258.

ing".[65] It was also driven by mere financial considerations, French expatriates being an expensive workforce.[66] In 1960, André Gamet, "the creator and organizer"[67] of the IPC, was proud to announce the future arrival of the first "Cameroonian Pasteurian":

> Day after day, the new nation is showing a growing interest in the young institute; one Cameroonian doctor, who had been trained during one year in our disciplines, has gone to the motherhouse to qualify for entrance into the great Pasteurian family. Two of his compatriots have already been enrolled for the next years to come.[68]

Prosper Etoundi Ntsama was this Cameroonian doctor. He left in October 1962 for the Pasteur Institute in Paris to follow the *Cours Pasteur.* He eventually qualified as a genuine "Pasteurian", along with a large promotion of French army doctors, academic scholars in tropical medicine, and other pupils from overseas Pasteur Institutes. When he returned in 1963 to the IPC, he was appointed head of the medical analysis department, and even began to teach in the school of technicians in 1965. Etoundi, at that time, was a figure of sincere

[65] "Capacity building", i.e., the reinforcement, through collaborative projects, of local skills and infrastructures, is nowadays one of the most commonplaces of international development literature.

[66] Although they were not as costly as they have been since the end of 1970s, they were already *hors-cadre* militaries, which mean that they were paid, with their expatriation grants, by the French Cooperation Service (or, before independence, by the territorial budget). A Cameroonian doctor, which would draw his considerably low salary from the Cameroonian Ministry of Health, was thus an interesting placement.

[67] As he was celebrated in historical reconstructions after his leave: "L'année 1964 a vu le départ . . . du Dr Gamet qui fut le créateur, l'organisateur et l'animateur de l'Institut. C'est grâce à son activité inlassable que cette Maison a pu prospérer et continuer la grande œuvre pastorienne en Afrique". H. Brottes, *Rapport sur le fonctionnement technique de l'Institut Pasteur de la République Fédérale du Cameroun*, 1965, 191.

[68] "L'intérêt que [ce jeune institut] éveille dans ce pays neuf grandit chaque jour ; un docteur en médecine camerounais, formé pendant un an à nos disciplines, est allé obtenir au sein de la maison mère ses titres d'accès dans la grande famille pasteurienne. Deux de ses compatriotes sont déjà inscrits pour les années à venir", p. 7. A. Gamet, "L'Institut Pasteur du Cameroun," *Bull. liais. A. A. E. I. P.* 21, 1964, 11–16.

commitment of Pasteurians to Cameroonian development. Was he heralding a new Pasteurian model?

The rise of Etoundi led to a reappraisal, or at least to a postponement of the extended Cameroonisation of the managing staff. Tensions culminated when Henri Brottes, the second director, had to be repatriated in 1966 for health reasons. Etoundi, who prided himself on impressive academic qualifications when compared to the other French doctors of the house, chose that moment to declare himself director. The French staff understood this as a coup. The Pasteur Institute in Paris reacted quickly, and sent the director of the Pasteur Institute in Dakar to "clear things out" and restore a French direction on the Institute. From then on, Etoundi, who was considered a menace, had to be kept out of the IPC: he was sent to France for "supplementary training" and in 1972 was cordially appointed Professor at the newly created Faculty of Medicine of Yaoundé, directed at that time by French doctors. The director of the IPC thought he had found "a solution to the Etoundi's case".[69]

The institutional tensions provoked by Etoundi's arrival as part of the scientific staff of the IPC were followed by a large-scale reform of public administrations and enterprises, still remembered as "Cameroonisation". Launched in 1974 by Pdt Ahmadou Ahidjo, the reform visibly sought to create and reallocate numerous bureaucratic positions (the famous "DG" and "SG" posts[70]) in order to integrate a new elite, often qualified in Europe, into the state apparatus. The IPC was hence included in a bigger institution of biomedical research, the Institut de Recherche Médicale et des Plantes Médicinales (IMPM) itself included in a central research agency (the ONAREST, under Prime Minister's authority). Expatriates were consequently told to give place, or to take part in research projects defined by the Cameroonian state, on the basis of "equal relations". Prosper Etoundi, as one of the most prominent figures

[69] Interview with former French director (Dir2), 11 March 2002, Paris.

[70] DG (*Directeur Général*) and SG (*Secrétaire Général*) are french equivalents for administrative ranks like CEO (Chief Executive Officer). These acronyms have a great popular value in Cameroon, as attested by the name of the most prestigious dish, the *Poulet DG* (literally, the "Chicken CEO").

of the medical scene, was unsurprisingly appointed director of the IMPM.

These were sufficient reasons to decide the IPC director, to *leave Cameroon* with the agreement of Paris. In April 1975, he removed the name of "Institut Pasteur" from the facade. The Pasteur Institute in Paris practically severed all relations, whether commercial or scientific, with its former Cameroonian branch and the building was renamed, under Etoundi's direction, the "Centre Pasteur". This name was a literal affirmation of emancipation from the French motherhouse. It also reflected the failure of the post-colonial assimilation policy—Parisian authorities did not allow Etoundi, though theoretically a perfect "Pasteurian", to use the name "Institut Pasteur". This can be heard in veiled terms in these words of a former French director:

> Dir 1: When it was Cameroonised, the Cameroonians did not want to keep the label "Institut Pasteur", and on the other hand, the Pasteur Institute in Paris didn't want to give the name "Institut Pasteur" to an institute that was not headed by a French person.
>
> GL: It really had to be headed by a *French person* ?
>
> Dir 1: By a French person or by someone trained in the Pasteur Institute of Paris. . . . But Etoundi had absolutely no qualification for . . . (silence).[71]

The year 1975 thus witnessed a major rupture. Taken as a political turn in Franco-Cameroonian political relations, it resembled a long delayed independence: a moment of forced "abdication of responsibilities" for the French, and, above all, a clear and optimistic assertion of Cameroonian sovereignty in the field of knowledge and development. Viewed from the Health Hill, it seemed brutal

[71] Interview with former French director (Dir1), 19 December 2002, Paris. "Dir1: Quand ça a été camerounisé, ils ont pas voulu garder l'appellation Institut Pasteur, d'une part, et d'autre part, Pasteur Paris n'a pas voulu garder . . . laisser le nom d'Institut Pasteur à un institut qui n'avait pas à sa tête un français (silence).

GL : c'était vraiment question de français.

Dir1 : Un français ou quelqu'un ayant été formé à l'Institut Pasteur de Paris. Or Etoundi n'avait absolument aucune formation de."

and unpredictable. The last director of the IPC bitterly remembers "Ahidjo laughing . . . while [he was] injecting him in the bottom" [72] a few days before the Cameroonisation reform—an image of post-colonial intimacy that could not predate a "nationalist rupture". Yet the rupture was not only a hitch of a complex Cameroonian political life; it was echoing more global changes, especially in the "Pasteurian world". For example, the whole policy of the Pasteur Institute overseas was by 1975 being remodelled, certainly in relation with Yaoundé events. Fifteen years after the African independences, the Pasteur Institute in Paris mentioned—for the first time—that the former colonies, until then seen as "insufficiently developed countries" with "insufficiently mature autochthons", [73] were now expressing a "legitimate ambition . . . to take a larger and larger, if not a preponderant part, in the functioning of their research organisms". Without ambiguities, the PI called for a "new style", and urged to "adapt to the realities of the present" [74] the policies of scientific cooperation. The year 1975 gave the impression of a general turn, from Yaoundé to Paris. [75]

Cameroonisation turned out to be a failure, if we believe that well-known and heavily symbolic story (here told by a personal doctor of Pdt Ahidjo), which took place in the privacy of the top of French and Cameroonian states:

> Ahidjo had diabetes, and did regular blood and urine exams [at the ex-Pasteur Institute]. For a urine exam, which had been sent under a false name, it had been answered: "Pregnancy test: positive". It gives you an idea of what happened to the Pasteur Institute. This is when Ahidjo

[72] Interview with former French director (Dir2), 11 March 2002.

[73] Institut Pasteur, *Rapport du conseil d'administration* (Paris: Institut Pasteur, 1968), Chapter IV.

[74] Institut Pasteur, *Rapport du conseil d'administration* (Paris: Institut Pasteur, 1975)

[75] It must be noted that 1975 had been a turn for nationalisation of research institutions (and of other institutions) in many former French colonies, notably Ivory Coast or Malagasy.

[called Journiac] and told him: "[the Institut Pasteur] cannot go on like that".[76]

Journiac and Ahidjo's ties dated back to the late fifties when they were respectively head of the colonial Health Service and prime minister of self-governing French Cameroon. By 1978, when the "pregnancy affair" probably occurred, General Journiac headed the medical division of the Parisian Ministry of Cooperation, and was thus influential enough to "send back the French people" in Cameroon—as Ahidjo explicitly asked him. Pasteurians were first sent for diagnosis: they described a disaster. According to their reports, research was abandoned, analyses were fanciful, and "clan tensions" divided the staff.[77] Audits described Etoundi as the incarnation of Cameroonian mismanagement: regionalist, lax and patrimonial. The therapy was clearly prescribed: French staff had to be sent back.

Though it is still remembered in Yaoundé as a difficult moment, Cameroonisation was also a success, if interpreted as an experiment testing the effectiveness of Cameroonians' skills. By severing all links with Cameroon, by brutally ending sixteen years of ritualised transmission between scientists, and by cutting off every penny from French cooperation, Pasteurians proved themselves once more to be remarkable experimenters: they were taking no chances while attempting to prove that they were indispensable. Meanwhile, they were tautologically defining Cameroonians, incarnated in Etoundi, as "culturally inapt" for the direction of a "cooperative research institute".

In 1980, an experienced and authoritarian French military doctor was sent to "sanitize" [*sic*] the institution, renamed the "Centre Pasteur du Cameroun". Relations with Paris were re-activated on an informal basis and half of the employees were sent to other medical institutions. "Whites are back", some regretted, as they feared

[76] Interview with Dir 1. 'Ahidjo avait, disons un diabète, il faisait des examens d'urine et de sang régulièrement. Dans l'examen d'urine qu'ils avaient envoyé sous un autre nom, on a répondu "Test de Grossesse positif". Ça vous donne une idée de ce qui est arrivé. C'est là que Ahidjo a dit à Journiac " ça peut pas continuer comme ça.'

[77] Carton n2 "Institut Microbiologie Cameroun/ Centre Pasteur/ Yaoundé", Archives de l'Institut Pasteur de DakarDarkar, Sénégal.

"Pasteur was becoming Johannesburg again".[78] But we should not be misguided: the Pasteur Institute in Paris was cautious—it did not allow the use of its brand name—and the laboratory had a new status that permitted an effective control by Cameroonian elites. Once considered by Cameroonian elites as "a law unto itself", the institution was now headed by a Board ("C. A.", Administration Council) often Cameroonian members, representing different ministers and Health institutions, while still directly depending on the Ministry of Health. Over the 1980s, the Board proved itself to be an efficient means for the Cameroonian medical elite to be incorporated into the institution and to share symbolically and financially some of its benefits. Still excluded from scientific work and direction, Cameroonians had thus gained true control over the Pasteurian institution (which they have exerted harshly, if we believe the regular complaints of their French partners). At the same time, they were able to benefit from professional opportunities in places free from the hierarchical control of expatriates, notably in the Faculty of Medicine or in the emerging field of "international co-operation" that was to drastically expand with the rise in AIDS cases.[79] In a sense, a new compromise was established between local elites and former colonisers, representing a third way, between years of unconvincing cooperation followed by a threatening "Cameroonisation". It achieved an arbitrage between their respective appetites.

Numerous Cameroonian doctors, pharmacists, and highly skilled technicians ("techniciens supérieurs") were integrated in the staff during the 1980s, and often benefited from training in France or in the Pasteurian network (Dakar, Bangui). But hierarchies were still clear, even though they had been redefined: assigned exclusively to the service of medical analyses—considered as a "burden", or as an unrewarding "alimentary task" by French doctors[80]—the

[78] Interview with retired laboratory technician (Cm2), 16 September 2003, Yaoundé.

[79] Fred Eboko, "Logiques et contradictions internationales dans le champ du sida au Cameroun," *Autrepart* 12, 1999, 123–40.

[80] This discourse turned out to be a constant feature of Pasteurian reports. For example, H. Brottes, *Rapport sur le fonctionnement technique de l'Institut Pasteur de la République Fédérale du Cameroun*, 1966, 27.

Cameroonians did not challenge the expatriates' positions as *researchers* and managers. In the meantime, their progression on the administrative scale was controlled by the "C. A.", so that the state elites were able to interfere inside the Pasteurian house, by making and unmaking Cameroonian's careers, a complex policy of ethno-regional (un)balancing. As the 1980s were times of abundance and munificence for the Cameroonian state, bonuses and medals were regularly distributed to the rather appeased and privileged staff. The Centre Pasteur du Cameroun (CPC) was a wealthy institution with growing profits, new equipment, and new buildings, and its local *grandeur* was eventually attested by the celebrated re-affirmation of its link with the Parisian motherhouse, on the occasion of the Pasteur Institute centennial in 1988, for example.

Starting from 1989, by contrast, the Centre Pasteur violently felt the combined effects of a drastic economic crisis of "structural adjustment" measures and of the devaluation of *Franc CFA*. The state subsidies and the local resources from the vaccine and analysis market dramatically fell, and the institution was virtually bankrupt by 1994. After several costly and contradictory audits financed by the French Cooperation agency, the Centre Pasteur remodelled its funding strategies. This consisted essentially in improving its competitiveness as a private laboratory, and by effective insertion into "big science" projects, generously funded by international backers, particularly in the field of HIV-AIDS. The internal functioning of the institute was also adjusted: in an oppressive atmosphere, the Centre Pasteur fired half of its subaltern staff, and cut by 50 per cent the salaries of the remaining employees.[81]

As the *conjoncture* (the popular word for "economic circumstances" used throughout French-speaking Africa) shook the institution, Cameroonisation became a burning issue. The French Cooperation agency was pushing toward Cameroonsation, in the name of generous principles such as local sovereignty and more realistically because of the cost of expatriates' salary. Cameroonian scientific figures also regularly asked, during the 1990s, for an opening of the "French fortress", insisting on their own capacities, attested by their

[81] Lachenal, "Le Centre Pasteur du Cameroun", 173.

international success in the field of AIDS research. The bastion was giving signs of crumbling, when, in 1996, a *civil* Pasteurian was, for the very first time, appointed director. In 1998, the CPC welcomed its first Cameroonian as a full time researcher, and began to train several PhD students in molecular biology. He provided them with travel grants for France, so that the former inequities of Pasteurian science seemed to be vanishing. Successively in 1996, 2000 and 2004, as the four-year contracts of expatriated directors were expiring, the Cameroonisation of the CPC therefore appeared more imminent than ever.

But no less ritually, the Cameroonisation was postponed: the Centre Pasteur du Cameroun has hitherto been directed exclusively by French Pasteurians, as if, despite major innovations in the management of cooperative work, the most symbolic change of all was impossible.

Culturalist prejudices have proved to be most convincing in preventing Cameroonisation: "Cameroonians are not ready for cameroonisation", "you know how Cameroonians manage things, it's a question of culture", "the problem is the pressure of the African family", "Cameroonians just cannot agree with each other".[82] These commonplaces are not merely statements of self-interested Pasteurians, or of regular consumers attached to the reliable medical services. For example, the subaltern staff of the Centre Pasteur almost unanimously warns: "tell them in Paris that we don't want anymore blacks as directors".[83] And Yaoundé's *vox populi*, with its unique blend of self-derision, resignation and pragmatism, generally acknowledges the risk of Cameroonising an institution that *effectively* works. The frequently invoked reason is an implacable and elusive tautology, "Cameroon is Cameroon";[84] this may well indicate that the Cameroonisation is, above all, an ontological question—a matter of maintaining or dismantling categories.

82 Interviews with French expatriate staff Coop 4, 8 April 2002, Coop 2, 16 April 2002, Coop 3, 17 April 2002, Yaoundé.

83 Interview with Member of the Cameroonian staff (Cm1), 15 April 2004, Yaoundé.

84 "Le Cameroun c'est le Cameroun" is a famous expression, used in a fatalistic and humorous way, for example, when commentating on famous corruptions, affairs and national failures, in business, football, or politics.

What, exactly, is Cameroon? Etoundi, of course, is in everyone's mind, as the very embodiment of the fact that "Cameroonians are . . . Cameroonians", i.e., not only culturally at risk for misappropriation of funds, public prevarication, or familial management, but also, as Mbembe has suggested, corporally expressing a *habitus* "hostile to continence, frugality, and sobriety":[85]

> [Etoundi] was a very ambitious man, who had not a few faults. . . . He was keen on women, he was keen on boore, he did not really fit in, one can say. . . . He didn't know how to manage or administrate the Pasteur Institute for its well being. Of course, for his own well-being . . . yes, he did have a sense of management.[86]

This depiction of Etoundi by one of his French colleagues echoes an "orientalist" medical literature. Indeed such texts could define, with the attributes of medical and administrative objectivity, Cameroonians as "sexually obsessed". For instance, in an IPC annual report, one of the 1980s directors saw in the large number of urine exams done in the Centre Pasteur, "how great an interest [Cameroonian] populations of both sexes have in all that concerns their genitalia", and even mentioned "the obsessive nature of sexual contamination for some patients".[87]

By a well-known mechanism, such discourses aim at clarifying boundaries and identities.[88] As he became an obsessive incarnation

[85] Mbembe, *On the Postcolony*, 110.

[86] Interview with Former French expatriate at the IPC (Coop1), 12 December 2003 Marseille (France). "Bon c'est quelqu'un qui avait les dents longues, qui avait pas mal de défauts. . .il aimait bien les femmes, il aimait bien la bibine, ça cadrait pas trop quoi. . . .Il avait aucun sens de la gestion, de l'administration pour le bien être de l'Institut Pasteur, bien sur. Pour son bien être personnel, oui, ça il connaissait bien."

[87] J. P. Albert, "L'intérêt, Ô combien grand, que portent les populations des deux sexes à tout ce qui appartient à l'appareil génital", in *Rapport d'activité. Centre Pasteur du Cameroun, 1980–1982*, 1982, B.3 ; J. P. Albert, "Le caractère obsessionnel que prend chez certains sujets la contamination par voie sexuelle", in *Rapport d'activité. Centre Pasteur du Cameroun, 1980–1982*, 1982, B.15.

[88] Edward W. Said, *Orientalism* (New York: Pantheon Books, 1978). The discourse about Africans' hypersexuality is a commonplace of colonial

of "Cameroonian culture", Etoundi also became a counter-example of the "pasteurian ethos"—de-socialisation, disinterest, self-containment—and the very justification of the presence in Cameroon of "exemplary Pasteurians". Such efforts are, above all, signs of *anxiety*: boundaries are indeed permeable and regularly crossed,[89] the control of the scientific label is uneven, and Pasteurians themselves are anxious about their own incontinence.

From the subalterns' side, "the Pasteurian ethos" has been smoothly appropriated: the local staff is generally pleased to testify that the Pasteurian ethic is "excellence, excellence and excellence".[90] But beyond the opportune reprise of the managerial injunction ("when you are a good and devoted technician, when you give accurate results, you say that you have the Pasteurian spirit"[91]), the Pasteurian label has also been re-routed: the head of Pasteur himself has been printed on local *pagne* cloth, just as have other post-colonial *big men*, presidents, bishops or football players, and proudly exhibited by Cameroonian staff along the streets during the numerous official parades. The august Pasteur has thus become a prestigious object of social identity, but simultaneously, as a plebeian sign, a grotesque one.

---

medicine literature. See Megan Vaughan, *Curing Their Ills: Colonial Power and African Illness* (Stanford: Stanford University Press, 1991), 131.

89 The intimate destabilisation of socio-racial categories in colonial settings has been recently analysed by Ann Laura Stoler, among others. See Frederick Cooper and Ann Laura Stoler, "Between Metropole and Colony: Rethinking a Research Agenda," in *Tensions of Empire: Colonial Cultures in a Bourgeois World*, ed. Frederick Cooper and Ann Laura Stoler (Berkeley: University of California Press, 1996), 1–58; Ann Laura Stoler, "Sexual Affronts and Racial Frontiers: European Identities and the Cultural Politics of Exclusion in Colonial Southeast Asia," in Cooper and Stoler, *Tensions of Empire*, 198–237.

90 Interview with Cameroonian member of the staff (Cm5), 10 April 2002, Yaoundé .

91 Interview with retired laboratory technician (Cm3), 19 September 2003, Yaoundé. "GL : Est ce que le nom de Pasteur participe à l'ambiance même ? Ca représente quoi ?

-Cm3 :Oui. C'est une divinité. C'est une divinité. Parce que bon celui qui travaille bien, il dit que j'ai l'esprit pasteurien. Quand tu es un bon technicien dévoué, tu donnes tout le temps de bons résultats, on dit que j'ai l'esprit pasteurien."

On the top of the hill, certified Pasteurians have also continuously flirted with the frontiers of obscenity. Compromises with local power are always compromising, and the baroque story of Ahidjo's pseudo-pregnancy has shown that, given its long-standing intimacy with power, Pasteurian science has to share with it the post-colonial "aesthetics of vulgarity"—obscenity as the language of power and of its ludicrous deconstruction.[92] Besides, regarding individual (mis)conducts, expatriates have been faced with the century-old colonial drive towards corporal exuberance and incontinence, called "bougnoulisation" in French colonial argot.[93] The confined and heated community of expatriates, fond of rumours and scandals, is an infallible detector of the permeability of racial and cultural boundaries. One striking example is the insinuation: "I've heard that the director is completely cameroonized". Eventually, if we are to account for the many narratives[94] about the recurrent "money affairs" involving genuine "French Pasteurians", or their various "escapades" we might conclude here that the Pasteur Institute has actually been *Cameroonised* all along.

Conclusion

Through the example of the IPC, we have tried to understand the post-colonial viability of Pasteur Institutes in Africa, and more broadly that of French medical cooperation, with all its political implications. "Franco-African familiarities" oriented and tinged France's international *déploiement* in the medical field. Conversely, medical corporation, and in particular the "Pasteurian brotherhood", appeared as a catalyst of ambiguous connivances at the top of French and African states. The history of the IPC is embedded in

[92] Mbembe, *On the Postcolony*.

[93] "Niggerisation" could be an English translation. Although "Bougnoule" was initially an anti-Arab insult, "bougnoulisation" has been frequently used in African settings.

[94] French directors have been regularly accused of misappropriating funds, particularly during the crisis (1988–96), by French expatriates as well as Cameroonian officials. These accusations have been discussed in various audits (Archives du Centre Pasteur du Cameroun).

the singular course of "La Coopération", understood both as an era and as a form of international connexion, bridging pre- and post-independence periods, and (former) colonial and metropolitan spaces. The post-war years shaped it: colonial policies of development gave the initial boost to institutions and relations that have made the French presence remarkably stable. The 1990s announced its end, or at least a rupture in the functioning of Franco-African medical institutions: France initiated a policy of *désengagement* with drastic budget cuts, while local scientists found elsewhere (in short-term collaborative research projects) positions that were inaccessible in French-held institutions such as the CPC. The multi-lateralisation of North-South collaborations, embodied at its best in the Cameroonian field of AIDS research, acted to weaken the old monopoly of institutions still drawing on a (always theoretical) Franco-African *face à face*.

The concept of "familiarity" has proved heuristic in making sense of the paradoxes of post-colonial French presence in Africa, stressing the need to envisage the informal nature of the Franco-African microcosm, the "convivial struggles" experienced in collaborative institutions, and the intimate undermining of hierarchies. The history of the IPC offers insight into such post-colonial intimacies, and helps to analyse them, as Achille Mbembe has proposed, as "a practice and a stylistic" of power.[95] Our focus on the Pasteur Institute of Cameroon also suggests that medical discourse and institutions not only has repercussions for a more general "aesthetics of vulgarity", but deeply inspired it.

Part of this inspiration could be found in medical and scientific practices *per se.* Focused on a microanalysis of politico-institutional negotiations and conflicts, our study has left aside the practical modalities of scientific and medical work. Further discussions should include this point. Medico-scientific practices may crystallise post-colonial obscenity, by defining, incorporating, and exploiting socio-racial inequities. They shall also underline the importance of *trans-national* circulations—of persons, biological materials, scien-

[95] Achille Mbembe, *De la post-colonie: Essai sur l'imagination politique dans l'Afrique contemporaine* (Paris: Karthala, 2000), 177.

tific techniques, managerial style—whose reach has notably been *inter-African*, like the careers of many colonial Pasteurians. It may be along these transnational nexuses that the science and politics of Franco-African familiarity were forged, and through their reconfiguration that they should be un-forged.

Glossary

Antipyrin	pharmaceutical
bakshees	tips
batta	gratuity given to hospital in-patients, usually money in lieu of hospital dieting
bayt al-adviya	drugstore
boka	scolding
dai	traditional Indian birth attendant, also employed as a wet-nurse
dār al-shafâ	house of healing
dār al-shafâ-ye jadid-e tupkhâneh	modern artillery hospital
Dawa	medicine
Dawa ya hospitali	hospital medicine
dawa ya kisasa	modern medicine
dawa ya kizungu	European medicine
Deutsch-Ostafrikanische Gesellschaft	the German Chartered Company for East Africa
dispensaire	dispensary in French
ejazeh-nameh	certificates
firman	authorisation from the Sultan
fowj	regiment
gâh	site or position
hakim	Muslim doctor
hammâm	baths
jarrâhân-e jaded	new surgeons
khâneh	house
khânqâh and *tekyeh*	houses where Sufis and dervish gathered
Kupimo	Swahili word for measuring
madrasa-ye 'âli	high school
madrasa-ye dār al-shafâ	the school belonging to the hospital
makatb	religious primary school

malik	owner
mariz-khâneh	the house of the ill
marizkhâneh-ye dowlati	State hospital
Medresa	Swahili Koran school
mganga	Healer in the South-east
Mosri	contagious
Motawalli	expenses of the administrator
mowqufât	endowments.
mudiriyyah	local governorate
Mukhtâ	person who is responsible for a local religious community or a village in their relationship with the Ottoman authorities.
Mumia	Latin word for mummy
mumiani	Swahili term that relate European institutions and their African staff to the criminal use of human bodies are well known in East Africa
murûr	Arabic seal
mwalimu	The Muslim Koran scholar and teacher
ngoma	one of the forms of healing with regard to spirits
Nowruz	The new Iranian year
ordu	camp
owqâf	charitable endowments
pharmacopolium	Latin word for the reports to Rome
Phenacetine	pharmaceutical
Poliklinik	dispensary in English
punkah	large indoor fan pulled by a cord
purdah	female seclusion
Qâdî	chief judge
Qanât	subterranean water irrigation
rajakariya	feudal system of compulsory labour
sahn	courtyard
samaj	society
sati	self-immolation by Hindu widows on their husbands' funeral pyres
shirk	strictly prohibited pagan practice
Spital	mission station for treatment
Taka	Bangladeshi currency unit
tanguze'il and *sichqâne'il*	Turkish years corresponding to 1272–73 /1855–56
Tashrih	explanation
tashrih-e jaded	modern anatomy

tebb-e 'amali	practical or manual medicine
tekyeh	place where one leans to repose
Tibb-ul-Nabbi	prophet's medicine
towliyat	the administration
wagariba	biomedical training in hygiene and surgical skills for the experts performing circumcision
waqf	endowments
waqf-nâmeh	set of rules established by the founder of the waqf as to how the endowed money should be spent
Yunani-Tibb[u]	Ionic medicine

Bibliography

Archival information and other primary sources are mentioned only in the footnotes in each essay.

Abasiekong, M. E. "Feminism and Hospital Admission in Rural Nigeria: A Case Study." *Social Science & Medicine* 15(B), 1981, 45–50.

Ackerknecht, Erwin H. *Medicine at the Paris Hospital, 1794–1848*. Baltimore: Johns Hopkins University Press, 1967.

Adams, Vicanne. *Tigers of the Snow and Other Virtual Sherpas: Ethnography of Himalayan Encounters.* Princeton, New Jersey: Princeton University Press, 1996.

Adhikary, Kamal. "Naming Ceremonies as Rituals of Development". *Studies in Nepali History and Society* 1, no. 2, December 1996, 345–64.

Adityanjee, Dr. "Medical Priorities and Practices in Nineteenth-Century British India". *South Asia Research* 5, no. 2, 1985, 167–83.

——. "Suicide Attempts and Suicides in India: Cross-Cultural Aspects". *International Journal of Social Psychiatry* 32, no. 2, 1986, 64–73.

Adolfsson, M., and Anna Berntsson. *Ceza, a Roundabout Way to the Goal: Three Decades of Medical Missionary Work in South Africa*. Ljungbergs Boktr., Klippan 1984.

Agamben, Giorgio. *Homo Sacer.* Torino: Giulio E inaudi editore, 1995.

Ahmed, Emajuddin. *Bureaucratic Elites in Segmented Economic Growth: Pakistan and Bangladesh.* Dhaka: University Press, 1980.

Alavi, Seema. *The Sepoys and the Company: Tradition and Transition in Northern India, 1770–1830*. New Delhi: Oxford University Press, 1995.

Alpers, Edward A. "Towards a History of the Expansion of Islam in East Africa: The Matrilineal Peoples of the Southern Interior". In *The Historical Study of African Religion with Special Reference to East and Central Africa,* ed. Terence O. Ranger and Isaria Kimambo, 172–201. London: Heinemann, 1972.

Anderson, L. R. "Society, Economy and Criminal Activity in Colonial Natal, 1860–1893". PhD thesis, University of Natal, Durban, 1993.

Anderson, N., and S. Marks. "Apartheid Health in the 1980s". *Social Science & Medicine* 27, 1988, 667–81.

Anderson-Morshead, Anne Elizabeth Mary. *The History of the Universities' Mission to Central Africa, 1859–1909*. London: UMCA, 1909.

Arjomand, Amir S. "The Law, Agency, and Policy in Medieval Islamic Society." *Comparative Studies in Societies and History* 41, no. 2, 1999, 263–93.

Arnold, David. *Colonizing the Body: State Medicine and Epidemic Disease in Nineteenth-Century India*. Berkeley: University of California Press, 1993.

——. "Disease, Medicine and Empire." In *Imperial Medicine and Indigenous Societies*, ed. David Arnold, 1–26. Manchester: Manchester University Press, 1988.

Aruzi, Nezâmi. *Chahar Maqâla.* Translated by E. G. Browne as *The "Four Discourses" of Nidhami-i-Arudi-i-Samarqandi*. London: Luzuc & Co., 1900.

Atkinson, Paul. *Medical Talk and Medical Work: The Liturgy of the Clinic*. London: Sage, 1995.

Attewell, Guy. "Authority, Knowledge and Practice in Unani Tibb in India, c.1890–1930". PhD, diss., University of London, 2004.

Austin, Alvyn J. *Saving China: Canadian Missionaries in the Middle Kingdom, 1888–1959*. Toronto: University of Toronto Press, 1986.

Azmi, Altaf Ahmad. *Basic Concepts of Unani Medicine: A Critical Study*. Hamdard Nagar/New Delhi: Jamia Hamdard, 1995.

Baldwin-Ragaven, Laurel, Jeanelle de Gruchy, and Leslie London. *An Ambulance of the Wrong Colour: Health Professionals, Human Rights and Ethics in South Africa*. Rondebosch: University of Cape Town Press, 1999.

Balfour, Margaret, and Ruth Young. *The Work of Medical Women in India.* London: Oxford University Press, 1929.

Bandarage, Asoka. *Colonialism in Sri Lanka: The Political Economy of the Kandyan Highlands, 1833–1886.* Berlin, New York and Amsterdam: Mouton Publishers, 1983.

Bandyopadhyay, Mridula, and Stewart MacPherson. *Women and Health: Tradition and Culture in Rural India.* Aldershot: Ashgate, 1998.

Bank, L. "Beyond Red and School: Gender, Tradition and Identity in the Rural Eastern Cape". *Journal of Southern African Studies* 28, no. 3, 2002, 631–49.

Bari, Abdul, and Hussain, Arshad. "Hakim 'Imâd al-Dîn Mahmûd Shirâzi and Risâla Bîkh-I Chini." *Studies in History of Medicine & Science* 17, no. 1–2, new series, 2001.

Barjesteh, and Eskandari-Qajar, eds. *Qajar Era Health, Hygiene and Beauty*. Rotterdam and Santa Barbara: Barjesteh & Co., 2003.

Barry, J., and C. Jones, eds. *Medicine and Charity before the Welfare State*. London and New York: Routledge, 1991.

Basu, Subho. "Emergence of the Mill Towns in Bengal, 1880–1920: Migration Pattern and Survival Strategies of Industrial Workers". *The Calcutta Historical Journal* 18, no. 1, 1995, 97–133.

Bayly, C. A. *Indian Society and the Making of the British Empire.* Cambridge: Cambridge University Press, 1993.

Baziak, A. T., and R. K. Denton. "The Language of the Hospital and Its Effects on the Patient". In *Social Interaction and Patient Care,* ed. J. K. Skipper and R. C. Leonard, 272–77. Philadelphia: J. B. Lippincott, 1965.

Begum, Najmir Nur. *Pay or Purdah: Women and Income Earning in Rural Bangladesh*. Dhaka: Winrock International Institute for Agricultural Development, 1987.

Beinart, William. *Twentieth-Century South Africa*. Oxford: Oxford University Press, 2001.

Bell, Heather. *Frontiers of Medicine in the Anglo-Egyptian Sudan, 1899–1940*. Oxford: Clarendon Press, 1999.

Benedict, Carol. *Bubonic Plague in Nineteenth-Century China*. Stanford: Stanford University Press, 1996.

Bodenstein, W. "Contemporary Approaches of Healing: African Medicine". *The Report of the Umpumulu Consultation*, 1967, 51–64.

Bonner, B., and L. Segal. *Soweto: A History.* Cape Town: Maskew Miller Longman, 1998.

Bonneuil, Christophe. "Development as Experiment." *Osiris* 14, 2001, 258–81.

Borsay, Ann. *Medicine and Charity in Georgian Bath: A Social History of the General Infirmary, c.1739–1830*. Aldershot: Ashgate, 1999.

Bowers, John Z. *Western Medicine in a Chinese Palace: Peking Union Medical College, 1917–1951*. Philadelphia: Josiah Macy, Jr. Foundation, 1972.

——. *When the Twain Meet: The Rise of Western Medicine in Japan*. Baltimore: Johns Hopkins University Press, 1980.

——, and Akiko K. Bowers. "Japanese Medicine in Manchuria: The South Manchuria Medical College". *Clio Medica* 12, no. 1, 1977, 1–15.

Boyd, Robin. *Church History of Gujarat.* Madras: The Christian Literature Society, 1981.

Bozzoli, Belinda. "Why Were the 1980s 'Millenarian'? Style, Repertoire, Space and Authority in South Africa's Black Cities". *Journal of Historical Sociology* 12, 2000, 78–110.

Brockliss, Laurence, and Colin Jones. *The Medical World of Early Modern France*. Oxford: Clarendon Press, 1997.

Brooks, Barbara. "Colonial Power and Public Health in Japanese-held Korea". Paper presented at the Association for Asian Studies Meeting, Washington, D.C., 5 April 2002.

Brouwer, Ruth Compton. *Modern Women Modernizing Men: The Changing Missions of Three Professional Women in Asia and Africa, 1902–69.*Vancouver: UBC Press, 2002.

Bruchhausen, Walter. "Practising Hygiene and Fighting the Natives' Diseases: Public and Child Health in German East Africa and Tanganyika Territory, 1900–1960". *Dynamis. Acta Hisp. Sci. Hist. Illus*. 23, 2003, 85–114.

——, and Volker Roelcke. "Categorising 'African Medicine': The German Discourse on East African Healing Practices, 1885–1918". In *Plural Medicine, Tradition and Modernity, 1800–2000.* Routledge Studies in the Social History of Medicine. Vol. 13, ed. Waltraud Ernst, 76–94. London: Routledge, 2002.

Buckingham, Jane. *Leprosy in Colonial South India: Medicine and Confinement*. London: Palgrave, 2002.

Bürgel, J. Christoph. "Secular and Religious Features of Medieval Arabic Medicine". In *Asian Medical Systems: A Comparative Study,* ed. Charles Leslie, 44–62. Delhi: Motilal Banarsidass Publishers, 1998. First published 1976.

Burns, Susan L. "From 'Leper Villages' to Leprosaria: Public Health, Nationalism and the Culture of Exclusion in Japan". In *Isolation: Places and Practices of Exclusion*, ed. Carolyn Strange and Alison Bashford, 104–18. London: Routledge, 2003.

Burrows, Edmund H. *A History of Medicine in South Africa up to the End of the Nineteenth Century*. Cape Town: A. A. Balkema, 1958.

Canguilhem, Gorges, ed. *The Normal and the Pathological.* New York: Zone Books, 1991.

Carmel, Alex . "A Note on the Christian Contribution to Palestine's Development in the 19th Century". In *Palestine in the Late Ottoman Period: Political, Social and EconomicTtransformation,* ed. David Kushner, 302–8. Jerusalem / Leyden: Yad Izhak ben-Zvi / E. J. Brill, 1986.

Cavallo, Sandra. "Charity, Power, and Patronage in Eighteenth-Century Italian Hospitals: The Case of Turin". In *The Hospital in History*, ed. Lindsay Granshaw and Roy Porter, 63–92. London: Routledge, 1989.

Chafer, Tony. *The End of Empire in French West Africa: France's Successful Decolonization?* Oxford: Berg, 2002.

Chakrabarti, Pratik. "'Neither meete nor drinke but what the Doctor alloweth': The Hospital amidst War and Commerce in Eighteenth-Century Madras". *Bulletin of the History of Medicine* 80, no. 1, Spring 2006, 1–38.

Chakravorty Spivak, Gayatri. *The Post-Colonial Critic: Interviews, Strategies, Dialogues.* New York and London: Routledge, 1990.

Chang, Cheng. *Xiandai Dongbei shi* [The History of the Contemporary North-East]. Haerbin: Heilongjiang jiaoyu chubanshe, 1986.

Chen, Edward I. "Gotô Shinpei: Japan's Colonial Administrator in Taiwan; A Critical Re-examination". *The American Asian Review* 13, no. 1, 1995, 29–59.

China Medical University, Information Center. "China Medical University (CMU): Survey," Shenyang, 2003, http://www.cmu.edu.cn/overview/overview.htm (accessed 1 August 2004).

Clark, David, ed. *Cicely Saunders: Founder of the Hospice Movement; Selected Letters, 1959–1999*. Oxford: Oxford University Press, 2005.

Clausen, Soren, and Stig Thogersen. *The Making of a Chinese City: History and Historiography in Harbin*. Armonk, NY: M.E. Sharpe, 1995.

Clayton, Andrew J. "Christianity and Islam in South-East Tanzania: A Study of Religious Appropriation Among Makonde". Diss., John Rylands University of Manchester, 1993.

Cohen, Amnon. *The Guilds of Ottoman Jerusalem.* Leyden / Boston / Cologne: Brill, 2001.

Collingham, E. N. *Imperial Bodies: The Physical Experience of the Raj, c.1800–1947.* Cambridge: Polity Press, 2001.

Collins, Treacher. *In the Kingdom of the Shah*. London: T. Fisher Unwin, 1896.

Comaroff, Jean, and John Comaroff. *Of Revelation and Revolution: The Dialectics of Modernity on a South African Frontier*. Chicago: Chicago University Press, 1997.

Cook, Harold J. "Global Economies and Local Knowledge in the East Indies: Jacobus Bontius Learns the Facts of Nature". In *Colonial Botany: Science, Commerce, and Politics in the Early Modern World,* ed. Londa Schiebinger and Claudia Swan, 100–18. Philadelphia: University of Philadelphia Press, 2005.

Cooper D., R. Hamilton and H. Mashaba. *Race Relations Survey, 1992/1993*. Johannesburg: SAIRR, 1993.

Cooper, Frederick. *Africa since 1940: The Past of the Present*. Cambridge: Cambridge University Press, 2003.

——. *Decolonization and African Society: The Labour Question in French and British Africa*. Cambridge: Cambridge University Press, 1996.

——, and Ann Laura Stoler. "Between Metropole and Colony: Rethinking a Research Agenda." In *Tensions of Empire: Colonial Cultures in a Bourgeois World*, ed. Frederick Cooper and Ann Laura Stoler. Berkeley: University of California Press, 1996, 1–58.

Coox, Alvin D. "The Kwantung Army Dimension". In *The Japanese Informal Empire in China, 1895–1937*, ed. Peter Duus, Ramon H. Myers and Mark R. Peattie, 395–428. Princeton: Princeton University Press, 1989.

Crawford, D. G. *A History of the Indian Medical Service*. 2 vols. London: Thacker & Co., 1913.

Cui, Dan. *The Cultural Contribution of British Protestant Missionaries and British-American Co-operation to China's National Development During the 1920s*. New York: University Press of America, 1998.

Currey, R. N. ed. *Letters and Other Writings of a Natal Sheriff, 1815–1876.* Cape Town: Oxford University Press, 1968.

Da Silva, Gracias, F. *Health and Hygiene in Colonial Goa, 1510–1961*. New Delhi: Concept Publishing, 1994.

Davies, Jack Neville Phillips. "The Development of 'Scientific' Medicine in the African Kingdom of Bunyoro-Kirara". *Medical History* 3, 1959, 47–57.

De Alarçon, Hernando Ruiz. Introduction to *Treatise on the Heathen Superstitions that Today Live Among the Indians Native to This New Spain*. Trans. and ed. J. R. Andrews and R. Hassig. Norman: University of Oklahoma Press, 1984.

De Beer, Cedric. "How Many Beds Does Baragwanath Hospital Need?" Occasional paper no. 10, Centre for the Study of Health Policy, Department of Community Health, Johannesburg, 1988.

——. *The South African Disease: Apartheid Health and Health Services*. Johannesburg: Southern African Research Service, 1984.

De Silva, Chandra Richard. *Sri Lanka: A History*. New Delhi: Vikas Publishing House, 1994.

De Silva, Kingsley M. *Social Policy and Missionary Organisations in Ceylon, 1840–1855.* London: Longmans, Green and Co. Ltd, 1965.

Deacon, H. "Insanity, Institutions and Society: The Case of the Robben Island Lunatic Asylum, 1846–1910". In *The Confinement of the Insane: International Perspectives, 1800–1965*, ed. Roy Porter and D. Wright, 20–53. Cambridge: Cambridge University Press, 2003.

Deacon, Harriet. "Medical Gentlemen and the Process of Professionalisation before 1890". In *The Cape Doctor in the Nineteenth Century: A Social History*, ed. Harriet Deacon, Howard Phillips and Elizabeth van Heyningen. Amsterdam/ New York: Rodopi, 2004, 85–103.

Del Vecchio Good, M. J. "Cultural Studies of Biomedicine: An Agenda for Research". *Social Science & Medicine* 41, 1993, 461–73.

DeLancey, Mark W., and Mbella H. Mokeba. *Historical Dictionary of the Republic of Cameroon*. Metuchen: Scarecrow Press, 1990.

Des Chene, Mary. Editorial, "In the Name of *Bikās*". *Studies in Nepali History and Society* 1, no. 2, December 1996, 259–70.

Digby, Anne. *Diversity and Division in Medicine: Health Care in South Africa from the 1800s*. Oxford, New York: Peter Lang Publishing, 2006.

——. "Early Black Doctors in South Africa". *Journal of African History* 46, 2005, 427–54.

——. "Self-Medication and the Trade in Medicine Within a Multi-Ethnic Context: A Case Study of South Africa from the Mid-Nineteenth to Mid-Twentieth Centuries". *Social History of Medicine* 18, no. 3, 2005, 439–57.

——, and Helen Sweet. "Nurses as Culture Brokers in Twentieth-Century South Africa". In *Plural Medicine, Tradition and Modernity, 1800–2000*, ed. Waltraud Ernst. London and New York: Routledge, 2001.

Dodwell, H. H. ed. *The Indian Empire, 1858–1918 and The Last Phase, 1919–1947 by R. R. Sethi.* The Cambridge History of India. Vol. 6. Cambridge: Cambridge University Press, 1964.

Doerr, Lambert, ed. *Peramiho, 1898–1998: In the Service of the Missionary Church.* Ndanda-Peramiho: Benedictine Publications, 1998.

Dreger, Alice Domurat. "The Limits of Individuality: Ritual and Sacrifice in the Lives and Medical Treatment of Conjoined Twins". *Studies in the History and Philosophy of Biology and Biomedical Science* 29, 1988, 1–29.

Duara, Pransenjit. *Sovereignty and Authenticity: Manchukuo and the East Asian Modern*. New York: Rowman and Littlefield Publishers, 2003.

Dubow, Saul. *Scientific Racism in Modern South Africa.* Cambridge: Cambridge University Press, 1995.

Duffin, Jacalyn. *To See with a Better Eye: A Life of R. T. H. Laennec*. Princeton: Princeton University Press, 1998.

Dwork, Deborah. *War is Good for Babies and Other Young Children: A History of the Infant and Child Welfare Movement in England, 1898–1918*. London: Tavistock, 1987.

Ebrahimnejad, Hormoz. *Medicine, Public Health and the Qajar State*. Leiden, Boston: Brill, 2004.

Echenberg, Myron J. *Black Death, White Medicine: Bubonic Plague and the Politics of Public Health in Colonial Senegal, 1914–1945*. Oxford: James Currey, 2002.

Eckart, Wolfgang U. "Malaria and Colonialism in the German Colonies New Guinea and the Cameroons: Research, Control, Thoughts of Eradication." *Parassitologia* 40, no. 1, 1998, 83–90.

——. "Medicine and German Colonial Expansion in the Pacific: The Caroline, Mariana, and Marshall Islands". In *Disease, Medicine, and Empire: Perspectives on Western Medicine and the Experience of European Expansion*, ed. Roy MacLeod and Milton Lewis, 80–102. London: Routledge, 1988.

Edgar, Robert R., ed. *An African American in South Africa.* Athens and Johannesburg: Ohio University Press, 1992.

——, and Hilary Sapire. *African Apocalypse: The Story of Nontetha Nkwenkwe; a Twentieth-Century South African Prophet.* Johannesburg: Witwatersrand University Press, 2000.

Elgood, Cyril. *A Medical History of Persia and the Eastern Caliphate.* Reprint, Amsterdam: APA-Pjilo Press, 1979.

——. Bahá-ul Douleh and His Quintessence of Experience". *Annals of Medical History* 10, 1938, 261–65.

——. *Safavid Medical Practice: Or, the Practice of Medicine, Surgery and Gynaecology in Persia Between 1500 AD and 1750 AD.* London: Luzac, 1970.

Ellis, Stephen. "Writing Histories of Contemporary Africa." *Journal of African History* 43, no. 1, 2003, 1–26.

Engels, Dagmar. "The Politics of Childbirth: British and Bengali Women in Contest, 1890–1930". In *Society and Ideology: Essays in South Asian History Presented to Professor K. A. Ballhatchet*, ed. Peter Robb, 222–46. Delhi: Oxford University Press, 1994.

Erdtsieck, Jessica. "In the Spirit of Uganga: Inspired Healing and Healership in Tanzania". Diss., University of Amsterdam, 2003.

——. *Pepo as an Inner Healing Force: Practices of a Female Spiritual Healer in Tanzania.* Amsterdam: Royal Tropical Institute, 1997.

Ernst, Waltraud. "The European Insane in British India, 1800–1858: A Case-study in Psychiatry and Colonial Rule". In *Imperial Medicine and Indigenous Societies*, ed. David Arnold, 27–44. Manchester: Manchester University Press, 1988.

——. "Idioms of Madness and Colonial Boundaries: The Case of the European and 'Native' Mentally Ill in Early Nineteenth-Century British India". *Comparative Study in Society and History* 39, no. 1, 1997.

——. *Mad Tales from the Raj: The European Insane in British India, 1800–1858*. London: Routledge, 1991.

Faaland, Just, and John Richard Parkinson. *Bangladesh: The Test* Case *of Development*. Dhaka: University Press, 1975.

Farley, John. *Bilharzia: A History of Imperial Tropical Medicine*. Cambridge: Cambridge University Press, 1991.

Finkler, K. "Diffusion Reconsidered: Variation and Transformation in Biomedical Practice; A Case Study from Mexico". *Medical Anthropology* 19, no. 1, 2000, 1–39.

Finzsch, Nobert, and Robert Jütte, ed. *Institutions of Confinement: Hospitals, Asylums, and Prisons in Western Europe and North America, 1500–1950*. Cambridge: Cambridge University Press, 1996.

Fisher, James F. *Living Martyrs: Individuals and Revolution in Nepal*. Delhi: Oxford University Press, 1997.

Fitzgerald, Rosemary. "'Clinical Christianity': The Emergence of Medical Work as a Missionary Strategy in Colonial India, 1800–1914". In *Health, Medicine and Empire: Perspectives on Colonial India*, ed. Biswamoy Pati and Mark Harrison, 88–136. New Delhi: Orient Longman, 2001.

——. "A 'Peculiar and Exceptional Measure': The Call for Women Medical Missionaries for India in the Later Nineteenth Century". In *Missionary Encounters: Sources and Issues*, ed. Robert A. Bickers and Rosemary Seton, 174–96. Richmond: Curzon Press, 1996.

——. "Rescue and Redemption: The Rise of Female Medical Missions in Colonial India During the Late Nineteenth and Early Twentieth Centuries". In *Nursing History and the Politics of Welfare*, ed. Anne Marie Rafferty, Jane Robinson and Ruth Elkan, 64–79. London: Routledge, 1997.

Fletcher, Grace Nies. *The Fabulous Flemings of Kathmandu: The Story of Two Doctors in Nepal*. London: Hodder and Stoughton, 1965.

Floor, Willem. *Public Health in Qasar Iran*. Washington D.C.: Mage Publishers, 2004.

Forbes, Geraldine. "Managing Midwifery in India". In *Contesting Colonial Hegemony: State and Society in Africa and India,* ed. Dagmar Engels and Shula Marks, 152–72. London and New York: I. B. Tauris, 1994.

——. "Medical Careers and Health Care for Indian Women: Patterns of Control". *Women's History* 3, no. 4, 1994, 515–30.

Forster, P. G. "Missionaries and Anthropology: The Case of the Scots of Northern Malawi". *Journal of Religion in Africa* 16, 1986.

Foucault, Michel. *The Birth of the Clinic: An Archaeology of Medical Perception*. London: Routledge, 1997 [1963].

——. Introduction to *The Normal and the Pathological*, ed. Canguilhem, 7–24.

——. *Madness and Civilisation: A History of Insanity in the Age of Reason*. New York: Vintage Books, 1988.

Fouché, G. "Mental Health in Colonial Pietermaritzburg." In *Pietermaritzburg: A New History of an African City*, ed. J. P. C. Laband and R. Haswell, 186–88. Pietermaritzburg: University of Natal Press and Shooter and Shuter, 1960.

Fox, Daniel M. *Health Policies, Health Politics*. Princeton: Princeton University Press, 1986.

Frank, P., T. I. Campbell, and C. G. Sheilds. "Social Relationship and Health: The Relative Roles of Family Functioning and Social Support". *Social Science & Medicine* 34, no.7, 1991, 779–88.

Freidson Eliot. *The Hospital in Modern Society*. London: The Free Press, 1963.

Fugikura, T. "Technologies of Improvement, Locations of Culture: American Discourses of Democracy and 'Community Development' in Nepal". *Studies in Nepali History and Society* 1, no. 2 December 1996, 271–311.

Fulton, Austin. *Through Earthquake, Wind and Fire: Church and Missions in Manchuria, 1867–1950: The Work of the United Presbyterian Church, the United Free Church of Scotland, the Church of Scotland and the Presbyterian Church of Ireland with the Chinese Church in Manchuria*. Edinburgh: Saint Andrew's Press, 1967.

Gelfand, Michael. *Christian Doctor and Nurse: The History of Medical Missions in South Africa from 1799–1976*. Sandton: Mariannhill Mission Press, 1984.

——. *Livingstone the Doctor, His Life and Travel: A Study in Medical History*. Oxford: Basil Blackwell, 1957.

Gerdener, G. B. A. *Recent Developments in the South African Mission Field.* Cape Town and Pretoria: N. G. Kerk-Uitgers, 1958.

Germain, C. P. *The Cancer Unit: An Ethnography.* Wakefield: Nursing Resource, 1979.

Giles, Linda. "Possession Cults on the Swahili Coast: A Re-examination of Theories of Marginality." *Africa* 57, 1987, 234–57.

——. "Spirit Possession and the Symbolic Construction of Swahili Society". In *Spirit Possession: Modernity and Power in Africa,* ed. Heike Behrend and Ute Luig, 142–64. Madison: University of Wisconsin Press, 1999.

——. "Spirit Possession on the Swahili Coast: Peripheral Cults or Primary Texts?" Diss., University of Austin, 1989.

Gluckman, Max. *Essays on the Ritual of Social Relations*. Manchester: Manchester University Press, 1962.

Goheen, R. H. H. "Indian Medical Missions: The Lessons of the Survey". *Conquest by Healing*, March 1929, 10–13.

Gordon, D. "Science, Superstition and Colonialism: Disease and Therapy at King Williams Town, Xhosaland, 1847–91". Unpublished paper.

Granshaw, Lindsay. "'Fame and Fortune by Means of Bricks and Mortar'? The Medical Profession and Specialist Hospitals in Britain, 1800–1948". In *The Hospital in History*, ed. Lindsay Granshaw and Roy Porter, 199–220. London: Routledge, 1989.

Gu, Mingyi et al. *Riben qinzhan Luda sishinian shi* [A Forty-year History of Japan's Occupation of Lushun and Dalian]. Shenyang: Liaoning renmin chubanshe, 1991.

Guha, Supriya. "'The Best Swadeshi': Reproductive Health in Bengal, 1840–1890". In *Reproductive Health in India: History, Politics, Controversies,* ed. Sarah Hodges, 139–66. Orient Longman: New Delhi, 2006.

H. H. W. B. "Perils and Pressures". *Saving Health*, September 1973, 45–46.

Hahn, Robert A., and A. D. Gaines. *Physicians of Western Medicine: Anthropological Approaches Theory and Practice.* Dordrecht: Reidel, 1985.

Hailey, William Malcolm. *East Africa: Uganda, Kenya, Tanganyika*. Native Administration in the British African Territories. Part 1. London: H. M. Stationary Office, 1950.

Haneveld, G. T. "From Slave Hospital to Reliable Health Care: Medical Work on the Plantations of Sumatara's East Coast". In *Dutch Medicine in the Malay Archipeligo, 1816–1942*, ed. G. M. van Heteren, A. de Knecht-van Eekelen and M. J. D. Poulissen. Amsterdam and Atlanta: Rodopi Press, 1989.

Hankins, Gerald W. *A Heart for Nepal: The Dr. Helen Houston Story.* Winnipeg: Windflower Communications, 1991.

Harper, Ian. "Capsular Promise as Public Health: A Critique of the Nepal National Vitamin A Programme". *Studies in Nepali History and Society* 7, no. 1, 2002, 137 –73.

——. "Mission, Magic and Medicalisation: An Anthropological Study into Public Health in Contemporary Nepal". Unpublished PhD thesis, University of London, 2003.

Harries, Lyndon. "Bishop Lucas and the Masasi Experiment". *International Review of Missions* 34, 1945, 389–96.

Harrison, Mark. "Disease, Discipline and Dissent: The Indian Army in France and England, 1914–1915". In *Medicine and Modern Warfare*, ed. Roger Cooter, Mark Harrison and Steve Sturdy. Amsterdam and Atlanta: Rodopi, 1999.

——. *A Great Independence of Mind: British Medicine in an Age of Commerce and Empire, c.1600–1830*. In preparation.

——. *Public Health in British India: Anglo-Indian Preventive Medicine, 1859–1914*. Cambridge: Cambridge University Press, 1994.

——. "Science and Medicine in Early Colonial India, c.1750–1820". In *The Oxford Companion to the History of the British Empire: India*, ed. Nandini Gooptu and Douglas M. Peers. Oxford: Oxford University Press, forthcoming.

——, and Michael Worboys. "A Disease of Civilization: Tuberculosis in Britain, Africa and India, 1900–1939". In *Migrants, Minorities and Health: Historical and Contemporary Studies*, ed. Laura Marks and Michel Worboys, 93–124. London: Routledge, 1997.

Hattersley, Alan F. *A Camera on Old Natal.* Pietermaritzburg: Shooter and Shuter, 1960.

Headrick, Rita, and Daniel Headrick, eds. *Colonialism, Health and Illness in French Equatorial Africa, 1885–1935*. Atlanta: African Studies Association Press, 1994.

Hecht, Gabrielle. "Rupture-Talk in the Nuclear Age: Conjugating Colonial Power in Africa." *Social Studies of Science* 32, nos. 5–6, 2002, 691–727.

Henrich, H. R."Training African Nurses". *Conquest by Healing*, December 1942, 54–56.

Herrick, Claire. "'The Conquest of the Silent Foe': British and American Military Medical Reform Rhetoric and the Russo-Japanese War". In *Medicine and Modern Warfare*, ed. Roger Cooter, Mark Harrison and Steve Sturdy, 99–131. Amsterdam: Rodopi, 1999.

Hewa, Soma. *Colonialism, Tropical Disease and Imperial Medicine.* Lanham: University Press of America, 1995.

Hobart, Mark. Introduction to *An Anthropological Critique of Development: The Growth of Ignorance*, ed. Mark Hobart, 1–30. New York and London: Routledge, 1993.

Hodges, Sarah, ed. *Reproductive Health in India: History, Politics and Controversies*. Hyderabad: Orient Longman, 2006.

——. "Women in Madras Presidency Health Policy, 1840–1890". Unpublished paper, University of Wisconsin, 1992.

Hoftun, Mark, William Raeper, and John Welpton. *People, Politics and Ideology: Democracy and Social Change in Nepal.* Kathmandu: Mandala Book Point, 1999.

Hogg, Jabez. *The Domestic Medical and Surgical Guide, for the Nursery, the Cottage, and the Bush: Giving the Best Advice, in the Absence of a Physician or Surgeon in Cases of Accident or Sudden Illness: Useful to Families, Emigrants, Travellers, Missionaries, Village Clergymen, and Sea Captains*. London: Ingram Cooke, 1853.

Hokororo, A. M. "The Influence of the Church on Tribal Customs at Lukuledi". *Tanganyika Notes and Records* 54, 1960, 1–13.

Holland, E. "State Medical Service for Native Rural Areas". *South African Medical Journal* 10, 1936, 387.

——, N. Haysom, A. Brodie, S. Javet, and M. Abel. "National Health Insurance and Medical Services for Rural Areas". *South African Medical Journal* 10, 1936, 249–56.

Holman, E. J. *A Report on the Medical Program of the Evangelical Lutheran Church in Southern Africa South Eastern Region, Natal Province, Republic of South Africa.* Dundee, South Africa: R. A. Burns and Co, 1967.

Horden, Peregrine. "The Earliest Hospitals in Byzantium, Western Europe, and Islam". *Journal of Interdisciplinary History* 35, no. 3, 2005, 361–89.

——. "The World of the Hospital: Comparisons and Continuities". In *The Impact of Hospitals, 300–200*, ed. John Henderson, Peregrine Horden and Alessandro Pastore. Oxford: Peter Lang, 2007.

Hulugalle, H. A. J. *British Governors of Ceylon.* Colombo: Arjuna Hulugalle Dictionaries, 2002.

Hunter, W. W. *Life of Brian Houghton Hodgson: British Resident at the Court of Nepal.* New Delhi and Madras: Asian Educational Services, 1991 [1898].

Huque, A. S. *Paradoxes in Public Administration: Dimensions of Development.* Dhaka: University Press, 1990.

Ikai, Shuhei. "Becoming Hospital Owners: The Evolution of Doctors in Japan from the 1870s to the 1930s". Unpublished paper.

Iliffe, John. *East African Doctors: A History of the Modern Profession*. Cambridge: Cambridge University Press, 1998.

Ishimoto, Rikizo. *Nan Man Igakudô jûnen shi* [Ten-year History of the South Manchuria Medical College]. Hôten: Nan Man Insatsusha, 1922.

Jabavu, D. D. T. *The Black Problem: Papers and Addresses on Various Native Problems*. Lovedale: Lovedale Press, 1920.

Jahan, Roushan. *Hidden Danger: Women and Family Violence in Bangladesh*. Dhaka: Women for Women, 1994.

Jamil, Ishtiaq. "Administrative Culture in Bangladesh: Tensions Between Tradition and Modernity". *International Review of Sociology* 12, no.1, 2002, 93–125.

Jansen, Marius B. "Japanese Imperialism: Late Meiji Perspectives". In *The Japanese Colonial Empire, 1895–1945*, ed. Ramon H. Myers and Mark R. Peattie, 61–79. Princeton: Princeton University Press, 1984.

Janzen, J. M. "Therapy Management: Concept, Reality, Process". *Medical Anthropology Quarterly* 1, no.1, 1987, 68–84.

Jaques, P. H., and Sam Fehrsen. "The Role of Mission Hospitals in Providing Health Care in South Africa". *Health Sector Reform: Coping Strategies and Professional Identity of Primary Health Care Clinicians*. Unpublished, discussion paper, c. 1997.

Jayawardena, Kumari. *Nobodies to Somebodies. The Rise of the Colonial Bourgeoisie in Sri Lanka.* London and New York: Zed Books, 2002.

Jeffery, Roger, Patricia Jeffery, and Andrew Lyon. "Only Cord-Cutters? Midwifery and Childbirth in Rural North India". *Social Action* 34, no.3, 1984, 229–50.

Jennings, Mike. "'This Mysterious and Intangible Enemy': Health and Disease Amongst the Early UMCA Missionaries". *Social History of Medicine* 15, 2002, 65–87.

Jewson, N. "The Disappearance of the Sick Man from Medical Cosmology, 1770–1870". *Sociology* 10, 1976, 225–44.

Jie, Xueshi. *Wei Manzhouguo shi* [History of the False Manzhouguo]. Beijing: Renmin chubanshe, 1995.

Jones, Margaret. "Infant and Maternal Health Services in Ceylon, 1900–1946: Imperialism or Welfare?" *Social History of Medicine* 15, no. 2, 263–89.

——. *Health Policy in Britain's Model Colony: Ceylon, 1900–1948.* New Delhi: Orient Longman, 2004.

Kakar, S. "Leprosy in British India, 1860–1940: Colonial Politics and Missionary Medicine". *Medical History* 40, 1996, 215–30.

Kark, Ruth. "The Contribution of the Ottoman Regime to the Development of Jerusalem and Jaffa, 1840–1917". In Kushner, ed., *Palestine in the Late Ottoman Period,* 46–58.

Kayser, Erling. "Medicine and Modern Philosophy: An Introduction". In *The Healing Church: The Tübingen Consultation, 1964*, ed. Frank Davey, 16–23. Geneva: World Council of Churches, 1965.

Keel, Othmar. "The Politics of Health and the Institutionalisation of Clinical Practices in Europe in the Second Half of the Eighteenth Century". In *William Hunter and the Eighteenth-Century Medical World*, ed. W. F. Bynum and Roy Porter, 207–58. Cambridge: Cambridge University Press, 1985.

Keen, P. "Surgical Problems in Bantu Practice". In *The African Nurse,* ed. T.N.E.D.G. Unpublished Seminar Series, 1961.

Khadka, Narayan. *Foreign Aid and Foreign Policy: Major Powers and Nepal.* Delhi: Vikas Publishing House Pvt Ltd, 1995.

Khan, Akbar Ali. *Discovery of Bangladesh: Exploration into Dynamics of a Hidden Nation.* Dhaka: University Press, 1996.

Khoury, Ghada Yusuf, ed., *The Founding Fathers of the American University of Beirut: Biographies.* Beirut: AUB Press, 1992.

Kinnosuke, Adachi. *Manchuria a Survey*. New York: Robert M. McBride & Company, 1925.

Kirkpatrick, Joanna. *The Sociology of an Indian Hospital.* Calcutta: Firma KLM Private, 1979.

Kitaoka, Shin'ichi. *Gotô Shinpei: Gaikô to bijon* [Gotô Shinpei: A Vision of International Politics]. Tokyo: Chûô Koronsha, 1988.

Knutson, P. J. *Partnerships in Mission: Mismeeting in Jesus Name?* Unpublished D. Theol. University of the Western Cape, Dept. of Theology, Cape Town, 1998.

Kotalova, Jitka. *Belonging to Others: Cultural Construction of Womanhood in a Village in Bangladesh.* Dhaka: University Press, 1996.

Kumar, Deepak. "Unequal Contenders, Uneven Ground: Medical Encounters in British India, 1820–1920". In *Western Medicine as Contested Knowledge*, ed. Andrew Cunningham and Bridie Andrews, 172–90. Manchester and New York: Manchester University Press.

Kumwenda, Linda Beer. "African Medical Personnel of the Universities' Mission to Central Africa in Northern Rhodesia". In *Healing Bodies, Saving Souls: Medical Missions in Asia and Africa*, ed. David Hardiman, 193–226. Amsterdam: Rodopi Press, 2006.

Lal, Maneesha. "'The Ignorance of Women Is the House of Illness': Gender, Nationalism and Health Reform in Colonial North India". In *Medicine and Colonial Identity*, ed. Mary P. Sutphen and Bridie Andrews, 14–40. London and New York: Routledge, 2003.

——. "The Politics of Gender and Medicine in Colonial India: The Countess of Dufferin's Fund, 1885–1888". *Bulletin of the History of Medicine* 68, no. 1, 1994, 29–66.

Landau, Jacob M. "The Educational Impact of Western Culture on Tradition Society in Nineteenth-Century Palestine". In *Studies on Palestine During the Ottoman Period,* ed. Moshe Ma'oz, 499–506. Jerusalem: The Magnes Press / Yad Izhak Ben-Zvi, 1975.

Lang, Séan. "Drop the Demon Dai: State Maternity Policy in Madras Presidency, 1840–1875". *Social History of Medicine* 18, no. 3, 2005, 357–78.

——. "Saving India Through Its Women". *History Today* 55, no. 9, 2005, 46–51.

Last, M. "Professionalization of Indigenous Healers". In *Medical Anthropology: A Hand Book of Theory and Method*, ed. T. M. Johnson and C. F. Sargent, 349–66. New York: Greenwood Press, 1990.

Latourette, Kenneth Scott. *A History of Christian Missions in China*. New York: The Macmillan Company, 1929.

Lattimore, Owen. *Manchuria: Cradle of Conflict*. New York: The Macmillan Company, 1935.

Lawrence, Susan C. *Charitable Knowledge: Hospital Pupils and Practitioners in Eighteenth-Century London*. Cambridge: Cambridge University Press, 1996.

Lazich, Michael C. "Seeking Souls Through the Eyes of the Blind: The Birth of the Medical Missionary Society in Nineteenth-Century China". In Hardiman, *Healing Bodies, Saving Souls,* 59–86.

Lee, R. P. L. "Comparative Studies of Health Care Systems". *Social Science & Medicine* 16, 1980, 629–42.

Leslie, Charles. *Asian Medical Systems: A Comparative Study*. Berkeley: University of California Press, 1976.

Lester, Allan. "The Margins of Order: Strategies of Segregation on the Eastern Cape Frontier, 1806–1850". *Journal of Southern African Studies* 23, no. 4, 1993.

Lewis, Frederick. *Sixty-Four Years in Ceylon*. New Delhi: Navrang, 1993.

Lewis, Jane. *The Politics of Motherhood: Child and Maternal Welfare in England, 1900–1939*. London: Croom Helm, 1980.

Liechty, Mark. "Selective Exclusion: Foreigners, Foreign Goods, and Foreignness in Modern Nepali History". *Studies in Nepali History and Society* 2, no. 1, June 1997, 2–68.

Lindell, Jonathan. *Nepal and the Gospel of God*. Kathmandu: Pilgrims Book House, 1997.

Lislerud, Rev. Rector Gunnar (Director). *The Report of the Umpumulu Consultation of the Healing Ministry of the Church*. Lutheran Theological College, Mapumulu, Natal, 19–27 September 1967. Unpublished Proceedings, 1967.

Litman, J. T. "The Family as a Basic Unit in Health and Medical Care: A Social Behavioural Overview". *Social Science & Medicine* 8, 1973, 495–519.

Liu, Kwang-Ching. "Early Christian Colleges in China". *Journal of Asian Studies* 20, no. 1, 1960, 71–78.

Liu, Shiyung. "Medical Reform in Colonial Taiwan". PhD, diss., University of Pittsburgh, 2000.

Liu, Zhongming. *Fengtian Yike Daxue (Liaoning Yi Xueyuan) jianshi* [A Brief History of the Mukden (Shenyang) Medical College]. Shenyang: Fengtian Yike Daxue, 1992.

Lo, Ming-cheng. "Between Ethnicity and Modernity: Taiwanese Medical Students and Doctors under Japan's *Kôminka* Campaign, 1937–1945". *Positions* 10, no. 2, 2002, 285–332.

——. *Doctors Within Borders: Profession, Ethnicity, and Modernity in Colonial Taiwan*. Berkeley: University of California Press, 2002.

Lock, Margaret M., and Deborah R. Gordon, eds. *Biomedicine Examined*. Dordrecht: Kluwer, 1988.

Lodge, Tom, and Bill Nasson. *All Here and Now: Black Politics in South Africa in the 1980s*. London: Hurst & Co, 1992.

Loughlin, K. "Spectacle and Secrecy: Press Coverage of Conjoined Twins in 1950s Britain". *Medical History* 49, no. 2, 2005, 197–212.

Lucas, William Vincent. "The Christian Approach to Non-Christian Customs". In *Christianity and Native Rites*, 4–38. London: Central Africa House Press, 1950.

Lyons, Maryinez. *A Social History of Sleeping Sickness in Northern Zaire, 1900–1940*. Cambridge: Cambridge University Press, 1992.

Macmillan, W. M. *Bantu, Boer, and Briton: The Making of the South African Native Problem*. Oxford: Clarendon Press, 1929.

MacPherson, Kerrie. *A Wilderness of Marshes: The Origins of Public Health in Shanghai, 1843–1893*. Hong Kong: Oxford University Press, 1987.

Macvicar, N. *Africa Tomorrow*? Johannesburg: SAIRR, 1947, 91.

——. "Doctors and the State". In *Science and Society in Southern Africa*, ed. S. Dubow. Manchester: Manchester University Press, 2000.

——. *English/Xhosa Nurses' Dictionary*. Lovedale: Lovedale Press, n.d.

——. "Native Health, General Survey and Hospitals". In *Native Health*, ed. N. Macvicar, D. Ryan and H. M. Bennett. Lovedale: Lovedale Press, 1940.

——. "Notes on Scurvy". *South African Medical Record*, 1906, 101–3.

——. *Outlines of Anatomy and Physiology for Nurses*. Lovedale: Lovedale Press, 1927.

——. Preface to *Health Reader for Standard Three*. Lovedale: Lovedale Press, 1911.

——. "Retiring Address". *South African Outlook*, 1938.

——. "Scurvy in Native Children". *South African Medical Journal*, 1931, 596–99.

——. *Side-lights upon Superstition*. Lovedale: Lovedale Press, 1939.

——. "The Training of the Native Hospital Nurse". *Christian Express*, 1919.

——. "Tuberculosis of Bones and Joints in Native Patients in the Ciskei". *South African Medical Journal*, 1935, 643–45.

Mager, Anne Kelk. *Gender and the Making of a South African Bantustan: The Social History of the Ciske, 1945–1959*. Oxford and Cape Town: James Currey, 1999, 1–5.

Mahone, Sloan. "The Psychology of the Tropics: Conceptions of Tropical Danger and Lunacy in British East Africa". DPhil diss., University of Oxford, 2004.

Malhotra, Anshu. "Of Dais and Midwives: 'Middle Class' Interventions in the Management of Reproductive Health in Colonial Punjab". In *Reproductive Health in India: History, Politics, Controversies*, ed. Sarah Hodges, 199–226. Orient Longman: New Delhi, 2006.

Maloney, Clarence. *Behaviour and Poverty in Bangladesh*. Dhaka: University Press, 1986.

Manderson, Lenore. *Sickness and the State: Health and Illness in Colonial Malaya, 1870–1940*. Cambridge: Cambridge University Press, 1996.

Mani, Lata. "Contentious Traditions: The Debate on Sati in Colonial India". In *Recasting Women: Essays in Colonial History,* ed. Kumkum Sangari and Sudesh Vaid, 90–118. New Delhi: Kali for Women, 1989.

Manshikai [Manchurian History Society], ed. *Manshû kaihatsu yonjûnen shi* [A Forty-year History of Manchuria's Development]. Tokyo: Manshikai, 1964.

Marcovich, Anne. "French Colonial Medicine and Colonial Rule: Algeria and Indochina". In *Disease, Medicine, and Empire: Perspectives on Western Medicine and the Experience of European Expansion*, ed. Roy MacLeod and Milton Lewis, 103–18. London: Routledge, 1988.

Marks, Lara V. *Metropolitan Maternity: Maternal and Infant Welfare in Early Twentieth-Century London*. Amsterdam and Atlanta: Rodopi, 1991.

Marks, Shula. *Divided Sisterhood: Race, Class and Gender in the South African Nursing Profession.* Johannesburg: Witwatersrand University Press, 1994.

——. "'Every Facility That Modern Science and Enlightened Humanity Have Devised': Race and Progress in a Colonial Hospital; Valkenberg Mental Asylum, Cape Colony, 1894–1910." In *Insanity, Institutions and Society, 1800–1914: A Social History of Madness in Comparative Perspective*, ed. J. Melling and B. Forsythe, 268–91. London: Routledge, 1999.

Mash, Rachel. "Margaret Fitzhugh Johnson, Doctor and Missionary, 1941–1963: Her Work and Family Life in the Context of Pre-independence and Post-imperial India". B.A., thesis, University of Brighton, 2001.

Mashaba, T. G. *Rising to the Challenge of Change: A History of Black Nursing in South Africa*. Cape Town: Juta and Co. Ltd, 1995, 17–20.

Matsusaka, Yoshihisa Tak. *The Making of Japanese Manchuria, 1904–1932*. Cambridge, MA: Harvard University Asia Center, 2001.

Matthews, Z. K. *Freedom for My People: The Autobiography of Z. K. Mathews; Southern Africa, 1901–1906,* ed. Monica Wilson. Cape Town: David Philip, 1983, 35.

Mayer, Johannes Gottfried, Bernhard Uehleke, and Kilian Saum. *Handbuch der Klosterheilkunde*. München: Zabert Sandmann, 2003.

Mbembe, Achille. *On the Postcolony*. Berkeley: University of California Press, 2001.

McCormack, Gavan. *Chang Tso-lin in North-east China, 1911–1928: China, Japan, and the Manchurian Idea*. Stanford: Stanford University Press, 1977.

McGilvray, James C. *The Quest for Health and Wholeness*. Tübingen: German Institute for Medical Missions, 1981, 50–51.

Mihaly, Eugene Bremer. *Foreign Aid and Politics in Nepal: A Case Study*. London, New York and Toronto: Oxford University Press, 1965.

Mills, James H. *Madness, Cannabis and Colonialism: The 'Native-Only' Lunatic Asylums of British India, 1857–1900*. London: Macmillan, 2000.

Minde, Max. "Early Psychiatry in Natal". *South African Medical Journal* 30, no. 12, 1956, 287–91.

Minden, Karen. *Bamboo Stone: The Evolution of a Chinese Medical Elite*. Toronto: University of Toronto Press, 1994.

Misra, Kiran. *BP Koirala: Life and Times*. New Delhi: Wishwa Prakashan, 1994.

Mitter, Rana. *The Manchurian Myth: Nationalism, Resistance, and Collaboration in Modern China*. Berkeley: University of California Press, 2000.

Molema, S. M. *The Bantu Past and Present*. Edinburgh: W. Green and Co., 1920.

Monro, Donald. *An Account of the Diseases which Were Most Frequent in the British Military Hospitals in Germany, from January 1761 to the Return of the Troops to England in March 1763*. London: A. Miller, D. Wilson and T. Durham, 1764.

Moorshead, R. Fletcher. *The Appeal of Medical Missions.* Edinburgh: Oliphant, Anderson and Ferrier, 1913.

Morley, D., J. Rohde, and G. Williams. *Practising Health for All*. Oxford: Oxford University Press, 1983.

Morris, P. "Soweto: A Brief History". *The Black Sash* 24, no. 2, 1981, 10–15.

Morrison, James Horne. *The Scottish Churches' Work Abroad*. Edinburgh: T. & T. Clark, 1927.

Mostert, N. *Frontier—The Epic of South Africa's Creation and the Tragedy of the Xhosa People*. London: Jonathan Cape, 1992.

Moulin, Anne Marie. "The Pasteur Institutes Between the Two World Wars: The Transformation of International Sanitary Order." In *International Health Organisations and Movements, 1918–1939*, ed. Paul Weindling. Cambridge: Cambridge University Press, 1995.

——. "Patriarchal Science: The Network of the Overseas Pasteur Institutes." In *Science and Empires*, ed. Patrick Petitjean, Catherine Jami and Anne Marie Moulin. Dordrecht: Kluwer Academic Publishers, 1992, 307–22.

Mudaliar, A. Lakshmanaswamy. *Maternity and Child Welfare*. Madras: Everyman's, 1922.

Muniruzzaman, T. *Politics and Security of Bangladesh*. Dhaka: University Press, 1994.

Murshid, Ghulam. *Reluctant Debutante: Response of Bengali Women to Modernisation, 1849–1905*. Rajshahi: Rajshahi University, 1983.

Myers, Ramon H. "Japanese Imperialism in Manchuria: The South Manchuria Railway Company, 1906–1933". In *The Japanese Informal Empire in China, 1895–1937*, ed. Peter Duus, Ramon H. Myers and Mark R. Peattie, 101–32. Princeton: Princeton University Press, 1989.

Napachihi, Sebastian Wolfgang. *The Relationship Between the German Missionaries of the Congregation of St. Benedict from St. Ottilien and the German Colonial Authorities in Tanzania, 1887–1907*. Ndanda, Peramiho: Benedictine Publications, 1998.

Nathan, Carl F. *Plague Prevention and Politics in Manchuria, 1910–1931*. Cambridge, MA: East Asian Research Centre, Harvard University, 1967.

Ndege, George O. *Health, State, and Society in Kenya*. Rochester, NY: University of Rochester Press, 2001.

Newbigin, Lesslie. "The Healing Ministry in the Mission of the Church". In Davey, *The Healing Church,* 8–15.

Newell, K. *Health by the People*. Geneva: WHO, 1975.

Nichter, M., and C. Nordstrom. "A Question of Medicine Answering: Health Commodification and the Social Relations of Healing in Sri Lanka". *Culture, Medicine, and Psychiatry* 13, 1989, 367–90.

Novak, James Jeremiah. *Bangladesh: Reflections on the Water*. Dhaka: University Press, 1994.

Ntantala, P. *A Life's Mosaic: The Autobiography of Phyllis Ntantala*. Bellville: Mayibuye Centre, 1992.

"Nursing as a Profession for Non-European Women". *The Health Magazine*, February 1942, 1–15.

"Obituary of Dr Macvicar". *Health Magazine*, 126, February 1950.

"Obituary: James Hyslop". *South African Journal of Science* 14, 1917–1918, 312–14.

Opland, J. "The Drumbeat of the Cross". In *Christianity in South Africa*, ed. R. Elphick and R. Davenport. Oxford: James Currey, 1997.

Otte, Solveig. *Isibani*: XIV, 1972, 3.

Packard, Randall. *White Plague, Black Labour: Tuberculosis and the Political Economy of Health and Disease in South Africa*. Los Angeles: University of California Press, 1989.

Paget, E. K. *The Claim of Suffering: A Plea for Medical Missions*. London, 1913.

Parker, Geoffrey. *The Army of Flanders and the Spanish Road, 1567–1659*. Cambridge: Cambridge University Press, 2004 [1972].

Pelis, Kim. "Prophet for Profit in French North Africa: Charles Nicolle and the Pasteur Institute of Tunis, 1903–1936." *Bulletin of the History of Medicine* 71, 1997, 583–622.

Perkin, Harold. *Origins of Modern English Society*. London and New York: Ark Paperbacks, 1986.

Perrins, Robert. "Doctors, Disease and Development: Engineering Colonial Public Health in Southern Manchuria, 1905–1931". In *Building a Modern Nation: Science, Technology and Medicine in Japan*, ed. Morris Low, 103–33. London: Palgrave Macmillan, 2005.

Perry, Cindy. *A Biographical History of the Church in Nepal*. Kathmandu: Nepal Church History Project, 2000.

Perry, Henry B. *Health for All in Bangladesh: Lessons in Primary Health Care for the Twenty-First Century*. Dhaka: University Press, 2000.

Pickstone, John V. "Dearth, Dirt and Fever Epidemics: Rewriting the History of British 'Public Health', 1780–1850". In *Epidemics and Ideas: Essays on the Historical Perception of Pestilence*, ed. Terrace O. Ranger and P. Slack, 125–48. Oxford: Oxford University Press, 1992.

——. "From Ferriar's Fever to Kay's Cholera: Disease and Social Structure in Cottonopolis". *History of Science* 22, 1984, 401–19.

——. *Medicine and Industrial Society: A History of Hospital Development in Manchester and Its Region, 1752–1946*. Manchester: Manchester University Press, 1985.

Pieris, Kamalika. *The Medical Profession in Sri Lanka, 1843–1980.* Colombo: Visidunnu Prakashakayo Ltd, 2001.

Pigg, Stacy L. "Inventing Social Categories Through Place: Social Representations and Development in Nepal". *Comparative Studies in Society and History* 34, 1992, 491–513.

Porter, Roy. "The Gift Relation: Philanthropy and Provincial Hospitals in Eighteenth-Century England". In *The Hospital in History*, ed. Lindsay Granshaw and Roy Porter, 149–78. London: Routledge, 1989.

——. *The Greatest Benefit to Mankind: A Medical History of Humanity from Antiquity to the Present.* London: Fontana Press, 1997.

Pottinger, George. *Sir Henry Pottinger: First Governor of Hong Kong.* Stroud: Sutton Publishing, 1997.

Prinsloo, N. M. "Conditions at Baragwanath Hospital". *South African Medical Journal* 72, 1987, 643.

Qadeer, Imrana, Kasturi Sen, and K. R. Nayar, eds. *Public Health and the Poverty of Reforms: The South Asian Predicament*. New Delhi: Sage, 2001.

Rabinowitz, B., and D. Demetriades. "Resuscitation". In Desmond Pantanowitz, ed. *Modern Surgery in Africa: The Baragwanath Experience*. Johannesburg: Southern Book Publishers, 1988.

Ramanna, Mridula. *Western Medicine and Public Health in Colonial Bombay, 1845–1895.* London: Sangam Books, 2002.

Ramasubban, Radika. "Imperial Health in British India, 1857–1900". In *Disease, Medicine and Empire: Perspectives on Western Medicine and the Experience of European Expansion,* ed. Roy MacLeod and Martin Lewis, 38–60. London/New York: Ramasubban, 1988.

Ranger, Terence O. "Godly Medicine: The Ambiguities of Medical Mission in South-east Tanzania, 1900–1945". *Social Science & Medicine*, 15B, 1981, 261–77.

——. "Missionary Adaptation of African Religious Institutions: The Masasi Case". In Ranger and Kimambo, *The Historical Study of African Religion,* 221–51.

Renshaw, Michelle. *Accommodating the Chinese: The American Hospital in China, 1880–1920*. New York: Routledge, 2005.

Rhodes, Lorna A. *Emptying Beds: The Work of an Emergency Psychiatric Unit*. Berkeley: University of California Press, 1995.

Rich, P. "Race, Science, and the Legitimization of White Supremacy in South Africa, 1902–1940". *The International Journal of African Historical Studies* 23, no. 4, 1990, 665–86.

Ringer, Monica. *Education, Religion, and the Discourse of Cultural Reform in Qajar Iran*. Costa Mesa, California: Mazda Publishers, 2001.

Ripley, Sydney Dillon. *Search for the Spiny Babbler: A Naturalist's Adventure in Nepal.* Kathmandu: Ratnar Pusthak Bhandar, 1978.

Risse, Günther B. *Hospital Life in Enlightenment Scotland: Care and Teaching at the Royal Infirmary of Edinburgh*. Cambridge: Cambridge University Press, 1986.

——. *Mending Bodies, Saving Souls: A History of Hospitals*. New York: Oxford University Press, 1999.

Robert, Dana. *American Women in Mission: A Social History of Their Thought and Practice*. Macon, Georgia: Mercer University Press, 1996.

Rogaski, Ruth. *Hygienic Modernity: Meanings of Health and Disease in Treaty-Port China*. Berkeley: University of California Press, 2004.

Rosenberg, Charles E. *The Care of Strangers: The Rise of America's Hospital System.* Baltimore: Johns Hopkins, 1995.

Rosenthal, Frantz. "The Physician in Medieval Muslim Society." In *Science & Medicine in Islam: A Collection of Essays*. Great Yarmouth, Norfolk: Variorum, 1991.

Ross, S. "Scurvy in Native Children". *South African Medical Journal*, 1931, 596–99.

Saayman, W. A. *A Man with a Shadow: The Life and Times of Professor Z. K. Mathews; A Missological Interpretation in Context.* Pretoria: University of South Africa, 1996, 27–28.

Sachs, L., and G. Tomson. "Medicine and Culture: A Double Perspective on Drug Utilization in a Developing Country". *Social Science & Medicine* 34, 1992, 307–15.

Sadowsky, Jonathan. *Imperial Bedlam: Institutions of Madness in Colonial Southwest Nigeria*. Berkeley: University of California Press, 1999.

Said, Edward W. *Orientalism*. New York: Pantheon Books, 1978.

Sakalo, W. "Letter from . . . Soweto, Baragwanath Hospital". *British Medical Journal* 1, no. 6165, 1979, 739–41.

Schendel, Gordon. *Medicine in Mexico: From Aztec Herbs to Betatrons*. Austin and London: University of Texas Press, 1968.

Schiebinger, Londa. *Plants and Empire: Colonial Bioprospecting in the Atlantic World*. Cambridge, MA: Harvard University Press, 2004.

Schölch, Alexander. "European Penetration and the Economic Development of Palestine, 1856–1882". In *Studies in the Economic and Social History of*

Palestine in the Nineteenth and Twentieth Centuries, ed. Roger Owen, 10–87. Oxford: St. Antony's College / McMillan Press, 1982.

Schulpen, Timotheus Wilhelmus Joseph. "Integration of Church and Government Medical Services in Tanzania: Effects at District Level". Diss., University of Nijmegen, 1975.

Searle, Charlotte. *The History of the Development of Nursing in South Africa, 1652–1960: A Socio-Historical Survey.* Pretoria: South African Nursing Association, 1980. First published 1965.

Selim, Monique. *The Experience of a Multinational Company in Bangladesh.* Dhaka: International Centre for Business Studies, 1995.

Sewell, Bill. "Public Health Concerns in a Manchurian Treaty Port". Paper presented at the conference, "Foreign Fevers and Colonial Cures: Disease and Medicine in the British, French and Japanese Empires", Acadia University, Canada, 23 August 2003.

Shaha, Rishikesh. *Modern Nepal: A Political History, 1769–1955.* Vols. 1 and 2. Kathmandu: Manohar, 1996.

Shapiro, K. "Doctors or Medical Aids: The Debate over the Training of Black Medical Personnel for the Rural Black Population in South Africa in the 1920s and 1930s." *Journal of Southern African Studies* 13, no. 2, 1987, 234–55.

Sharma, Shridhar. *Mental Hospitals in India.* New Delhi: Directorate General of Health Services, 1990.

Sharma Subedi, Madhusudan. *Medical Anthropology in Nepal.* Kathmandu: Udaya Books, 2001.

Shepherd, R. H. W. *Lovedale South Africa: The Story of a Century, 1841–1941.* Lovedale: Lovedale Press, 1941.

——. *A South African Health Pioneer.* Lovedale: Lovedale Press, 1952, 81–84, 128.

Shrestha, Nanda. *In the Name of Development: A Reflection on Nepal.* Kathmandu: Educational enterprise (P) Ltd, 1999.

Siddiqui, Kamal. *Towards Good Governance in Bangladesh: Fifty Unpleasant Essays.* Dhaka: University Press, 1996.

Sigerist, Henry. "An Outline of the Development of the Hospital". *Bulletin of the History of Medicine* 4, 1936, 573–81.

Sinn, Elizabeth. *Power and Charity: The Early History of the Tung Wah Hospital.* Hong Kong: Oxford University Press, 1989.

Skerry, Christa A., Kerry Moran, and Kay M. Calavan. *Four Decades of Development: The History of U.S. Assistance to Nepal.* Kathmandu: USAID Nepal, 1992.

Skota, T. D. M. *The African Yearly Register.* Johannesburg: R. L. Esson, 1931.

Smith, J. "Baragwanath: The Squalor of Segregation". *British Medical Journal* 298, 1989, 773–74.

Spence, Jonathan. *To Change China: Western Advisers in China, 1620–1960.* New York: Penguin Books, 1980.

Stanley, John. "Professionalising the Rural Medical Mission in Weixian, 1890–1925." In Hardiman, *Healing Bodies, Saving Soul,* 115–36.

Stirling, Leader. *Come Over and Help Us—A Doctor in Africa.* Dar es Salaam: AMREF, 1995.

Stoler, Ann Laura. "Matters of Intimacy as Matters of State: A Response." *Journal of American History* 88, no. 3, 2001, 893–97.

——. "Sexual Affronts and Racial Frontiers: European Identities and the Cultural Politics of Exclusion in Colonial Southeast Asia." In Cooper and Stoler, *Tensions of Empire,* 198–237.

Stransky, Thomas F. "The Austrian Hospital at Tantur, 1869–1918". In *Austrian Presence in the Holy Land in the 19th and Early 20th Century: Proceedings of the Symposium in the Austrian Hospice in Jerusalem on March 1–2, 1995,* ed. Marian Wrba, 98–121. Tel Aviv: Publication of the Austrian Embassy in Tel Aviv, 1996.

Summers, Anne. "The Costs and Benefits of Caring: Nursing Charities, c.1830–1860." In *Medicine and Charity Before the Welfare State*, ed. J. Barry and C. Jones, 133–148. London and New York: Routledge, 1991.

Swanson, Maynard. "The Sanitation Syndrome: Bubonic Plague and Urban Native Policy in the Cape Colony, 1900–1919." *Journal of African History* 18, 1977, 387–410.

Swantz, Lloyd W. *The Medicine Man Among the Zaramo of Dar es Salaam.* Uppsala: Scandinavian Institute for African Studies and Dar es Salaam University Press, 1990.

Swantz, Marja Liisa. *Ritual and Symbol in Transitional Zaramo Society with Special Reference to Women.* Studia Missionalia Uppsaliensia 16. Lund: Glerup, 1970.

Swartz, Sally. "The Black Insane in the Cape, 1891–1920." *Journal of Southern African Studies* 21, no. 3, 1995, 399–415.

——."Changing Diagnoses in Valkenberg Aylum, Cape Colony, 1891–1920: A Longitudinal View." *History of Psychiatry* 6, 1995, 431–51.

——. "Colonialism and the Production of Psychiatric Knowledge in the Cape, 1891–1920". PhD thesis, University of Cape Town, 1996.

Sweet, Helen. *Medicine with a Mission: The Role and Development of Missionary Nursing and Medicine in KwaZulu Natal, c. 1920–1980?* Monograph in preparation.

——. "'Wanted: 16 Nurses of the Better Educated Type'—Provision of Nurses to South Africa in the Late Nineteenth and Early Twentieth Century." *Nursing Inquiry Special Issue* 11, no. 3, 2004, 176–84.

——, and Anne Digby. "Race, Identity and the Nursing Profession in South Africa, 1850–1958." In *New Directions in the History of Nursing*, ed. B. Mortimer and S. McGann, 113–20. Routledge: London, 2005.

Switzer, L. *Power and Resistance in an African Society*. Madison: Wisconsin University Press, 1993.

Takahashi, Aya. *The Development of the Japanese Nursing Profession: Adopting and Adapting Western Influences*. London: Routledge Curzon, 2004.

Tan, Yi, ed. *'Jiu Yiba' kangzhan shi* [A History of the War of Resistance]. Shenyang: Liaoning renmin chubanshe, 1991.

Terziuglu, Arslan. "The History of Istanbul Medical Faculty." *Istanbul tip fakültesi mecmuasi*, 63, 2000.

Thomson, J. D., and G. Golding. *The Hospital: A Social and Architectural History*. New Haven: Yale University Press, 1975.

Tinker, Hugh. *A New System of Slavery: The Export of Indian Labour Overseas, 1830–1920.* London: Oxford University Press, 1974.

Tsai, H. H. "Dugald Christie, CMG, FRCS, FRCP Edin: Scottish Medical Pioneer in Manchuria (1883-1923)". *Scottish Medical Journal* 34, 1989, 443–44.

——. "Scottish Women Medical Pioneers: Manchuria, 1894–1912". *Scottish Medical Journal* 37, 1992, 56–59.

Turner, Bryan S. *Medical Power and Social Knowledge*. London: Sage, 1987.

United Mission to Nepal. *Celebrating 45 Years in Nepal*. Kathmandu: UMN, 1999.

United Nations. *The Common Country Assessment: Bangladesh*. Dhaka: The University Press, 2000.

Uragoda, C. G. "General Teaching Hospital (1)". *Ceylon Medical Journal* 36, no. 2, 1991, 27–32.

——. *A History of Medicine in Sri Lanka: From the Earliest Times to 1948*. Colombo: Sri Lanka Medical Association, 1987.

Van Alphen, J., and Anthony Aris, eds. *Oriental Medicine: An Illustrated Guide to the Asian Arts of Healing*. Boston: Shambala, 1995.

Van Dijck, Jose. "Medical Documentary: Conjoined Twins as a Medical Spectacle". *Media, Culture and Society* 24, no. 4, 2002, 537–56.

Van Donzel, E., ed. *Encyclopaedia of Islam*. Boston: Brill. 1998.

Van Ginkel, Rob. "Writing Culture from Within: Reflections on Endogenous Ethnography". *Etnofoor* 7, no. 1, 1994, 5–23.

Vaughan, Megan. *Curing Their Ills: Colonial Power and African Illness.* Stanford: California University Press, 1991.

Vess, David. *Medical Revolution in France, 1789–1796*. Gainesville: University Presses of Florida, 1975.

Vlassoff, Carol. "The Status of Women in Rural India: A Village Study". *Social Action* 32, October–December 1982, 380–407.

Von Arni, Eric Gruber. *Hospital Care and the British Standing Army, 1660–1714*. Aldershot: Ashgate, 2006.

Walls, A. F. "The Heavy Artillery of the Missionary Army: The Domestic Importance of the Nineteenth-Century Medical Missionary." In *The Church and Healing*, ed. W. J. Sheils, 287–97. Oxford: Basil Blackwell, 1982.

Walt, Gill. "Health Care in the Developing World, 1960–2001". In *Caring for Health: History and Diversity*, ed. Charles Webster, 253–94. Milton Keynes: Open University Press, 2001.

Walter, Bernita. *Sustained By God's Faithfullness: The Missionary Benedictine Sisters of Tutzing*. 2 vols. St Ottilien: EOS, 1992.

Wang, Bingzhong, trans., and ed. *Manzhou kaifa sishinian shi* [A Forty-year History of the Development of Manchuria]. Shenyang: Dongbei lunxian sishinian shi Liaoning bianxie zu yi, 1987.

Weiner, Dora. *The Citizen-Patient in Revolutionary and Imperial Paris*. Baltimore: Johns Hopkins University Press, 1993.

Weisberg, D. "Physician's Private Clinic in a Northern Thai Town: Patient Healer Collaboration and the Shape of Biomedical Practice". *Culture, Medicine and Psychiatry* 8, 1984, 165–86.

Wells, James. *Stewart of Lovedale.* London: Hodder and Stoughton, 1909.

Welpton, John. *A History of Nepal.* Cambridge: Cambridge University Press, 2005.

Wembah-Rashid, John A. R. *The Ethno-History of the Matrilineal Peoples of South-east Tanzania.* Acta Ethnologica et Linguistica 32 Series Africana 9. Wien: Stiglmayr, 1975.

Werner, Christoph. *An Iranian Town in Transition: A Social and Economic History of the Elites of Tabriz, 1747–1848*. Wiesbaden: Harassowitzt Verlag, 2000.

White, Luise. *Speaking with Vampires: Rumor and History in Colonial Africa.* Berkeley: University of California Press, 2000.

WHO. *Apartheid and Health*. Geneva: WHO, 1983.

Whyte, Susan Reynolds. "Anthropological Approaches to African Misfortune: From Religion to Medicine". In *Culture, Experience, and Pluralism: Essays on African Ideas of Illness and Healing*, ed. Jacobson-Widding and David Westerlund, 289–301. Uppsala: Acta Universitatis Upsaliensis, 1989.

Wilkinson, John. *The Coogate Doctors: The History of the Edinburgh Medical Missionary Society, 1841 to 1991*. Edinburgh: The Edinburgh Medical Missionary Society, 1991.

Wills, Trevor. "The Segregated City." In *Pietermaritzburg: A New History of an African City*, ed. J. P.C. Laband and R. Haswell, 33–45. Pietermaritzburg: University of Natal Press and Shooter and Shuter, 1988.

——. "Segregation, Separation and Desegregation: Pietermaritzburg since 1910." In *Receded Tides of Empire: Aspects of the Economic and Social History of Natal and Zululand since 1910*, ed. B. Guest and J. Sellers, 283–309. Pietermaritzburg: University of Natal Press, 1994.

Wilson, F. *Migrant Labour in South Africa*. Johannesburg: South African Council of Churches, 1972.

Wilson, F., and D. Perrot, eds. *Outlook on a Century: South Africa, 1870–1970*. Braamfontein: Lovedale Press, 1973.

Wilson, George Herbert. *The History of the Universities' Mission to Central Africa*. London: UMCA, 1936.

Wilson, Monica. "Cooperation and Conflict: The Eastern Cape Frontier". In *The Oxford History of South Africa*, ed. M. Wilson and L. Thompson. 2 vols. Oxford: Oxford University Press, 1969.

Wong, Timothy Man-kong. "Local Voluntarism: The Medical Mission of the London Missionary Society in Hong Kong, 1842–1923". In Hardiman, *Healing Bodies, Saving Souls*, 87–114.

Worboys, Michael. "The Spread of Western Medicine". In *Western Medicine: An Illustrated History*, ed. Irvine Loudon, 249–63. Oxford: Oxford University Press, 1997.

Wright, Marcia. *German Missions in Tanganyika, 1891–1941: Lutherans and Moravians in the Southern Highlands*. Oxford: Clarendon Press, 1971.

Wylie, Diana. *Starving on a Full Stomach*. Charlottesville: Virginia University Press, 2001.

Yarshatater, Rshan, ed. *Encyclopaedia Iranica*. Costa Mesa, California: Mazda Publishers, 1993.

Yip, Ka-che. *Health and National Reconstruction in Nationalist China: The Development of Modern Health Services, 1928–1937*. Ann Arbor: Association for Asian Studies, 1995.

Young, Carl Walter. *Japanese Jurisdiction in the South Manchuria Railway Areas*. Baltimore: The Johns Hopkins Press, 1931.

Young, John. *Paul Brand and His Leprosy Work*. London: SCM Press, 1980.

Young, Louise. *Japan's Total Empire: Manchuria and the Culture of Wartime Imperialism*. Berkeley: University of California Press, 1998.

Contributors

Philippe Bourmaud

Philippe Bourmaud completed his PhD in history from Aix-en-Provence University. In his doctoral thesis, he studied the training and practice of medicine within a context of medical pluralism in the late Ottoman Middle East. His academic interests also include healthcare and health insurance in contemporary Israel and the Palestinian occupied territories. Bourmaud currently teaches contemporary history at Lyon 3 University. Email: p_bourmaud@yahoo.fr

Walter Bruchhausen

Walter Bruchhausen is Senior Lecturer in "History, Anthropology and Ethics of Medicine", Vice-Director of the Institute for the History of Medicine, University of Bonn. He has studied medicine, theology, philosophy *of* medicine/health care ethics and anthropology in Bonn, Würzburg and Glasgow. Some of his research projects include: "Past and Present Medical Pluralism in South-eastern Tanzania", and "Catholicism and Issues of Health Care in the Second German Empire". Email: Walter.Bruchhausen@ukb.uni-bonn.de

Anne Digby

Anne Digby is Research Professor in History at the Centre for Health, Medicine and Society at Oxford Brookes University. She has published widely in the social history of medicine focussing her research on Britain and, more recently, on South Africa. Digby's books include *Madness, Morality and Medicine* (1985); *Making a Medical Living* (1994); *The Evolution of General Practice in Britain, 1850–1948* (1999); and *Diversity and Division in Medicine: Healthcare in South Africa from the 1800s* (2006). Currently, with colleagues from the University of Cape Town, Digby is working on the history of Groote Schuur Hospital, Cape Town—where the world's first heart transplant took place—for a book to mark the seventieth anniversary of the institution next year. Email: adigby@brookes.ac.uk

Hormoz Ebrahimnejad

Hormoz Ebrahimnejad is Wellcome Trust Lecturer in History, School of Humanities at the University of Southampton. He has published widely on the history of medicine and public health in nineteenth-century Iran, examining particularly theoretical and institutional aspects of medical modernisation. Ebrahimnejad's current research is on the modernisation of medicine in Iran from the nineteenth century onwards, with particular focus on the role of military, state and charitable hospitals in the development of modern medicine. Email: h.ebrahimnejad@soton.ac.uk

David Hardiman

David Hardiman is Professor of History at the University of Warwick. He is a founder-member of the Subaltern Studies group, and has published several articles in Subaltern Studies, and edited one of the volumes. Some of Hardiman's famous works are—*Peasant Nationalists of Gujarat: Kheda District, 1917–1934* (1981), *The Coming of the Devi: Adivasi Assertion in Western India* (1987), *Feeding the Baniya: Peasants and Usurers in Western India (1996), Gandhi in His Time and Ours* (2003), and *Histories for the Subordinated (2006).* Recently he has been working on mission medicine in India, and his book *Missionaries and Their Medicine: A Christian Modernity for Tribal India* was published in 2008. Email: D.Hardiman@warwick.ac.uk

Ian Harper

Ian Harper is trained in both medicine and social anthropology, and currently lectures at the University of Edinburgh, where he is also the programme co-director for studies in Medical Anthropology. For three and a half years he managed a tuberculosis control project in Nepal, and for two years worked with NGOs throughout India in supporting community health programmes. His experiences of practicing medicine and public health in such diverse cultural and political situations led him to study medical anthropology. From August 1998 to March 2000 Dr Harper researched into the social relations around, and the effects of, a series of public health programmes in Nepal. He is currently researching as a member of an interdisciplinary team on a project titled "Tracing Pharmaceuticals in South Asia". Email: iharper@staffmail.ed.ac.uk

Mark Harrison

Mark Harrison is Professor of the History of Medicine and Director of the Wellcome Unit for the History of Medicine, University of Oxford. He has published widely on the history of disease and medicine, especially in relation to the history of war and imperialism from the seventeenth to the twentieth centuries. His publications include *Public Health in British India: Anglo-Indian Preventive Medicine, 1859–1914*; *Climates and Constitutions: Health, Race, Environment and British Imperialism in India, 1600–1850;* and *Health, Medicine and Empire: Perspectives on Colonial India.* He is currently working on the history of medicine and British imperial expansion, c.1700–1850, the history of medicine during the First World War and on the relationship between disease and commerce. Email: mark.harrison@wuhmo.ox.ac.uk

Simonne Horwitz

Dr Simonne Horwitz completed her DPhil on the history of Baragwanath Hospital, Soweto, South Africa at the University of Oxford in 2006, where she studied as a Rhodes Scholar. She is currently Assistant Professor at the University of Saskatchewan, Canada. Her areas of research focus on the history of medicine in South Africa with a specific focus on leprosy and the history of hospitals and their staff. Email: simon.horwitz@usask.ca

Margaret Jones

Margaret Jones is a Research Fellow at the Wellcome Unit for the History of Medicine, University of Oxford. She has worked and published extensively on the history of Western medicine in Sri Lanka. She is currently working on the history of public health in the British West Indies. Jones's first book *Health Policy in Britain's Model Colony, Ceylon, 1900–1948* was published in 2004, and her second title *The Hospital System and Health Care: Sri Lanka, 1815–1960* will be published in 2009. Email: margaret.jones@wuhmo.ox.ac.uk

Guillaume Lachenal

Guillaume Lachenal is a lecturer at the Department of History and Philosophy of Science at the University of Paris Diderot, Paris. He has completed his PhD thesis in History of Science at the University of Paris 7 on "Biomedicine and Decolonisation in Cameroon, 1944–1994". He now works on the interactions between medicine, Catholicism and politics in the French-African world.
Email: lachenal@univ-paris-diderot.fr

Seán Lang

Seán Lang is Senior Lecturer in History at Anglia Ruskin University, where he completed his PhD on state maternity provision in nineteenth-century British India. He is an experienced history teacher, and is currently conducting research on royal patronage for Indian medical institutions in the nineteenth century. Email: sean.lang@anglia.ac.uk

Julie Parle

Julie Parle is Associate Professor of History at the University of KwaZulu-Natal, South Africa. Her first book titled, *States of Mind: Searching for Mental Health in Natal and Zululand, 1868–1918* was published by UKZN Press in 2007. She has also published on the history of witchcraft and gender in Southern Africa; on the history of suicide; and on the difficulties of teaching science to disadvantaged students. Parle is currently co-authoring a critical history of McCord "Zulu" Hospital in Durban, and is engaged in a study of the role of families in psychiatric patient committal in South Africa from 1916–1960. Email: parlej@ukzn.ac.za

Robert Perrins

Robert John Perrins is the Dean of the Faculty of Arts, at Acadia University in Nova Scotia, Canada, where he is also the Director of the North-East Asia Research Centre, and Professor of History. A specialist in the histories of modern China and Japan, Perrins served as editor of the *China Annual Facts and Figures Handbook* (Academic International Press) from 1999 to 2005. He is a member of the editorial boards for the journal, *The Social History of Medicine,* as well as H-NEAsia. In 2006, as a visiting research fellow at the Centre for the Social History of Health and Healthcare at the Universities of Strathclyde and Glasgow Caledonia he conducted research on the history of the United Free Church of Scotland's mission to Manchuria. He is currently working on a major research project that explores the history of plague in modern Asia. Email: robert .perrins@acadiau.ca

Helen Sweet

Helen Sweet has worked and published extensively on the history of medicine and nursing in South Africa and in the UK. Her first book written with Rona Dougal, *Community Nursing and Primary Healthcare in Twentieth-Century Britain* was published by Routledge in 2007; and her second, *Medicine with a Mission: The Role and Development of Missionary Nursing and Medicine in KwaZulu Natal,* c. *1920–1980* is in preparation for publication in 2010. Dr Sweet has worked on two previous Wellcome-funded research projects. The first focused on the historical development of general practice medicine in Great Britain, 1851–1948, whilst the second explored the concept of medical pluralism in the South African Cape, from the early nineteenth to mid-twentieth centuries. She is also a registered nurse and midwife. Email: helen.sweet@yahoo.co.uk

Shahaduz Zaman

Shahaduz Zaman is a medical anthropologist and a public health physician. He studied Medicine and Public Health in Bangladesh, and Medical Anthropology in the Netherlands. Zaman worked as Associate Professor and MPH Programme Coordinator at James P. Grant School of Public Health, BRAC University, Bangladesh. Currently he is working at Institute of Health and Society, Newcastle University, UK. Email: zaman567@yahoo.com

Index